•••••••••••••••

FOURTH EDITION

An Introduction to Human Services

Marianne Woodside
Tricia McClam

•••••••••••••••

University of Tennessee

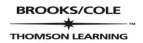

BROOKS/COLE

THOMSON LEARNING

Australia • Canada • Mexico • Singapore • Spain • United Kingdom • United States

BROOKS/COLE

™

THOMSON LEARNING

Sponsoring Editor: *Julie Martinez*
Editorial Assistant: *Cat Broz*
Marketing: *Caroline Concilla/Megan Hansen*
Assistant Editor: *Jennifer Wilkinson*
Project Editor: *Kim Svetich-Will*
Production Service: *Carlisle Communications*
Manuscript Editor: *Terry Lang*
Permissions Editor: *Sue Ewing*

Interior Design: *Terri Wright*
Cover Design: *Roy R. Neuhaus*
Cover Photo: Photo Disc, PhotoEdit/Michael Newman,
  Felicia Martinez, Jonathan Nourok
Photo Editor: *Terri Wright*
Print Buyer: *Vena Dyer*
Compositor: *Carlisle Communications*
Printing and Binding: *Webcom*

For more information about this or any other Brooks/Cole product, contact:
BROOKS/COLE
511 Forest Lodge Road
Pacific Grove, CA 93950 USA
www.brookscole.com
1-800-423-0563 (Thomson Learning Academic Resource Center)

Printed in Canada

10   9   8   7   6   5   4   3   2   1

Library of Congress Cataloging-in-Publication Data
Woodside, Marianne.
    An introduction to human services / Marianne Woodside, Tricia McClam.—4th ed.
      p. cm.
    Includes bibliographical references and index.
    ISBN 0-534-36879-4
    1. Human services. 2. Human services—United States. 3. Social workers—United
States. I. McClam, Tricia. II. Title.

HV31 .W66 2002
361—dc21   2001025032

Contents

· ·

Chapter 2: A History of Helping   42

Chapter 3: Human Services Today   86

Chapter 4: **Models of Human Service Delivery   134**

●●

• •

PART THREE: *The Practice of Human Services*   244

Chapter 7: **The Helping Process**   246

Chapter 8: **Working Within a System   288**

Chapter 9: **Professional Concerns   332**

Preface

In writing the first three editions of this book, our goal was to offer instructors a textbook choice devoted entirely to human services—not psychology, sociology, or social work. We addressed the definition of the term *human services* in its broadest sense and described a variety of clients, the generalist human service professional, and the interaction between helper and client. We approached human services as a profession that, although newly established, continues to grow and develop. Our goals remain the same for this fourth edition of *An Introduction to Human Services,* but we have revised the book in ways that we believe improve it.

Our revisions are based upon the feedback we received from faculty and students during the review process. Many other revisions resulted from our own research and teaching; they document the changing face of the environment in which human services are delivered. Part One defines the concept of human services. The focus of Chapter 1 continues to be on the principles that define human services. The case of Almeada and baby Anne has been revised to better represent the human service delivery system and climate that exist today. Chapter 2 combines a history of helping with a history of the human service movement; this combination allows thoughtful integration of human services into a long-standing historical context and updates developments to the present time. We added time lines throughout the chapter to help students understand the chronology of events. Chapter 3 offers a look at the current influences on human services: technology, managed care, the international dimension, and resolution-focused helping. This chapter was revised to reflect the impact that these influences continue to have on human services. Chapter 4 concludes Part One by introducing three models that contribute to our understanding of human services. We have updated the models to mark the changes that have occurred during the last decade. Updated case studies illustrate each model.

Part Two continues to focus on the participants in the delivery of human services—the helper and the client—and includes new information about client populations. Chapter 5 adds a new discussion on "clients" as individuals, small groups, and populations. A new case study has been added to illustrate these concepts. Chapter 6 explores the helper as the human service professional. To enhance this discussion, the human service roles have been added to this chapter. Part Three begins with Chapter 7 which introduces the helping process. This chapter was revised to focus on working with both individuals and groups. There are new inserts and updated case vignettes to facilitate student understanding of the helping process. Chapter 8 has been revised to include an ecological approach to understanding the context of the client's world and worker's environment. There are numerous figures, tables, and vignettes to help students learn about the influence of the environment upon client issues and helping responses. Chapter 9 continues to focus on ethical issues. A section has been added to introduce students to the day-to-day challenges they face as they work in the human service context.

There are two new additions to each chapter. Students are encouraged to use the internet to explore human service issues introduced in the text. Included in each chapter is a list and summary of relevant websites. We hope that these will serve as the beginning or enhancement of the search for additional information about human services. We have also added summary points throughout each chapter. Students can use these summary points to check their understanding of main ideas and to support their preparation for class discussions and other assignments.

Features

Two unique features of the book remain. The first is that the book continues to be introductory rather than encyclopedic. It presents basic information that students need to know about the human service field and encourages the use of other books, electronic materials, media resources, and other sources to enrich students' knowledge of the introductory course content. This knowledge will be more attractive to students when it is applied to case studies, books, current events, and audiovisual materials. In this book, you will find brief case studies, primary sources, and suggested additional readings for each chapter. The instructor's manual that accompanies the text also identifies videotapes, movies, websites, and nonfictional accounts of clients. All these resources can enhance student understanding of human services. We encourage you to use these resources and to let us know of others that you discover on your own. Please note that by the very dynamic nature of the Web, URLs are subject to change. Therefore, while weblinks in this text were selected with care, some links that were active at the time of publication may no longer be functional.

A second unique feature of the book is the International Focus sections. As the cultural composition of the United States continues to shift, human service professionals must be prepared to work effectively with culturally diverse clients. At the introductory level, our goal is to expand student awareness in order to incorporate a global dimension into the human service field. Each International Focus section is related in some way to the content of the chapter and provides an opportunity for thought and discussion about the international dimension of human services and how it influences practice in the United States.

Acknowledgments

Many friends and colleagues have contributed both to our growth as human service educators and to the writing of the fourth edition of this book. We are particularly grateful to our colleagues in the National Organization for Human Service Education and the Council for Standards in Human Service Education for their support, feedback, and contributions throughout the years.

We would especially like to thank our students, and the students, in other programs throughout the country, who use our book, for we have learned much from them about human services. Introductory students continue to be a favorite group for us to teach because of their enthusiasm and interest in the helping professions.

Many people provided assistance in this endeavor. Among them are John Ray, Charlotte Duncan, Linda Harrell, Karen Welch, Debi Whiteaker, Susan Sutton, and Rhonda Green. Our families have also encouraged us during this endeavor, and we are grateful for their patience and support.

The reviewers whose constructive comments helped us improve the manuscript include: Dr. Mary Kay Kreider, St. Louis Community College-Meramec; Dr. Marianne H. Mitchell, Indiana University; Dr. Pamela M. Kiser, Elon College; Professor Maria Markovics, Hudson Valley Community College; Professor Barbara G. Mitchell, M.A., C.S.P., Cambria County Area Community College, East; Dr. Stephanie Barnes, Northern Kentucky University; Daniel W. Anger, Ph.D., B.C.S.

We would also like to thank the staff at Brooks/Cole for all their work with this manuscript. This includes our editor, Julie Martinez, as well as Kim Svetich-Will, project editor; Cat Broz, editorial assistant; and Sue Ewing, permissions editor.

—Marianne Woodside
Tricia McClam

About the Authors

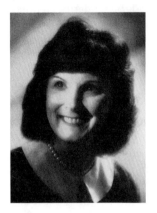 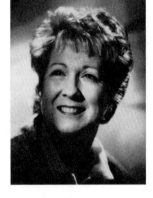

Marianne Woodside   Tricia McClam

As practitioners and instructors, we have been involved in human services for the past 30 years. As a result, we have experience both in delivering services and in preparing those who are learning to do so. From our years as practitioners in public schools and in rehabilitation settings, we have gained an understanding of helpers' commitment to their clients, their work, and their professions. In recent years, we have conducted in-depth interviews with practitioners and clients in an effort to better understand the methods of delivering services, the interaction between clients and human service professionals, and the changing context of service delivery. In recognizing the complexity of clients' lives and the complicated problems they sometimes face, we have developed more effective communication skills, a realistic understanding of helping using the human service model, and an appreciation of the problem-solving process that is based on the strengths of clients and their environments. These were valuable skills and understandings for us as practitioners. As instructors, we have discovered the importance of developing them in our students if these new practitioners are to become effective human service professionals.

Our work as educators has also contributed to our understanding of the evolving field of human services. As we develop curriculum with our colleagues, conduct research in human service education, participate in national and regional human service organizations, and travel and study internationally, we continue to be students ourselves. Concepts such as serving the whole person, using an interdisciplinary approach, training the generalists, and empowering clients have become basic to our work with beginning students.

An Introduction to Human Services

QUESTIONS TO CONSIDER

1. What are the perspectives for defining human services?

2. How has human services evolved in the last 50 years? What factors influenced its development?

3. How has society responded to the needs of people throughout history?

4. What are the current trends in human service delivery today? What is projected for the future?

5. What is the model most often used in human service delivery? How is it influenced by other models?

PART ONE

Defining Human Services

Human services may be a question mark to you as you begin this book. It is a difficult concept to define. Some think of it as the activities of workers who try to meet the needs of people. Others think of local and state agencies that used to be called departments of welfare or social services; today, many such agencies are departments of human services. Still others consider human services a profession for which a person receives special training.

Part One is titled "Defining Human Services." If you think of human services as a puzzle, the chapters in this part will provide you with the pieces necessary to understand this difficult and complex concept. Each piece will give you a different perspective from which to consider human services. Chapter 1 introduces Almeada, a client who needs help from the human service delivery system. Through Almeada's experience, this chapter examines both scholarly and professional definitions. Chapter 2 provides an historical overview of helping, and a 20th-century perspective on the recent emergence of human services as a profession. Chapter 3 describes current influences on human service delivery and considers the future of such services. Chapter 4 describes three models of service delivery and includes a case study to illustrate each one.

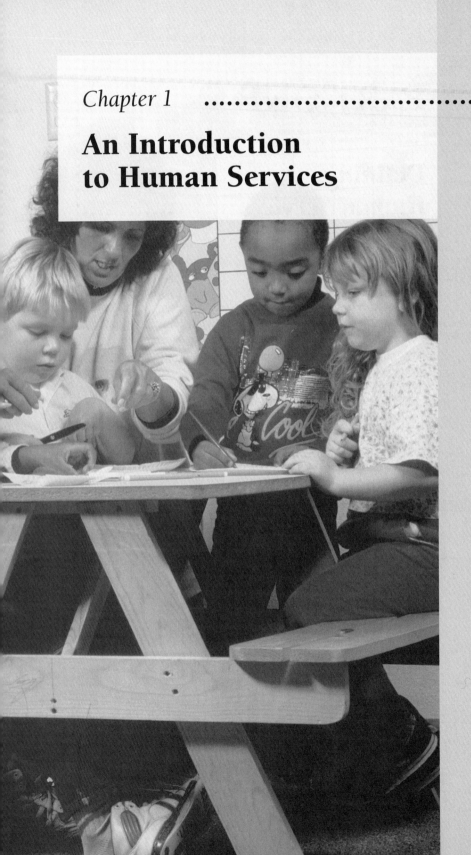

Chapter 1

An Introduction
to Human Services

One of the first questions you will probably ask as you pick up this book is "What is human services?" This question has come up often in the last several decades as the field has changed and restructured. The purpose of this chapter is to help you gain an understanding of the term. The definition of *human services* is derived from six perspectives: (1) the themes and purposes of human services, (2) the interdisciplinary nature of human services, (3) the dual focus of client and helper, (4) management principles, (5) professional roles, and (6) professional activities. Understanding and integrating these diverse perspectives will help you formulate a definition of human services.

This chapter introduces the themes and purposes of human services as described by scholars and prominent leaders in the field. The six themes presented summarize the principles that guide the delivery of human services. A case study of Almeada, a young mother who is living in a large city with her baby daughter, Anne, illustrate these concepts. We also describe the interdisciplinary nature of human services and examine human services from the dual focus of the client and helper. Important ideas to consider here are the nature of the client, the client's environment, and the interaction between the client and the helper.

Another important and defining characteristic of the human service delivery system is the management principles used by human service providers as they continually work to improve services to clients. The fourth perspective on human services introduces roles of professionals and nonprofessionals. Finally, a description of the professional activities of human service helpers illustrates their commitment to helping the client by providing needed services within a supportive environment.

Together, the six perspectives presented in this chapter will help clarify what human services is. They will also provide a basic understanding that will serve as a framework for the remainder of the book.

 ## Themes and Purposes of Human Services

The first perspective from which human services can be defined is a scholarly one. Scholars approach the definition of human services by describing the themes and purposes that guide human services; these themes and purposes have emerged over the past four decades. Those presented in this section represent the ideas of a range of scholars writing in the field today and include concerns with problems in living, the increase in problems in our modern world, the need for self-sufficiency, and the goals of social care, social control, and rehabilitation. A case study of Almeada and her daughter, Anne, illustrates these themes.

Problems in Living

Human beings are not always able to meet their own needs. Human services has developed in response to the need of individuals, groups, or communities for assistance to live better lives. Examples of such people are often publicized in the media: the very young; the elderly; people with limited physical or mental capabilities; victims of crimes, disasters, or abuse; people with acquired immune deficiency syndrome (AIDS), and many others. Assisting individuals is an example of the helping interaction. Families and groups also receive the attention of human service professionals, as do communities and larger geographic areas.

Anne, a 1-year-old child, lives with her mother, Almeada, in a housing project in Chicago. Their home is a dirty, rat-infested, one-room apartment that offers little beyond protection from the weather. Almeada, 17 years old, works six days a week for a local clothing manufacturer for minimum wage. She spends day after day in a large, hot, noisy workhouse, sewing sleeves in dresses and shirts. Almeada feels lucky to have this job, since the plant has downsized twice. Most of her friends who work do so in the fast-food industry or in local supermarkets in the area.

This summer, baby Anne is watched by a 10-year-old neighbor, Andy, from 7:30 A.M. until 5:30 P.M. Andy takes Anne to the playground each day and watches her while he plays with his friends. When she needs a nap, he puts her down to sleep on the only grassy spot. He changes her once a day at noon and feeds her a bottle of watered juice, a bottle of watered milk, and cut-up hot dogs. The playground is located in a rough neighborhood and is the hangout for one of the many street gangs in the area. Almeada leaves the house at 7:00 A.M. and does not return until 6:30 P.M. During the hours that Andy is not watching Anne, she is alone in her bed in the apartment. Almeada knows that she needs help for herself and Anne. Before she moved from her old neighborhood, Almeada had been seeing a child welfare worker, Barbara Bailey. She plans to call Ms. Bailey tomorrow from work and hopes Ms. Bailey will be able to give her some ideas about where to go for help in this new part of the city.

Baby Anne cannot take care of herself. She is one of the many individuals who require human services just to have the necessities of life. Anne lacks adequate food, housing, and developmental opportunities. She is in danger because she does not receive appropriate supervision during the day. There is also some question as to whether Almeada can take care of herself properly. She is only 17, works long hours for little pay, and has the major responsibility of raising a child, although she is little more than a child herself.

Human services recognizes problems such as Almeada's as *problems in living.* As part of this recognition, the focus is not on the past but rather on improving the present and changing the future. Doing so involves directing attention to the client, the environment, and the interaction between the two. Individuals grow and develop through the life cycle, encountering problems in living such as adolescent rebellion, parenthood, midlife crises, caring for aging parents, and death and dying. Many difficulties in living arise in connection with families and communities; these may involve relating to children, spouses, and parents; maintaining progress in education; sustaining performance at work; and assuming responsibility for the very young or the very old. An important aspect of problems in living is the difficulty individuals encounter in interacting with their environments. If unemployment is high, finding work is not easy; if friends and relatives abuse drugs and alcohol, abstaining is difficult; if parents and peers do not value education, choosing to stay in school is problematic. Human services addresses problems in living, with a focus on both the individual or group and the situation or event. These problems occur throughout the life span.

Anne's mother, Almeada Smith, was 16 years old when Anne was born. Almeada received her early schooling in Chicago, but quit attending school regularly when she was in the fifth grade. She was held back in the first grade and again in the third grade because she had not mastered basic math and reading skills. Her parents did not think education was important; in fact, they did not require that she attend school at all. They were both alcoholics, continually unemployed and dependent on Almeada to structure their family life. By the time Almeada was 10, she had discovered that life was more pleasant away from home. After school, she would spend long hours playing with her friends on the streets; nights, she would spend with girlfriends. She became sexually active at the age of 12 under pressure from her friends, who ridiculed her until she became "one of the gang." At the time she became sexually active, she knew about AIDS but did not understand it as a problem for her.

Between the ages of 12 and 16, Almeada was in constant turmoil, wondering how and where to live her life. She received advice as well as pressure from parents, friends, and teachers to do what they wanted. Occasionally, she was asked to join special programs at school, but her parents would not give their permission. No one was particularly interested in what she wanted to do. She was entangled in a troublesome adolescent rebellion in which she rejected parents and teachers and accepted peers as models. Relating to peers brought unwelcome pressure to go along with the gang.

In responding to the needs of clients, human service professionals are encountering an increasing number of problems to be solved, a rise that many experts attribute partly to a changing culture and lifestyle. This broad increase in problems is another theme in human services.

The Growing Number of Problems in the Modern World

Human services has emerged in response to the growth in human problems in our modern world (Mehr, 1998). Life is complicated by several factors new to the last half of the 20th century. A growing number of people feel alienated and isolated from their neighborhoods and communities. No longer can they count on family and neighbors to share everyday joys and sorrows and assist in times of trouble and crisis. Households are in constant transition, as people leave family and friends to seek new job opportunities. Schools, churches, and recreation centers still provide meeting places, but because of the constant turnover, newcomers are welcoming newcomers. Stress is a hallmark of today's world. We worry about how to feed, clothe, and shelter children, families, adults, and the elderly. Illiteracy, a lack of employable skills, and unemployment rates or a low-wage employment add to people's feelings of helplessness and hopelessness, particularly in a technological age. The lifestyles that were once assured with a good education are no longer guaranteed. People may be trained for jobs that are being phased out or no longer exist. New technology may also cause many to lose their jobs. The world appears smaller as we have increased our capability for global communication. As more information is available, more choices appear possible. At the same time, new sources of worry are the problems of overpopulation, malnutrition, urbanization, and the environment of the planet. There is also threat of nuclear war, terrorism, civil wars and genocide, and religious and social conflict. The media bring vivid pictures of all these problems into the home through television, radio, and the Internet.

For the past two years, Almeada has felt the weight of daily living problems. When she was 16, she discovered she was pregnant, and she received this information with mixed feelings. She was familiar with the problem of pregnancy because many of her friends had been pregnant. They often discussed choices, but to Almeada there was only one choice: to have the baby and take care of it. She tried to seek help from a reproductive health agency but was frightened when she had to walk through a picket line of abortion protesters to get there. Of course, she could not expect much support from her parents, who were the only family she had ever known. She could not expect help from the father of her unborn baby or any of the other males in her life; most were just passing through the neighborhood. She was not sure where she would live or how she would support herself, but she knew that she would make it.

Almeada lives in a complex world with little support. An effective human service delivery system will teach her to use the skills she needs to manage her own life and survive the difficult challenges that face her. This self-sufficiency is another theme of human services.

Self-Sufficiency

For many human service professionals, the key to successful service delivery is providing clients, or consumers of human services, with the opportunity to be self-sufficient. Economic self-sufficiency strengthens an individual's self-esteem. When these individuals are able to contribute financially to meeting their own basic needs for food, clothing, and shelter, they gain a certain degree

●●●●●●●●●●

🌐 INTERNATIONAL FOCUS
The Sexual Exploitation of Children

The First International Congress was held August 27–31, 1996, in Stockholm, Sweden, to discuss the child sex trade and to begin advocacy for children who are its victims. The conference was organized by UNICEF, the Swedish government, and a Bangkok-based advocacy group called End Child Prostitution in Asian Tourism (ECPAT). Experts report that in Asia, over 1 million children a year are forced into sexual exploitation and that large numbers of children suffer this abuse in other parts of the world. Children are moved from city to city and country to country by sex traders, and many are used by men who believe they have less risk of contracting AIDS from having sex with a younger partner. According to expert Christine Beddoe, "In many developing countries, children are sent into the sex industry to earn money, since prostitution, in the short term, tends to be more lucrative than just about any other type of labor. And all over the world, children who live on the streets often turn to prostitution or are lured into sexual exploitation as a way to survive" (Barr, 1996a, p. 1). In more prosperous countries, many of the children who are exploited are "in flight from sexual abuse that usually began at home" (Daum, 1996, p. 19). For these children, sex for money gives them power that they never had at home.

Advocates believe that the key to attacking the sexual exploitation of children is the recognition that children are individuals who have human rights. In 1989, the United Nations Convention on the Rights of the Child promoted the concept of children's rights by stating that "every child has a right to live a life free of sexual exploitation and other abuses" (Barr, 1996b, p. 9). This idea is frightening to many adults, especially in countries where devotion to the family is considered primary or children are considered the property of their parents. The Convention states that children will not be protected until we believe that we must respect and nurture them.

SOURCE: Adapted from "World Activists Meet to Combat Child Sex Trade," by C. W. Barr, August 28, 1996a, *The Christian Science Monitor,* pp. 9–11; "Getting Adults to Think in New Ways," by C. W. Barr, September 16, 1996b, *The Christian Science Monitor,* pp. 9–11; "Sexually Exploited Children in Canada: The Law Is Not on Their Side," by K. Daum, September 17, 1996, *The Christian Science Monitor,* p. 19.

of independence, but they may still need some assistance. One important facet of moving clients to self-sufficiency is to empower them to make decisions and assume responsibility for their actions. Human services is committed to giving individuals and groups sufficient assistance to allow them to help themselves. Clients are encouraged to be independent and gain control of their lives as soon as they are able. They gain the beliefs in themselves or the efficacy to make the changes needed to become self-sufficient.

It was difficult for Almeada to become economically self-sufficient when she was 16, barely educated, and pregnant. She had little parental guidance or support and few skills. She was forced to move back home to live with her parents and seek the little help they could give her. In fact, she began taking care of them again. She got a job as a cashier at the local grocery store. Almeada saved a few dollars a week and bought groceries for the family with the rest. Her parents tried to borrow money from her to buy alcohol; they took her money if she brought it home.

In the early days of her pregnancy, Almeada's life became routine. She worked from 8 A.M. to 5 P.M., walked home, prepared dinner, and visited with her friends later at night. Her advancing pregnancy changed her relationships with some of her friends because she did not have the stamina or the desire to share their evening activities. Even as her life changed, she was determined that no one would interfere with it; she did not want help. Almeada wanted to make her own decisions. Despite that fiercely independent attitude, she would soon need assistance.

Almeada was somewhat self-sufficient because she was working and her parents provided housing. As her pregnancy advanced, however, she had to quit work and rely on others. She also needed prenatal care, parenting skills, and an opportunity to assess her decision to keep the baby. Although economic self-sufficiency is a key for many clients, it would clearly be only a beginning for Almeada.

Social Care, Social Control, and Rehabilitation

Human services serves three distinct functions: social care, social control, and rehabilitation (Neugeboren, 1991). *Social care* is assisting clients in meeting their social needs, with the focus on those who cannot care for themselves. The elderly, children, persons with mental disabilities or mental illness, and victims of crime, disasters, or crises are populations who might need social care.

Social control differs from social care in two fundamental ways: who receives the services and under what conditions they receive them. Social care is given to those who cannot provide for themselves (either temporarily or in the long term). In contrast, most recipients of social control are able to care for themselves but have either failed to do so or have done so in a manner that violates society's norms for appropriate behavior. Often, society rather than the individual determines who receives social control services. The purpose of such services is to restrict or monitor clients' independence for a time, because the clients have violated laws of the community. Children, youth, and adults in the criminal justice system are clients of social control.

Rehabilitation is the task of returning an individual to a prior level of functioning. What creates the need for rehabilitation? An individual who was once able to live independently becomes unable to function socially, physically, or psychologically. The inability to function can be caused by a crisis, a reversal of economic or social circumstances, an accident, or other circumstances. Rehabilitative services, which are designed to enable the individual to function near or at a prior level of independence, can have a short- or long-term focus. Veterans, persons with physical disabilities, and victims of psychological trauma are among those who receive rehabilitative human services.

In actuality, separating these three functions of human services is often difficult. Many clients have multiple problems, so social care, social control, and rehabilitation may be occurring at the same time.

Almeada finally became involved in the human service system in mid-autumn, when she was seven months' pregnant. She refused to go to school. Her parents let her continue to work at the neighborhood store—in fact, they encouraged her to. Her friends often missed school as well, so she saw them every day when they came to the grocery store to do their shopping. At evening, they all gathered at a shop in the neighborhood.

Two new programs were started at Almeada's school to provide more comprehensive support to many of its students. One program—Students, Parents Are Receiving KARE (SPARK)—targeted students who had irregular attendance, low math and reading scores, no discipline record, and positive teacher reports. In the fall, the school officials noted that Almeada, who qualified for this new program, had not returned to school after the summer vacation. The second program—Students Parents Each Are Special (SPEAS)—provided health care and other services to teen mothers. The case manager of SPARK, Barbara Bailey, visited the most recent address on the school records and found Almeada's father at home. He was in a drunken stupor and was unable to give Barbara information about Almeada. When Ms. Bailey talked to the neighbors, they suggested she try the grocery store where Almeada worked. Ms. Bailey found Almeada in the middle of her daily shift and made an appointment to pick her up after work and take her home.

In the next few months, Barbara Bailey provided social care for Almeada and then for her baby, Anne. The school offered Almeada several options for continuing her education: She could receive homebound instruction until and after the baby was born; she could come back to school; or she could attend a special night school for potential dropouts who work during the day. Ms. Bailey also referred Almeada to the SPEAS program. Almeada attended prenatal care class taught by a local teacher one night a week at the school. Because of Almeada's youth and lack of parental support, Ms. Bailey discussed with Almeada the options of keeping the baby or placing it for adoption. She also took Almeada to the health clinic located in the school to discuss these options further. Almeada remained sure that she wanted to keep her child. Ms. Bailey introduced Almeada to the welfare worker who was available on school grounds one day a week. Almeada rejected welfare as an option.

Once the baby was born, Almeada needed rehabilitative assistance but, instead, returned to work immediately. She expected her parents to care for Anne while she was gone, but her parents refused to baby-sit. Almeada was afraid that one day they might harm Anne out of their own frustration. Her parents could not stand to have the baby in the home because they had to compete with her for attention. Instead of receiving rehabilitative services, Almeada moved to a new neighborhood, rented a one-room apartment, and found a new job working in a garment factory six days a week. In her new neighborhood, Almeada was again without human services support.

The story of Almeada's struggles and need for assistance is just one of many about individuals who cannot meet their own needs without assistance from others. A common element seen in all human services is that these services help individuals, families, and groups with their problems. There would be little need for these services if people did not need assistance and support from others. The term *human services* encompasses the variety of helping services that addresses the range of problems that people experience.

The themes and purposes of human services—problems in living, increasing problems, self-sufficiency, and social care, social control, and rehabilitation—contribute to a definition of human services. Examining the interaction between the human service professional and the client also helps define human services. (See Table 1-1.)

TABLE 1-1   ✦   SUMMARY POINTS: ALMEADA'S CASE

- Both Almeada and baby Anne experience problems in living because their needs for adequate food, housing, and education are not met.
- Almeada's world is complex and she had little support during her pregnancy and after Anne's birth.
- Self-sufficiency was easier for Almeada when she was working, but her needs soon outgrew her resources.
- Social care provided Almeada with several choices to continue her education.
- Social control was not part of Almeada's case history because she maintained her independence throughout the pregnancy.
- Following Anne's birth, Almeada returned to work, moved, and found a new job rather than receive rehabilitative services.

WEB SOURCES
Find Out More About Meeting Almeada's Needs

http://community.michiana.org/famconn/teenpred.html

This website was developed by The Family Connection, a family agency in St. Joseph's County, Indiana, that provides comprehensive services to children and families. The website provides a summary of the services offered, state and local statistics, a description of welfare reform programs, and the community systems that are available within the county and within the state. In addition, there is an excellent list of recommended readings and links to related sites.

http://www.aecf.org/kidscount/kc1999/overview.htm

The Annie E. Casey Foundation website provides available data and analysis on critical issues affecting disadvantaged children and families. There are full texts of reports on issues that face children as well as a KIDS COUNT 1999 survey that tracks the status of children nationally and state by state.

http://www.agi-us.org/pubs/journals/2911597.html

This website is for a research journal, *Family Planning Perspectives*. This particular site covers Vol. 29, No. 3, May/June 1997, and is entitled "Teenage Abortion and Pregnancy Statistics by State, 1992." It is written by Stanley K. Henshaw. In this article he documents the national problem with teenage pregnancies.

http://www.acf.dhhs.gov

This website is for the Department of Health and Human Services. This department administers the major federal programs that provide services for children and families, such as Head Start and Temporary Assistance to Needy Families (TANF). This site has information about these programs as well as fact sheets and statistical information relating to children and families.

http://www.childrennow.org

Children Now disseminates information on children's issues, especially children and the media. This site has statistics on the status of children, polls on children's attitudes, research on television and the media, the *Media Now* newsletter, action alerts, and many links to sources of statistics, education, safety, parenting, government, and more.

http://www.familiesandworkinst.org

This site is developed by the Families and Work Institute, a national nonprofit research, strategic planning, and consulting organization that conducts policy and worksite research on the changing workforce and changing family/personal lives. It includes summaries of their publications on work–family issues, such as child care, family-friendly employers, and work–family programs and policies, as well as links to other sites.

http://www.futureofchildren.org

This site disseminates timely information on issues related to children's well-being.

···· The Interdisciplinary Nature of Human Services

The study of human service delivery, an understanding of the professionals who deliver services, and familiarity with the clients who are recipients of services requires the integration of knowledge from a wide variety of academic disciplines. These disciplines include but are not limited to sociology, psychology, and anthropology. Each discipline brings a unique perspective to the understanding of the nature of the individual, families, and groups of people. In addition, they focus upon the context of the environment in which "daily living" occurs and the interaction between the two.

While Barbara Bailey was working with Almeada, she knew that it was important to understand as best as she could about Almeada and her environment. The program in which Ms. Bailey received her training required her to take a large number of social science courses. According to her instructors, in order to understand the complexities of human behavior within the social environment, the study of sociology, psychology, and anthropology is helpful.

Sociology, as a discipline, examines the ways in which human societies influence the people who live in these societies. In other words, sociology assesses the individual and the broader culture, and tries to account for and understand the differences within human culture. Some of these differences are described very simply: "The Chinese wear white to funerals, whereas people in the United States prefer black. People in England and the United States say a watch 'runs' whereas the Spanish say it 'walks' and the Germans say it 'functions' " (http://www.macionis.com/whatis.htm). Sociology helps human service professionals understand elements of life that affect living such as family structure, family roles, gender, race, and poverty.

According to the American Psychological Association, "Psychology is the study of the mind and behavior. The discipline embraces all aspects of the human experience—from the functions of the brain to the actions of nations, from child development to care for the aged. In every conceivable setting from scientific research centers to mental health care services, 'the understanding of behavior' is the enterprise of psychologists" (APA, 1999). Many individuals believe that psychology helps explain "what makes people tick." It examines how people think, feel, and behave and explores why they think, feel, and behave in the ways in which they do. Numerous theories try to address how and why people act and think as they do. These theories analyze behavior and mental processes from the physiological, behavioral, cognitive, and psychodynamic perspectives. As they study psychology, students use these theories to develop a better understanding of people.

Anthropology studies the cultural, physical, and social development of humans and the variation in their customs and beliefs. A critical component of the study of anthropology is fieldwork. Anthropologists often live at the site they are studying as they try to learn about human groups and the role of culture in the lives of the individuals within these groups. Bronislaw Malinowski, a well-known anthropologist, explains fieldwork:

> Living in the village with no other business but to follow native life, one sees the customs, ceremonies and transactions over and over again, one has examples of their beliefs as they are actually lived through, and the full body and blood of actual native life fills out soon the skeleton of abstract constructions. . . . As to the actual method of observing and recording in fieldwork these imponderabilia of actual life and of typical behaviour. . . . The main endeavor must be to let facts speak for themselves. (Malinowski, 1984, p. 18, 20)

Today anthropologists study culture in its broadest sense. Not only are they studying about such groups who live in remote areas of the globe, but also they are studying individuals in mainstream culture in diverse settings. Similar to the tasks of the organizational psychologist, anthropologists are working in the business environment and studying topics such as the culture of work, employee relations, and human resources. In other words, they are learning about employee problems on the job by learning about employee perceptions and behavior. Directly related to human services are projects that help bring more clarity about the client served. For example, one project may focus on individuals with AIDS. Another may explore the life and problems of the homeless in contemporary society.

As Barbara Bailey tried to think about Almeada and her new life with baby Anne, she realized that the young woman's life would change as she moved away from her neighborhood, her friends, and her parents—and Barbara Bailey was worried about her. For many years Barbara has been able to use the information she learned in school to understand her clients and the situations they face. Almeada would be struggling to care for baby Anne and herself without a social support network or formal human services. Even though Almeada was strong and determined, the difficult environment within which she was living would present challenges that would be difficult to meet without help.

The work of human service delivery is an interdisciplinary endeavor that requires knowledge of individuals, an understanding of society and its relationship to individual and family life, and a view of the culture in which people live. Helpers like Barbara Bailey often work with clients who are very different from themselves. By integrating disciplines such as sociology, psychology, and anthropology, human service professionals can better understand the nature of their clients and their environments. This allows them to relate to their clients more effectively.

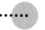 ## Dual Focus on Client and Helper

The delivery of human services involves both the client and the helper. The process of helping is client oriented as the helper focuses on assisting clients meet their needs. To do this, the helper performs many roles and assumes a wide variety of responsibilities. Let us look at Almeada and her human service worker, Barbara Bailey, to see the dual focus in action.

When Barbara Bailey first approached Almeada, she talked at length with Almeada about her situation. As her case manager, Barbara had contacted Almeada to learn whether she would come back to school and to help her with problems that were barriers to her school attendance. After they talked, it was obvious that Almeada faced many problems. Barbara planned to work with Almeada, baby Anne, and Almeada's parents if they would accept the help. First, Barbara wanted to introduce Almeada to services available at school, because Almeada and her parents were familiar with the school context.

Thirty years ago, a worker in Barbara Bailey's position would have focused on school-related issues; she would not have assessed Almeada's needs in other areas or referred her to other services. She might have told Almeada about other human service agencies, but Almeada would have had to contact them on her own. Today, human service professionals assist the whole person and empower clients to help themselves. Barbara Bailey was not able to meet all Almeada's needs, but she did work actively to connect her with other human service agencies in and outside of the school setting. In fact, multiple services at school reflect a current trend in human services to integrate client services. Barbara Bailey was providing assistance to Almeada and Anne who need help with their social, psychological, and economic problems. As a case manager, she also was coordinating the care that Almeada and Anne received.

As a human service professional, Barbara Bailey has the skills to develop a relationship with Almeada. In this situation, much of Ms. Bailey's success as a case manager is dependent on her personal interaction with Almeada and her ability to use professional skills such as active listening, observation, and assessment to establish a relationship. She is also able to apply her problem-solving skills to address the needs of Almeada and Anne. Using the problem-solving process, she initiates human service delivery by considering the relationship of her client with the environment and other professionals in the human service delivery system.

Barbara Bailey, the human service professional who helped Almeada, was a very effective helper. First, although she was employed by the school system, she was able to work with other professionals to develop a plan of assistance for Almeada and Anne, using the existing human service organizations for their benefit. Second, Barbara had the ability to engage in problem solving with Almeada and to recommend alternatives. She took a special interest in Almeada, provided a structure for Almeada's service plan, and linked Almeada with other organizations. For Barbara Bailey, Almeada was an important person, and one to be treated with respect and dignity.

The Client and the Client's Environment

Individuals who receive help do not exist in a vacuum; they are active participants in many different systems that influence their circumstances. Services to the client must be delivered with an understanding of the client's world and with the client's participation. To be effective, the human service professional must ask the client questions about present conditions, current stresses and relationships, and everyday events. The helper listens to the client, always attempting to see a situation through the client's eyes. Questioning and listening should help the human service professional understand the client's world. The helper must show both a strong commitment to the client and concern for the client's well-being. The helper also assists the client in identifying personal strengths and weaknesses and developing new skills and abilities to enhance personal development.

Human service professionals also function as educators. As educators, these professionals help clients develop certain skills to increase their intellectual, emotional, and behavioral options. The client is a complex individual with many intellectual, emotional, and behavioral possibilities. Clients feel better about themselves when human service professionals treat them as thinking, feeling, and acting human beings who are capable of change. If the human service professional believes in and promotes change, then change will be easier for the client.

In many situations the human service professional helps the client learn how to use the problem-solving process. According to McClam and Woodside (1994), "The purpose of performing the teaching role is to empower the client to solve future problems independently of the human service professional or agency." This leads to clients who begin to operate with increasing independence and self-esteem.

Almeada now lives in her new neighborhood with her daughter, Anne, and works six days a week in a garment factory. She knows she needs help. Because her major contact has been with human service professionals in another neighborhood, she does not really know whom to call, so she calls her previous case manager, Barbara Bailey. Ms. Bailey is delighted to hear from Almeada again and is alarmed at her plight. Almeada talks of her current work and child care situation in depressed and hopeless terms. Almeada seems to feel that she has limited options, and Barbara wants to refer Almeada to a source that can help increase those options. She tells Almeada

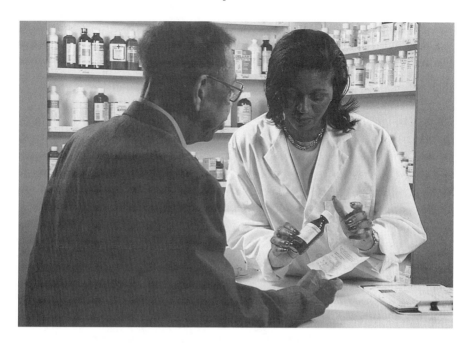

that she will make a few phone calls and then call her back. Barbara also wants to bolster Almeada's confidence in herself. As she gathers information about Almeada's move, her new employment, and her care of Anne, she praises Almeada's responsibility and maturity. She helps Almeada see how she has been a successful problem solver. She also praises Almeada's calling her and reaching out for help. Ms. Bailey knows that any positive change Almeada can make will help solve the rest of the problems.

A function of the human service professional is to help clients develop their ability to assess fundamental needs and to focus on the problems early in the helping process. Abraham Maslow, a psychologist, described a hierarchy of human needs that begins with basic physical needs and rises through higher levels to address safety and security needs, social belonging needs, self needs, and finally, self-actualization needs at the highest level. He stressed that addressing higher-level needs is difficult unless an individual's basic needs have been met (Maslow, 1971). In other words, if a child is hungry or very tired, or an adult is very scared, that child or that adult will have difficulty focusing on needs related to belonging or self-actualization. Clients are often so overwhelmed by their situations that they do not know how to identify what they need or where to begin to look for help or solutions. A good place to start is with the most basic needs, which are often the simplest to address and give the client satisfaction early in the helping process.

• • • • • • • • • •

 A Pioneer in Human Services

Dr. Harold McPheeters, a psychiatrist by training, is considered a key figure in the development of human service education. After serving as an administrator in the department of mental health in two states, he joined the Southern Regional Education Board (SREB) in 1965 as director for the Commission on Mental Health and Human Services and director of health programs.

His work began with a planning grant to bring together mental health professionals and community college officials to explore the feasibility of educating mental health practitioners in two-year colleges. That grant provided the groundwork for 20 years of research and training in the mental health and human service field. Defining the concept of the generalist worker, providing support for training mental health/human service professionals, developing a certification program for workers, and beginning an approval process for training programs were efforts completed under Dr. McPheeters's leadership and support. Before his retirement from the SREB in September 1987, Dr. McPheeters wrote (at our request) the following definition of human services, based on his 30 years of experience in the field. His definition integrates many of the ideas that have been presented.

> I never came up with an absolute definition of human services. Originally, our work began with the associate degree programs that were training people to work in some aspect of mental health. However, it soon became apparent that the graduates of those programs and the graduates of other programs that were titled according to other human service fields, such as child care workers, youth service workers, and aging program workers, were all finding employment in a variety of human service fields—not just in the narrow subspecialty areas of mental health, addiction, aging, and so on. So the terminology began to change to "human services" although no very precise definitions were applied. . . . Human services works with those same problems and people, but with a blend of primarily psychological and sociological theories and principles. Human services also has an eclectic approach to collaborating with whatever approaches (for example, medical) are needed to help people solve their problems. I suppose my definition would be something like this: Human services is the occupation/profession that uses a blend of primarily psychological and sociological theories and skills in preventing, detecting, and ameliorating psychosocially dysfunctioning people and in helping them attain the highest level of psychosocial functioning of which they are capable.

As an educator, the helper also teaches clients to recognize how their physical and interpersonal environments affect them. Clients are responsible for their own thoughts and behavior. Sometimes, however, clients are unable to make changes because their environments do not support such changes. Clients must be taught to determine the influence their environments have on their lives and to assess when and how their environments can be changed. Sometimes, such changes are very difficult or impossible.

In summary, an important conception of human services is the dual focus of the helper and the client. The helper is committed to developing a relationship with the client that facilitates problem solving within the client's own environment. Many times the human service professional is also an educator who is teaching the client important skills that can be used long after the potential help has ended.

Management Principles in Human Service Delivery

Understanding how services are delivered is an important part of defining human services. Three principles of management related to the delivery of services characterize the profession today: networking to develop a human service umbrella, forming teams and partnerships to provide service, and using case management to facilitate client growth. These management strategies help professionals provide more effective and efficient assistance to clients as well as enhance their own work environment.

Networking to Develop a Human Service Umbrella

Human services is not a single service delivery system, but a complex web of helping agencies and organizations whose primary goal is to assist people in need. It encompasses a variety of services that include but are not limited to child, youth, and family services; corrections; mental health; public health; crisis intervention; and education (see Figure 1-1).

Karin Eriksen (1981), a founding scholar in human service education, notes that "human services is often called the umbrella for our society's professions which are involved either directly or indirectly in promoting and reinforcing satisfying, healthy living and community cohesiveness" (p. 8). Going beyond the metaphor of the umbrella, Eriksen herself describes human services as a "bridge" between people and systems. One function of bridging is to narrow the gap between the services being offered and the needs of the individuals who are receiving those services.

Another bridging responsibility is to link human service agencies. Agencies and organizations share the common goal of assisting people in need. In the past, there has been little coordination, and the result has been overlapping worker responsibilities and competition for resources. Today, as service delivery philosophy changes and resources become scarce, agencies are limiting services, tightening eligibility criteria, and focusing on short-term interventions. Only increased communication, cooperation, and collaboration

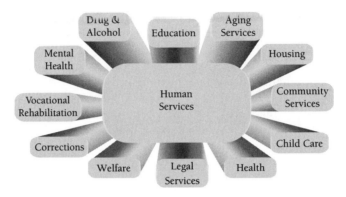

Figure 1-1 ✦ Human service network

SOURCE: Adapted from *Human Services Today,* by K. Eriksen, p. 7. Copyright © 1981 by Reston Publishing.

among helpers and agencies can promote effective service delivery. Networking is one way that service providers work together to serve clients.

Barbara Bailey wants to help Almeada in her new neighborhood, and she knows that finding a good entry into the system is critical. Ms. Bailey worries that, without the right help, Almeada will be lost in the human service delivery system. She needs to find another worker who is familiar with Almeada's neighborhood human service system and knows the formal and informal linkages that need to be made to deliver multiple services. She is looking for a worker who will help Almeada move between the many agencies whose services she will require. Almeada needs the support of those who provide child care and teach parenting skills. In addition, she needs assistance in improving her work skills and her health. Vocational development and public health services are rarely offered together. Coordination, monitoring, and evaluation are key services that are needed. Where will Barbara Bailey locate such a professional?

For Almeada or any other client to assume the responsibility of negotiating, the networking would be difficult; human service professionals must build the bridges between agencies, organizations, and services. Working together to provide services for the good of the client is often called "teaming" and is another management tool used for delivering good quality services to the client.

Forming Teams and Partnerships to Provide Services

Working as a team to provide services is part of the history of human services. Developers of the human service movement from early in its history stressed the importance of working with other professionals to assist the client in receiving services. More recently, the concept of working as a team has ex-

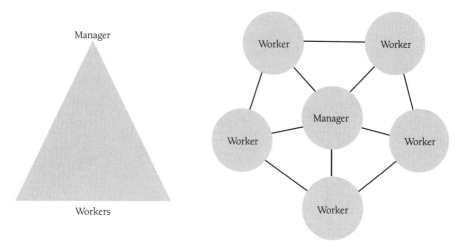

Figure 1-2 ✦ **Traditional organizational pyramid and new empowerment circle organization**

SOURCE: From *Empowerment: A Practical Guide for Success,* by C. Scott and D. Jaffe, p. 13. Copyright © by Crisp Publications.

panded, and "teaming" has become a common approach to organizing the work of an agency or organization.

The advent of teaming follows a progression in management philosophy. In the 1950s, managers were "learning to be friendly." In the 1960s, the trend was to be sensitive to the needs and motivations of one's employees, and in the 1970s, managers began asking employees for help. In the 1980s, managers were initiating meetings to hear from their employees, and in the 1990s, shared ownership between managers and workers was promoted (Scott & Jaffe, 1991). Today, at the beginning of the 21st century, the concept of partnership is being encouraged. Let us look at both teaming and partnership in human services and see how they are applied.

What exactly is the teaming concept? What principles do members of the team follow to deliver quality services? How does teaming improve services to the client or consumer? According to Foegen (1999), teaming, or empowerment, is a management concept based primarily on the changing role of the employee. Employees are encouraged to make more decisions and take responsibility with others for serving clients effectively. Responsibility and decision making in a human service context are better represented by a circle than by a pyramid. The circle illustrates the equality of responsibility among the team members (see Figure 1-2).

The following principles underlie the teamwork concept that makes this new management strategy so successful:

1. The customer is central to the planning and delivery of services. This basic principle guides the setting of goals, the intervention, and the

evaluation of services. It is not only important in teaming but is also a central philosophical principle of human services.

2. Members of the team must work together cooperatively. The team, not the individual, is the work unit, and all work is considered a joint effort. The successes of each individual are celebrated by the team, and everyone is committed to making the team more effective.

3. There is continual communication between the members of the team. This is a critical component of teamwork. To ensure cooperation and shared problem solving within a challenging environment, each member of the team needs to understand continually the status of other members' work, especially as the work of each is interdependent with that of the others.

4. All team members share responsibility, authority, and accountability. This concept is represented by the circle shown in Figure 1-2. The organization's commitment to giving its professionals the skills to assume this type of responsibility is at the heart of the teaming concept ("Selfish Managers," 1999).

After talking to several child and youth services offices, Barbara Bailey contacted Hernando Alvarez, a case manager in the child services division of the state department of human services. He recommended that Almeada call their office and schedule a meeting with an intake worker. Their office, just recently reorganized to be more customer oriented, was open for intake and service from 7 A.M. to 10 P.M. Mondays through Thursdays and on Saturdays from 8 A.M. until noon. Almeada would be assigned to a case manager who would not provide services but would coordinate them. In addition, four other workers would help plan, implement, and evaluate work with Almeada. A backup case manager would also know Almeada's case in detail and be available to support her if her primary case manager was absent. This particular team treats the entire human service delivery system as a larger team. They cooperate with each organization, sharing problems and finding creative solutions that benefit clients. One warning that Mr. Alvarez gave was the uncertainty of their agency's funding because of the evaluation of welfare return efforts. He hopes that Almeada does not get lost in the possible changes. At the conclusion of her conversation with Mr. Alvarez, Barbara Bailey felt she could make a good referral for Almeada, and she made a promise to herself to contact Hernando Alvarez in two months to check on her client's progress.

As stated in the case of Almeada, a major purpose of teaming is to improve the delivery of services to clients or consumers of the services. Teaming also makes the work of the organization more positive for the professionals involved. Teaming is intended to create an atmosphere that encourages creativity and problem solving and lessens tension in the workplace as it increases team spirit and motivation (Korine, 1999). The following quotation summarizes the team effort: "When you find yourself part of a group of people who are equally committed to the same mission, when you see that you are appreciated for your special qualities, when you know that your fellow team members care about you and your performance as much as they care about their own . . . it's a team" (Brown, 1992, p. 20).

There are also concerns that are currently being raised about teamwork. For example, teamwork does not seem to work unless all employees are engaged. It also takes good managers to teach and guide members of a team. Some workers want authoritarian leadership and seem to move to organizations where that type of leadership exists (Collins, 1999; Foegen, 1999; Mittler, 1999).

Even though there are some difficulties involved in using teams, the primary beneficiary of teaming in a human service setting is the client. The team approach yields more efficient and more effective service. As suggested in the case of Almeada, many professionals, functioning as a group, are working together to provide creative, coordinated services. Such teams are able to evaluate their own performance and make changes to improve their service delivery.

Partnerships are also emerging as a way that organizations in the human service delivery system can work together to serve their clients more completely. These partnerships are formed when two or more human service organizations agree to work together toward common goals. In addition, partnerships form with corporations, businesses, and government entities as those organizations outside the human service delivery system see benefits in supporting the social service sector. The goals of establishing partnerships are several (Snyder, 1996):

- Help promote an understanding of the challenges faced by all involved or concerned with providing human services to those in need.
- Provide an opportunity to access talent and expertise beyond each organization.
- Provide more cost-effective services.
- Increase awareness of broader issues and influence the planning and goal setting for all organizations and agencies involved.

Partnering requires many of the same qualities of teaming: a high degree of cooperation, a commitment of time, and a high level of trust. When partnering is successful, there is mutual gain for each of the parties involved.

The concept of partnership has emerged as a way for human service organizations to relate to each other for several reasons. Many of them are financial. As the cost of service provision increases and available financial resources decrease, many organizations are finding that they can provide services more cost effectively when they work with other agencies. Partnerships have also been encouraged by the increasing pressure to be accountable for resources expended. Agencies find that combining their resources and expertise enables them to provide better services to their clients.

One good example of a partnership exists in a rural West Virginia community. Simonton Windows is a Ritchie County manufacturer of vinyl windows. A primary goal of this company is not only to provide jobs and a good working environment for its employees, but also to be good citizens in the community. This company provides generous donations to local schools, supports city and county civic efforts, and provides special services to the elderly ("A Caring Company," 1998). Another example of a unique partnership is found in New York State. In an effort to meet several unrelated needs, New York operates a recycling center at a correctional facility. This facility services the surrounding area and provides employment training opportunities for inmates (Farrell, 1997).

Hernando Alvarez contacted Almeada the day after he talked with Barbara Bailey. Rather than place the burden of contacting the state department of human services (DHS) on Almeada, he went to see her at her workplace. He explained that Ms. Bailey had called him and that he was interested in working with Almeada to decide what services she needed and to help her find a way to access those services. Because the department had partnerships with many businesses and industries, he was able to schedule a time when he could meet with Almeada at her business site. Her employer had a small office for DHS workers and encouraged his employees to use the services the agency made available. Hernando knew that some services could be provided very quickly; others would evolve more slowly.

Hernando Alvarez and other DHS workers increased their ability to work effectively with clients through their partnership agreements with many local corporations and businesses. For DHS and other agencies, partnerships are usually established at the organizational level and are marked by a general statement of agreement that two or more organizations will work together. The text of the agreement contains language similar to the following: "This statement represents an acknowledgment by Organization A and Organization B of their mutual interest in forming a joint, long-term cooperative relationship whose purpose would be to encourage interaction between the two organizations." Later, the organizations work together to find specific projects and activities that would invite mutual support, and in Almeada's case her employer encourages DHS to support his employees.

Just as teaming and partnerships have emerged as powerful tools to improve the delivery of human services, another tool, the role and responsibility of case management, is emerging as a way to expand services available to meet the needs of the multiproblem or long-term client.

Case Management

Several factors make case management a viable alternative for service delivery today (Woodside & McClam, 1998). One is the shift from large, state-operated institutions to smaller, community-based facilities. This shift gives special importance to interorganizational coordination, a team approach, and helping professionals with a concern for the whole person because services are not being assessed or delivered in one comprehensive system.

A second factor is the categorical public funding of the past, which resulted in highly complex, redundant, fragmented, and uncoordinated services. The resulting system is burdensome for people with complex problems who are least able to act as advocates for themselves. In many cases, multiproblem clients are assigned a different worker within a given agency for each service and different workers in different agencies. Often there is no central worker who knows and understands the client's total situation or who is responsible for planning and coordinating treatment strategies.

A third factor is the very nature of human service work today. Service providers increasingly find themselves with a dual role: providing direct services and coordinating services from other agencies and/or professionals. Thom Prassa likens having a caseload to being an air traffic controller, coordinating and sometimes juggling many different cases. On a case-by-case basis, he often feels like he is "parachuting into a fire. We put out fires all the time: suicide attempts, arranging placements, paperwork, talking with parents, and so forth" (personal communication, July 10, 1994). This dual role can create problems in terms of time management, effective and efficient service delivery, and quality assurance.

According to Woodside and McClam (1998), the goal of case managers is to teach those who need assistance to manage their own lives but to support them when expertise is needed or a crisis occurs. In reality the use of case management is expanding rapidly into areas unheard of five years ago. Long-term care involving work with individuals encountering problems associated with aging, mental illness, disability, and mental retardation use case management as a method of coordinating and delivering services (Kane, Degenholtz, & Garske, 1999; Kane, 1999). A new use of case management is to link it with outreach functions to service targeted populations such as prenatal care for low-income, inner-city women and grandparents raising grandchildren (Loveland-Cook, Selig, Wedge, & Gohn-Baube, 1999).

What exactly do case managers do? They gather information, make assessments, and monitor services. In addition, they arrange services from other agencies, provide advocacy service, and assume responsibility for allocating scarce resources and providing quality assurance. They also provide direct services. Many human service professionals believe that being a case manager means they will do whatever they must to help their clients.

The case management structure affects both coordination of services and client access to services. Given the fragmented state of service delivery and claims of coordination that are not borne out in practice, what is needed is interorganizational and interagency coordination that does not shuffle clients

from one office to another. Exchanging resources rather than clients would ensure that clients do not get lost in the system or become frustrated with service delivery. Another necessary structural change is the establishment of a
single point of access rather than entry points at each agency. Another approach is to introduce clients to an array of community services. True coordination and integration allow clients to proceed through central intake, have
their needs assessed, and be assigned to providers.

Part of preparing for case management is learning to be proactive. Problems
today call for professionals who understand the need for case management and
have the skills to perform effectively in that role. As case manager positions increase, human service professionals will be ready to assume that responsibility;
but equally important, those trained as case managers will help develop organizational structures in which case management can work. We need professionals within the human service system who are able to promote these
changes. The management principles described in the preceding paragraphs define the emerging context in which human services are being delivered. Equally
important to understanding human services is knowing the broad range of
agencies and organizations that provide these services. (See Table 1-2.)

TABLE 1-2   ◆   SUMMARY POINTS: ALMEADA'S CASE

- Integrating different social science perspectives helps human service professionals
  understand clients and their environments.
- Barbara Bailey illustrates the importance of integrating and coordinating services as she
  teaches Almeada about problem solving and the influence of her environment on her life.
- Barbara Bailey's networking skills are useful in locating a human service professional who
  is knowledgeable about services in Almeada's new neighborhood.
- Almeada benefits from the creative, coordinated services provided by Hernando Alvarez
  and his team.
- A case management approach to Almeada's situation involves both providing and
  coordinating services.

Outcomes Evaluation

The environment of human services today reflects a consumer and community demand for competence, integrity, and accountability. Scarce resources
are being spent to provide help to individuals, families, and communities.
Outcomes assessment or evaluation assists in providing effective and efficient
services, determining best practices, and demonstrating what has been
achieved. The primary goals of outcomes evaluation are meeting accountability demands, facilitating decision making and planning, and improving
programs and services for the people served. Traditional questions that are
asked are as follows (Sherman, 2000):

- Why do we do what we do?
- What do we intend to do?

- Did we do what we said we were going to do?
- What were the results?

An outcomes evaluation provides information so that programs can be improved, maintained or redirected, or discontinued.

Human service agencies use several types of outcomes evaluation models. The traditional model uses an outside or in-house evaluator to establish the criteria or data that will be collected and used to describe the program, its staff, participants, and the gains made by the participants as a result of the services rendered. For example, a welfare-to-work program assessment might include demographic data concerning participants, descriptions of education and training received, time in the program, liaison services provided, time between education and employment, type of employment and salary, and length of time remaining employed.

A second model used in outcomes assessment is action evaluation (Rothman, 2000). This evaluation process provides feedback and data to funding sources, agency personnel, and participants throughout the provision of services. The evaluator actually begins with the process of goal setting by facilitating communication among those involved in the project to begin a dialogue among these different groups to determine similar, unique, and conflicting goals. During the initial process, goals are established by consensus, and the outcome measures directly relate to these goals. For example, a community group wants to establish affordable housing in a nearby community. Action research process works for consensus of goals (such as to provide jobs for youth in the area, develop a community action council, build housing) and involves all in the process.

A third model of outcomes assessment is empowerment evaluation (Fetterman, 2000). The goal of this model is to foster both the improvement and self-determination of participants. The methods of the model help individuals become independent problem solvers and decision makers. In other words, "it is designed to help people help themselves and improve their programs using a form of self-evaluation and reflection" (Fetterman, 2000). Empowerment evaluation occurs when administrators, frontline professionals, and clients all participate in determining outcomes of services delivered. Instead of using an outside evaluator to determine what gains have been made, those who know best provide information. For example, clients are asked to complete surveys, questionnaires, and interviews designed to explore exactly what the experience of the program was for them. They also make recommendations concerning what worked for them and how they would like services changed. They are encouraged to move beyond the expectations that professionals are the only ones who can help them with their problems.

 ## Roles of the Human Service Professional

The human service professional provides services in a variety of settings. To respond to the many settings and the diversity of clients these settings represent,

the helper needs a broad based education and a willingness to adapt to changing roles and circumstances. There are two principal types of human service
providers: the generalist and the nonprofessional.

The Generalist

The concept of the generalist is fundamental to human services. It describes
the kinds of skills the professional has and the types of functions the professional performs. The term *generalist* has not always been associated with human services; the concept has evolved over the last few decades. Early in the
history of human services, the term referred to a person who worked within
a specific discipline, such as psychology or psychiatry. Professionals in these
disciplines performed many functions: interviewing, diagnosis, therapy, and
follow-up. As a generalist, the professional performed all the duties expected
of a member of that particular profession.

As the role expanded, the term took on a new meaning, connected to a
specific client group. Generalists performed duties and had the skills to work
with only one group. For example, youth mental health workers specialized in
working with children. This would include working with individuals and with
groups in educational, recreational, and counseling situations. Such workers
would also be familiar with social, biological, and developmental problems of
children and adolescents; they would also understand the importance of working with the family.

A third emerging concept of the generalist is most representative of human services today. The human service generalist has the knowledge, values, and skills to perform several job functions in most human service settings. The generalist also understands how these functions fit with client
and agency goals. For example, a helper trained to conduct interviews,
write social histories, and define a treatment plan should be able to perform
those responsibilities with the elderly, young children, or persons with
mental retardation.

The human service generalist works with the client using both micro- and
macroperspectives (Cimmino, 1999). The micro system is represented by the
individuals in the client's environment and might include family, friends,
teachers, coworkers, and individuals within the human service delivery system. The macro system is represented by the organizations, agencies, communities, and neighborhood locales in which the client interacts. For example, if
the human service professional is working with the individual client using the
microperspective, then the professional is interviewing the client, establishing
rapport, and engaging in planning and problem solving. Using the macroperspective, the same professional works with the client to understand his or her
larger environment. This might include learning how to use the human service bureaucracy to convert needs into political action or to understand how
school relates to the neighborhood.

It is interesting to examine follow-up studies of graduates of human
service programs to see the development of the generalist concept as well as

the broadening definition of human services. Early studies compiled by the Southern Regional Education Board indicated that graduates of human service programs were getting jobs in state hospitals, educational settings, mental health centers, children's agencies, and general hospitals. Three-fourths of the jobs were in mental health agencies. Although these graduates were performing a wide range of services, most were indirect services dealing with patients and other staff members. Their job functions were client advocacy, community consultation, and collecting basic research data—in other words, working from the macroperspective. (Southern Regional Education Board, 1979).

Studies of graduates of human service programs since 1972 differ significantly from the earlier surveys. The results reflect a diversity of employment settings for graduates, including state hospitals, mental health centers, centers for the developmentally disabled, schools, child and family services centers, correctional facilities, nursing homes and other service facilities for the aging, abuse prevention and treatment centers, recreation centers, centers for people with physical disabilities, crisis intervention units, child- and elder-abuse prevention and treatment centers, group homes, and specialized fund-raising organizations. The job functions of these graduates include direct service activities, group and individual counseling, patient advocacy, interviewing, referral, gathering and recording information, treatment planning, discharge, follow-up, grant writing, fundraising, and administration. These responsibilities reflect work within both the micro- and the macroperspectives.

Future job opportunities for human service graduates are expected to be excellent (*Occupational Outlook Handbook,* 1998) and will continue to reflect the generic nature of helping. "The number of social and human service assistants is projected to grow much faster than the average for all occupations between 1996 and the year 2006—ranking among the most rapidly growing occupations" (p. 155). In fact, for two years in a row, *U.S. News & World Report* included human service responsibilities in the 20 hot job tracks in its *1998 Career Guide* and its *1999 Career Guide* ("20 Hot Job Tracks," 1997; "20 Hot Job Tracks," 1998). Many of the professions also emphasize the expanding elderly population. Today, the fastest growing population is centenarians.

Just as the role of the generalist human service worker has evolved over the past four decades, the role of the nonprofessional helper has changed and expanded. This change is described next.

The Nonprofessional

In the past decade two categories of helpers have made significant contributions to the human service delivery system: volunteers and self-help groups. Today, volunteers contribute considerable staff power within the human service sector. According to the Independent Sector website (http://www.indepsec.org), volunteerism in the United States, and globally, is experiencing

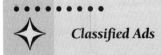

Classified Ads

Resident Care Assistant
Assistant Living Facility
Now accepting applications at Health Care Facility
Hours are 7 A.M.–5 P.M.
Education: Required AA or BA in human services or related degree.

Child Care Teachers
Needed to love and nurture children ages 8 weeks to 5 years.
Full-time and Part-time Positions Available.
Education: Required AA in child care education. BA in child and family
or human services or psychology preferred.

Counselor
Needed for in-home treatment program assisting families, children, and
adolescents. Position requires a minimum of a BA in social work or related field. MA preferred. Minimum of 2 years experience with children
and families. Responsibilities include individual and family therapy,
treatment planning, clinical and case management.

Counselor
Outpatient substance abuse treatment program needs a full-time counselor.
Degree or certification in a behavioral science field required.

Probation and Parole
Need responsible individual to work with youth on parole. BA required.
Must take state exam. Preference given to those with experience working
with youth.

an increase in both the number of those volunteering and in the time spent
volunteering. In 1991, 12.4 million individuals volunteered their time, and in
1996 this number increased to 60.6 million. In 1991, the average number of
hours per year volunteered by an individual was 166.4 and by 1996 this had
increased to 182.0. By 1998 an estimated 109.0 participated in volunteer activities (Independent Sector, 2000).

Typically, we think of volunteers as people who give their time without any
pay, but early scholars on volunteerism such as Ellis and Noyes (1978) maintain that this definition is overly simplistic today. Elements of an accurate def-

inition of *volunteer* are (1) that people give their time of their own free will, (2) that they do so because of a feeling of social responsibility, and (3) that they show little concern for monetary profit. The third element allows for some form of reward or reimbursement that is much less than the actual value of the service provided. For example, volunteers may be reimbursed for mileage incurred in transporting clients.

People volunteer for various reasons: to work with people, to meet people, to gain job references, or to help others. Whatever the reason, retaining volunteers involves matching the tasks assigned them with their motivations. For example, a person who wants to work with people would probably not be happy if assigned to a filing job. Volunteers are valuable resources, particularly in times of decreased funding. They personalize services, can be good advocates, and bring new skills and interests and a high level of enthusiasm to an agency setting. Today, the number of volunteers is growing among young working professionals.

In fact, the number of organizations that broker volunteers for various agencies has increased. For example, cities provide these coordinating services and advertise through newspapers, local TV stations, and the World Wide Web. A coordinating agency tries to simplify volunteering. In a sense, it tries to "sell" the volunteer experience by asking questions such as:

- So you want to explore a career area?
- Do you like helping others?
- Would you like to meet new people?
- Do you know you have something to offer others?

Volunteers can find jobs for as intense a commitment or as small a commitment as they would like to make. One such agency focuses on volunteering on an impromptu basis. Instead of asking for a two-hour commitment from a volunteer each week, the network links the volunteer and the organization on a more short-term basis. Calls are made to a central organization a week prior or even the day of the volunteering effort, and the volunteer is given a choice of direct service activities such as painting buildings, selling tickets for fund-raising events, or reading to children (Sack, 1995).

Another approach to using volunteers is to provide long term, intensive training to volunteers and to integrate these individuals into the human service delivery system. There is a body of knowledge that has developed around establishing and managing volunteer efforts and many agencies have a specific staff member assigned to coordinate volunteers. These coordinators solicit committed volunteers, invest time and other resources in training, and schedule and evaluate the volunteer efforts. One such agency is CONTACT, a 24-hour phone help line that first provided its services in 1963 in Sydney, Australia. The first contact center in the United States opened in Dallas, Texas, in 1967. Today there are 82 accredited centers in the United States providing 24-hour-a-day, seven-days-a-week care by phone to the lonely, the troubled, and the depressed.

●●●●●●●●●

◆   *"Bunny" Brichetto*

"Doing for others makes me happy." This has been "Bunny" Brichetto's life motto and is still the motivating factor that keeps him hopping from morning until night. His day begins at his desk creating some of the 400 greeting cards he mails each year; then he and his wife, Martha, skip over to the Golden Age Retirement Village in east Knoxville to serve lunch to senior citizens who are enrolled in the Senior Nutrition Congregate Meals Program; and finally in the afternoon, he bounds over to the First Christian Church to plan the next program or day trip for their seniors. (You would never guess this energetic, enthusiastic gentleman will be 80 years old this summer!)

Bringing smiles to others is a constant occupation for this Bunny. Back in the 1950s, he sold popcorn for 10 cents a bag at the theater he owned. He added a personal touch by drawing a bunny and having a rubber stamp made to stamp each bag—and thus began his "hare mail" tradition. Recipients of his special cards always know who the sender is because of his bunny mailman stamp. He has a unique talent for matching the card with the receiver. Many a lonely, homebound, elderly person has had their day brightened by the cheerful card he sent. He has recruited other stampers in the area to help him design the cards and expand his outreach.

Each week for eight years, Bunny and Martha delivered Mobile Meals to homebound seniors. He joined with other concerned volunteers and community leaders in 1998 to establish Friends of Mobile Meals, a group formed to help the Senior Nutrition Program staff find ways to eliminate the list of over 200 seniors who needed meals but could not be served because of lack of funds. From this group, the ADOPT A SENIOR fund-raising campaign was started. The community support dollars from this effort helped the program serve those seniors on the waiting list, and it continues to help the program expand the number of homebound elderly it serves.

At a Friends of Mobile Meals meeting, another area of service was mentioned. The Senior Nutrition Congregate Program no longer had funds available to pay a staff person to serve meals daily at the Golden Age Retirement Center. Several of these folks were in wheelchairs or on walkers. They really needed the social contact in the dining room where the meals were served, but the program was in a dilemma as to how to continue their service. Bunny contacted his wife and they volunteered to serve meals there three days a week. They would also help recruit volunteers for the other two days. Within six months, they had recruited and trained another couple to work when they were volunteering at their church or the hospital.

Bunny leaped into action when he and Martha arrived at the Golden Age Center. Whenever he saw a need among the residents, he searched

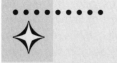

for a resource to help. He planned an ice cream social, providing the ice cream, toppings, and cake along with fruit for the diabetics. The seniors were delighted! Then he planned a pancake breakfast with he and his wife serving as chefs. He used these social gatherings to encourage the seniors who were not already eating in the dining room to enroll in the Senior Nutrition Program. Thus, they would benefit from the hot nutritious meals and it would be a reason for them to get dressed, come outside their apartment walls, and meet other residents. This strategy worked! New participants were enlisted and spirits soared at the towers.

"Mr. and Mrs. Bunny have lifted the morale of the entire apartment complex," exclaims Nettie Anderson, the apartment manager. "Their smiles, their positive attitudes, and their upbeat approach to life have transformed this place. Bunny takes pictures of the clients involved in activities and posts them on the bulletin boards. When the vegetable man isn't coming, he brings a load of bananas and distributes them in the building. (Those who have high blood pressure need potassium daily, he explained.) They are always bringing surprises: pencils, mugs or cups, caps, flowers or plants, etc. They also check in with the shut-ins to see if they have an errand to be done. They recycle newspapers from all the residents for their church recycling bin. For the residents who cannot come downstairs and bring the papers, they go to their apartments and pick them up. Now, other seniors are following their example and collecting papers from their neighbors. In fact, the Bunnies have helped create a community atmosphere of helping each other."

Like the Energizer bunny, this Bunny is always on the move. He is in charge of the senior class at First Christian Church and plans a potluck and special program monthly. Together, Bunny and Martha visit the nursing homes and hospitals for their church each week. Their list also includes seniors from the Golden Age Retirement Center.

Bunny Brichetto loves people and is happiest when he can bring a smile to a weary face or share the load of someone in need. When anyone mentions slowing down, he just flashes a "Bunny" grin and says he's too busy! His compassion, his humor, his ability to assess a situation and render immediate help, his steadfastness, his bubbly personality, and his integrity keep him reaching out to others, especially the frail elderly. He is making a difference daily in their quality of life. The Senior Nutrition Program is incredibly blessed to have Bunny as a special volunteer.

SOURCE: Jennifer Oakes, Senior Nutrition Program Volunteer Coordinator, Office on Aging, CAC, Knoxville, Tennessee, 2000. Reprinted by permission.

Another category of helpers who are assisting human services to respond to today's challenges is *self-help groups*. These groups consist of laypeople from all walks of life who come together to create a mutual support system to meet their own needs. Members share a common problem; they consider themselves peers; and they organize separately from human service organizations. The purposes of such groups include helping with chronic problems or general problems in living, raising consciousness, securing political rights, and providing support for behavior changes. Over half a million such groups are currently providing support for people with similar problems. Examples include Mothers Against Drunk Driving (MADD) and Alcoholics Anonymous (AA).

Self-help groups have multiplied for several reasons. First, individual members have needs that are not met by traditional sources. This situation often arises when fiscal constraints force agencies to trim budgets, personnel, and services. Second, there has been a decline of support from family, church, and neighborhoods as well as a decline in personal involvement with these institutions. A third reason is that self-help groups are very effective in meeting needs. Those involved are able to articulate clearly the needs of the target group and can establish support rather easily as the others involved have similar experiences and difficulties.

Self-help groups also have emerged as a way in which clients can develop a clearer sense of identity and competence. Within the context of a self-help group, clients are able to gain control over their own lives and begin to help themselves and others (Dickerson, 1998). As social issues have changed, self-help groups have developed around new issues and problems. These include support for caregivers for dementia and Alzheimer's patients, community safety, sandwich generation, and others (Jansson, Almberg, Grafstroem, & Winblad, 1998; Porter, 1998; Sadler & Morty, 1998).

One unique approach to self-help/mutual aid is represented by the voluminous amount of material available that was prepared by individuals who have themselves been clients in the human service delivery system. These individuals have developed materials designed to describe their own struggles and experiences or provide guidelines, directions, or instructions about how to ameliorate such circumstances. Much of this material is found on the Web. We suggest that material of this nature be reviewed critically by asking the following questions: Who is the author? What is the author's purpose? Does this information correlate with what experts say about the subject? One such example is a website prepared by Jennifer G., a 23-year-old college student who has suffered from depression since she was 15. Her expressed goal for creating the website is to help others with depression feel less isolated and alienated. The site contents include an autobiography, a glossary of mental health terms, a bill of rights for clients, self-injurer's loss of rights, helpful quotes, a web page of "hot" links to other sources, a discussion on the stigma associated with depression, recommended readings with a "hot" link to amazon.com, and a distraction survey provided for those who suffer from depression and want to engage in a positive activity (http://members.aol.com/zuzubailie/siteinfo.html).

Even practicing psychologists are using this type of material as a component of their therapy by recommending autobiographies written by mental health patients (Clifford, Norcross, & Summer, 1999). Those most recommended include *An Unquiet Mind* (Jamison, 1995), which tells of the struggle of a full professor of medicine who has suffered from manic depression since her teenage years. She describes her own world of madness, her darkness days, and how this illness has affected her life. Another book that is often recommended is *Nobody Nowhere,* (1994), Donna Williams' account of her battle with autism. She provides insights not only to those who experience autism, but also to parents, teachers, and clinicians who work with the autistic.

The other helpers (volunteers and self-help) described here have been welcomed by professionals. Perhaps the most immediate reason for their acceptance is that all agencies face financial constraints at one time or another, and this can lead to a shortage of professionally trained workers. Some agencies may have an uneven distribution of mental health professionals with respect to race, social class, and place of birth; the utilization of nonprofessionals can remedy this problem. Nonprofessionals also have been willing to work in places and with populations that professionals find unattractive.

Activities of the Human Service Professional

The professional activities of the human service helper are often discussed in the professional literature and are defined by the helper's relationship with clients and other professionals, academic training, ethical standards, continuing education, and measured competence. Human service professionals often work with individuals who have few material possessions and little emotional support and who need many professional services and much professional care. The human service professional is often the first to provide support when the client enters the system. Clients become involved with helpers because they hope for a better existence. They view human service professionals as important people with special information and skills to help them identify and work toward their goals.

A human service professional's activities include academic training founded on a systematic body of knowledge. Academic preparation for human services takes either two or four years, depending on the training program. This intense training, academically and experientially based, focuses on the acquisition of knowledge and skills pertinent to human service systems, workers, and clients. The training is also systematic. It begins with the study of introductory concepts of human services, then explores types of clients, problems, and methods of addressing those problems, and culminates in supervised field experiences. The body of knowledge on which the training is based is interdisciplinary, drawn from other helping fields including psychology, criminology, rehabilitation, counseling, and social work. Human service field practice is unique in its diversity of settings and populations; however, the basic helping skills and methods of addressing client needs are both unique to human services and borrowed from other helping professions. Trained as generalists, human service professionals are thus taught knowledge and skills that can be transferred to diverse settings and populations. Fullerton (1999) describes it as follows:

> The theories we use in human services vary along many dimensions. They range in scope from comprehensive explanations of human behavior to theories regarding very specific behaviors. They range in perspective from biological to psychological to sociological explanations of the human condition. They vary considerably in the degree to which they have been empirically tested, and they vary in terms of their applicability across age, gender, race, or cultures. (Fullerton, 1999, p. 75)

Practitioners need such flexibility to deal with the complex individuals and environments they encounter.

The good relationship the human service professional has with other social service professionals is a measure of the status of human services. Other helpers work with human service professionals side by side in a professional setting. For some, this professional is the one individual who is specifically designated to focus on the client's mental health and to coordinate social care. In a nursing home, for example, the human service professional admits the client, takes a social history, monitors and facilitates the client's adjustment, coordinates services with family needs, counsels the client during troubled times, and attends treatment team meetings with the staff to discuss the client's admission, progress, and discharge. Other professionals include physical therapists, physicians, nurses, and pharmacists who focus on the client's physical health. These professionals look to the human service worker to address the client's mental health needs, which may involve support or referral to a specialist. In other settings, the human service worker is one of many mental health professionals. In a mental health institution, for example, psychiatrists, psychiatric nurses, psychiatric social workers, psychologists, human service workers, and psychiatric technicians all focus on the mental health of the client. Each of these workers has a particular function within this setting, and each relies on the others to perform their appropriate tasks effectively. For clients and other social service providers, the work of human service professionals is essential.

Ethical standards also define professional human service activities. Human service professionals are committed to the ethical treatment of clients and the development of ethical relationships with coworkers, other professionals, and the system. Ethical standards guide this behavior. Because clients are the central focus in human services, their treatment and rights are of great concern, including issues of confidentiality and respect for the client's values, heritage, beliefs, and self-determination. Human service professionals are usually bound by two sets of ethical standards: those developed by human service professionals and educators and those developed specifically for the populations they serve. See Chapter 9 for the Ethical Standards of Human Service Professionals.

Another important professional activity of human service professionals is continuing education. A commitment to continued learning and development while working in the field is essential for such professionals. This continuing education takes many forms. According to follow-up studies of human service program graduates, many seek advanced degrees. More than half the graduates of two-year programs seek a bachelor's degree—most often in human services, psychology, sociology, criminal justice, or related fields. Graduates of four-year human service programs seek master's degrees in social work, public health administration, nursing, counseling, educational psychology, rehabilitation, and related fields. Human service professionals also continue their education by belonging to professional organizations. Many of these organizations are related to the specific fields in which their members work or the specific population they serve (Woodside, McClam, & McGarrh, 1993). A final way human service professionals grow and develop is through in-service training. Many agencies sponsor seminars on current social or policy issues, on skill development, or on professional issues. Agencies that do not offer such seminars often encourage their workers to attend seminars sponsored by others.

Competence in human services is certified by awarding two-year, four-year, or advanced degrees in human services; however, competence is not supervised by a national organization. In 1982, the National Commission for Human Service Workers was incorporated "to provide a national system for voluntary registration and certification of human service workers" (National Commission for Human Service Workers, 1982, p. 1). The commission has disbanded, but there is now some interest in reestablishing registration and certification standards.

In the mid-1990s, a project was undertaken by the federal government to establish standards for a number of emerging professions. The Human Service Research Institute was given the responsibility for researching the current status of human service occupations and describing the contemporary workplace within the human service delivery system. This project developed for human service practitioners skill standards, activities the professional assumes, and practical outcomes of the work. The result of this study is a document, *The Community Support Skill Standards: Tools for Managing Change and Achieving Outcomes,* that more clearly defines the work of human service professionals (Human Services Research Institute, 2000).

In summary, human service professionals are concerned about and participate actively in training, ethical commitment, continuing education, and registration and certification. It is a relatively new occupation involved in professional activities of value to those who receive its service. (See Table 1-3.)

TABLE 1-3   ✦   SUMMARY POINTS: PROFESSIONAL ACTIVITIES

- Acquire the knowledge and skills that can be transferred across settings and populations.
- Establish good working relationships with other professionals.
- Abide by the ethical standards that guide professional behavior.
- Pursue continuing education opportunities to learn and develop as a professional.

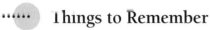 ## Things to Remember

1. Human services has developed in response to the need of individuals or groups for assistance to live better lives.
2. Because human services recognizes client needs as problems in living, it does not focus on the past but seeks to improve the present and change the future.
3. Human services has emerged as a response to the increase in human problems in our modern world.
4. Human services provides three distinct functions: social care, social control, and rehabilitation.
5. Human services uses an interdisciplinary approach to understanding clients, helpers, and the context.
6. Human services consists of those services that help people with their problems.
7. The dual focus of client and helper guides the delivery of services.
8. Certain management principles influence delivery and reflect the value of focusing on the client.
9. The interaction between the client and the human service system also defines human services.
10. The services provided are designed to improve an individual's well-being.
11. In the successful delivery of services, the client develops new insights, skills, and competencies.
12. The field of human services is respected by its clients and other helping professions.
13. Human service work is a profession committed to ethical standards and continuing education.

Additional Readings: Focus on Poverty

Zucchino, D. (1997). *Myth of the welfare queen: A Pulitzer prize–winning journalist's portrait of women on the line.* New York: Touchstone.
The author, a journalist, spent a year sharing the lives of two "welfare mothers" in Philadelphia to gain a look at their day-to-day existence.

Finnegan, W. (1998). *Cold new world: Growing up in a harder country.* New York: Random House.
An intimate report of the lives of some families who are not thriving in the new American class structure: a 15-year-old drug dealer in New Haven, Connecticut; a sleepy Texas town transformed when crack arrives; Mexican-American teenagers in Washington State unable to locate their immigrant parents and trying to find an identity in gangs; and jobless, young white supremacists in a downwardly mobile Los Angeles suburb.

Kotlowitz, A. (1998). *The other side of the river: A story of two towns, a death and America's dilemma.* New York: Doubleday.

Two Michigan towns separated by the St. Joseph River, one a primarily white, prosperous community and the other an impoverished black community, are the setting for an investigation of a death that becomes a screen onto which each community projects its resentments and fears.

Simon, D., & Burns, E. (1997). *The corner: A year in the life of an inner-city neighborhood.* New York: Broadway Books.

This true story describes one year in the life of an inner-city neighborhood in West Baltimore by focusing on a handful of people who struggle to survive (and escape) the drug market that fuels their world.

Chapter 2

A History of Helping

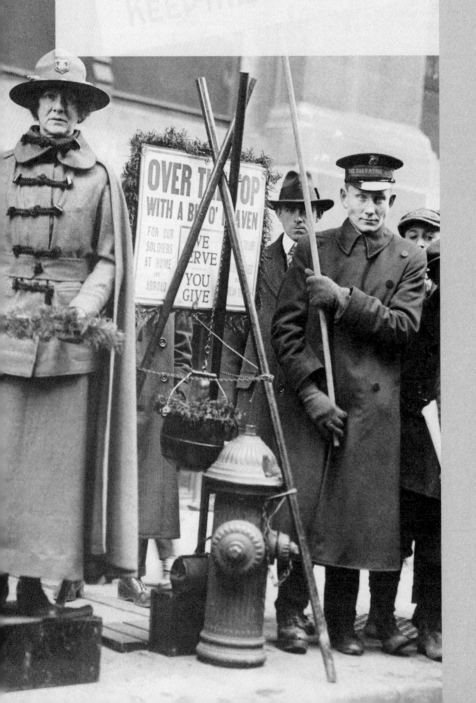

Chapter 2 presents an overview of the history of helping to provide insight into the emergence and growth of services to people in need. This chapter traces the changing beliefs about who is "less fortunate" and examines the different categorizations of less fortunate people throughout history. The categories familiar to us today—the poor, persons with mental impairments, and criminals—have not always been used. What is central to a definition of *less fortunate,* both then and now, is consideration of the "have-nots" in society, who meets their needs, and how those needs are met. In addition, we examine the emergence and growth of the human service movement. This chapter assists us further in defining human services.

 ## Early History

Until the Middle Ages, people believed that mental illness was caused by evil spirits, and early forms of treatment focused on ridding the body of these demons. One treatment used was trephining the skull (using a crude saw to remove circular discs of bone). This hole in the head allowed evil spirits to escape. Another popular method of treatment was exorcising evil spirits through religious rites. Persons with mental illness were feared because their supposed possession by spirits was perceived as a link with the supernatural. Other attempts to control the demons included chaining, beating, starving, and bleeding the unfortunate human host (NIMH, 1971).

Hippocrates, a physician in the third century B.C., was one of the few professionals who used the scientific approach to explain and treat problem behavior and mental illness. He believed that problem behavior was a function of natural illness and that mental disorders had natural causes. In other words, evil spirits were not probable causes of mental illness. He believed that mental illness could be caused by brain disease, heredity, and head injuries. Hippocrates was also able to distinguish between different types of mental problems; among his most significant contributions were labels for illnesses such as *melancholia* and *epilepsy,* which are still used in mental health today. His work marks the beginning of the medical model of service delivery.

200 B.C.	Hippocrates influences
Early History	Mental illness, evil spirits
1500s	St. Thomas, St. Francis—First human service workers
1500–1600s	England protects mentally impaired
1601	First Elizabethan Poor Law
1700s	Almshouses established
1773	State hospital opened in Williamsburg, VA
1792	Pinel's humane treatment of the mentally ill

Early History Timeline

Until the 1500s, the Catholic Church was chiefly responsible for providing human services. Religious figures such as St. Thomas Aquinas and St. Francis of Assisi are considered by some to be the first human service professionals (Eriksen, 1981). Under the Church's guidance, many institutions were founded for the poor, orphans, the elderly, and people with disabilities. At this time, deviant behavior was perceived as a sickness, and asylums were established to house those who were so labeled. After A.D. 1500, the power of the Church declined and that of government increased, producing conflict between church and state.

In addition to services provided by the Church, the needy in England also received attention from the government. (In fact, the English Crown's right and duty to protect persons with mental impairments had existed from the 13th century.) For persons with mental impairments, two categories were established: (1) natural fools or idiots and (2) those who were non compos mentis. *Idiots* became the preferred term for the first category, which included people with retarded intellectual development whose condition was permanent, present at birth, or both. The second category, *non compos mentis,* was the umbrella term for all other mental disabilities. By the 15th century, the term *lunatic* had replaced non compos mentis.

Diagnoses of mental illness were determined by inquisitions (unrelated to those established by the Catholic Church), which were conducted by a government official and a jury of at least 12 men (Neugebauer, 1979). The following questions were asked in the investigation:

- Was the person an idiot or a lunatic?
- When, how, and in what manner was the individual lucid?
- What lands and other property did the individual own?

The Crown's rights and duties were determined by these diagnoses. It was the king's duty to protect an idiot's lands and property and to provide the individual with the necessities of life; and the king was entitled to all the revenues from those lands. More extensive protection was provided for lunatics at no charge to the individual, because the revenues of a lunatic's estate were used to support the person and his or her family during the time of the illness. Of course, this system provided no help to the many lunatics who had no estate.

Before the Middle Ages, feudal lords had assumed responsibility for much of the care of poor and sick people who lived on their lands. During the Middle Ages, needy people received aid from three sources. Human service institutions (such as orphanages) continued to assist specific populations. The Church also provided services directly to the needy and donations to other service providers. Late in this period, governments began to adopt innovative legislation, which provided the framework for human services for many years to come.

Several types of institutions provided services during the Middle Ages. One important source of aid to the needy was hospitals. Not only did they provide medical assistance to the ill, but they also fed and housed tired travelers, orphans, the elderly, and the poor. These institutions were usually attached to monasteries, and their capacity ranged from a dozen to several hundred patients.

A second type of institution, the insane asylum, was established in Europe during the 15th and 16th centuries. These institutions represented some concern for the care and housing of people with mental illness, but the patients did not receive effective treatment, and their living conditions were poor. The following excerpt (Friedrich, 1976, p. 49) describes the conditions at London's Bethlehem Hospital, an institution typical of the asylums established during that time:

> London's Bethlehem Hospital, better known as Bedlam, founded in the thirteenth century as a priory, converted in the fourteenth century into a hospital, given by Henry VIII to the City of London in 1547 as Britain's first insane asylum, became, within a few decades, little more than a dungeon. Women were chained by the ankles to one long wall. Men were liable to be attached by the neck to a vertical bar. One man was kept that way, even in the eighteenth century, for twelve years.

Relief for the poor was the responsibility of the Church during the Middle Ages. Church authorities at the diocese or parish level administered relief to feed and protect the poor within their districts. The money available for their care was sufficient to meet the needs in these local districts (Trattner, 1999). In ministering to the poor, the Church served in the capacity of a public institution, and the tithe was considered a public tax. Scholars have suggested that the system run by the Church was the model for the secular system established later by the Elizabethan Poor Law of 1601. The care of the poor by the Church altered as the nature and incidence of poverty changed with the socioeconomic conditions. Specifically, the decline of feudalism, the growth of commerce, and the beginning of industrialization made it necessary to find new ways of assisting those in need. The poor, the unemployed, the disabled, widows, dependent children, the elderly, people with mental retardation, and people with mental illness who were previously cared for on the feudal estates by the feudal lords now had no place to

---

TABLE 2-1   ◆   SUMMARY POINTS: EARLY METHODS OF TREATMENT

- Trephining the skull involved using a crude saw to remove circular disks of bone.
- Exorcising evil spirits was a religious rite to rid the body of their presence.
- Hippocrates believed that mental illness was a disease.
- Institutions were founded for the poor, orphans, the elderly, and people with disabilities
- Asylums housed those with deviant behavior.
- Inquisitions determined diagnosis of mental illness as non compos mentis or idiots.
- Poor relief was the responsibility of the Catholic Church during the Middle Ages.
- The Elizabethan Poor Law was passed to mount a large-scale attack on poverty.

go. Most wandered around, often settling in cities that were ill equipped to handle them. (See Table 2-1.)

A new type of economy and the employment needs of the incipient industrial revolution also affected a number of poor people. The growth of commerce encouraged the development of a money economy, based on capital investments, credit, interest, rent, and wages. This system was very different from the rural economy, which depended on the bartering of goods and services. As the poor could no longer survive by bartering and had little money, they often could not afford food, housing, and clothing. Compounding their problems was the development of the factory system, which required large groups of people with specialized skills. Employment of these workers was seasonal, cyclical, and beyond their control. To be able to care for oneself, one had to be employed by those who controlled the resources.

The pressures of the poor in the cities created the need for a large-scale attack on poverty and prompted the passage of the Elizabethan Poor Law of 1601. This legislation was critical in the history of human services. It guided social welfare practices in England and the United States for the next 350 years by specifying who was to provide what services to those in need. For example, parents were legally responsible for their children and grandchildren, and children were responsible for the support of parents and grandparents. One harsh feature was the punishment of vagrants who refused to work by imprisonment, whipping, stoning, or even execution. More significant, however, was the acknowledgment in the legislation that the state had a responsibility to relieve need and suffering and that the disadvantaged not only deserved assistance but also had a legal right to it.

The law included three main features. The first was compulsory taxation to raise funds to help the needy. The administration of this money resembled the Church's system developed during feudal times. Government representatives, called "overseers of the poor," managed the distribution of money in each parish or county. Second, dependents were classified according to their ability to work: children, the able-bodied, and the "impotent poor" (adults unable to work). Relief was provided to each group: Dependent children were apprenticed or indentured; the able-bodied worked or were punished; and the lame, the blind, and other poor people unable to work received home or institutional relief. Third, the responsibility for the sick, the poor, and others in need rested first with the family. If the family could not provide assistance, the government was responsible for doing so.

An interesting amendment to the Elizabethan Poor Law, added 60 years later, was the Law of Settlement. This law established a residency requirement for determining eligibility for assistance. The requirements of needy people wandering from town to town seeking food and shelter overburdened many towns and districts. This law helped the districts plan for the number they would serve. (See Table 2-2.)

By the end of the 18th century, a dramatic change in the care of persons with mental illness occurred. A move toward more humane treatment of those in mental institutions began in 1792 when Philippe Pinel unchained

The Elizabethan Poor Laws

The Elizabethan Poor Laws were passed as a response to the increasing number of poor in Great Britain. During earlier times the lords were directly responsible for the care of their tenants. But the feudal system began to crumble and the tenant farmers lost their land. Having no source of relief, they drifted to the cities and larger towns. Few of this population had the skills to earn a living wage, and as their numbers increased, pauperism became a national problem. The first attempt to correct this problem was the enactment of voluntary alms to be collected in each parish. When this enactment did not alleviate the problems, an act was passed that required severe punishment for vagabonds and relief for the poor. This act led to an attempt to discriminate between the criminal population and the poor. Finally, the Poor Law of 1601 provided a clear definition of the "poor" and articulated services that they were to receive. This legislation is the foundation for the current social welfare system existing today in Great Britain. The following describes the law.

POOR LAW OF 1601

By this act two or more "substantial householders" were to be yearly nominated by the justices of the peace to serve as overseers of the poor in each parish. The overseers were to raise

> weekly or otherwise, by taxation of every inhabitant, such competent sums of money as they shall think fit, (a) for setting to work the children of all such whose parents shall not be thought able to keep and maintain them; (b) for setting to work all such persons, married and unmarried, having no means to maintain them, and who use no ordinary and daily trade of life to get their living by; (c) for providing a convenient stock of flax, hemp, wool, thread, iron, and other ware and stuff, to set the poor on work; (d) for the necessary relief of the lame, old, impotent, blind, and such other among them being poor and not able to work. Children whose parents cannot maintain them are to be apprenticed till the age of four-and-twenty years in the case of boys and twenty-one years or the time of marriage in the case of girls. The overseers may, with the leave of the Lord of the Manor, erect houses for the impotent poor on any waste or common.

No provision is made for the erection of any house in which work may be done, and it was evidently intended that the flax, hemp, and

other raw material should be worked up at the houses of the poor. But an act of 1576 had already empowered the justices of each county to erect "houses of correction" in which "such as be already grown up in idleness and so rogues at this present" should be set to work under strict prison discipline; and the justices were now ordered to commit to these places, or to the common jail, those who refused to work on materials provided by the parish. What they had to expect at the houses of correction may be seen from one of the rules of the Suffolk House for the year 1589:

> Item—it is ordered and agreed upon that every strong or sturdy rogue at his or her first entrance into the said house shall have twelve stripes upon his bare skin with the said whip provided for said house; and every young rogue or idle loiterer six stripes with the said whip in form aforesaid. And that every one of them, without fail, at their first coming into the said house, shall have put upon him, her, or them some clogs, chain, collars of iron, ringle, or manacle, such as the keeper of the said house shall think meet.

The new act was only gradually carried out. In 1622, "A Wellwisher" complained, in a tract called "Grievous Groans for the Poor," that

> tho the number of the poor do daily increase, there hath been no collection for them, no not these seven years, in many parishes of this land, especially in country towns; but many of those parishes turneth forth their poor, yea and their lusty laborers that will not work, or for any misdemeanor want work, to beg, filch, and steal for their maintenance, so that the country is pitifully pestered with them; yea, and the maimed soldiers that have ventured their lives and lost their limbs on our behalf are also thus requited. . . . So they are turned forth to travel in idleness (the highway to hell) . . . until the law bring them unto the fearful end of hanging.

SOURCE: Excerpt from *The New Encyclopedia of Social Reform*, by W. Bliss, pp. 918–920. Copyright © 1908 by Funk and Wagnalls.

TABLE 2-2 ✦ SUMMARY POINTS: ELIZABETHAN POOR LAW OF 1601
• Compulsory taxation to raise funds to help the needy.
• Classification of dependents according to ability to work: children, the able-bodied, and the "impotent poor."
• Responsibility for those in need was first with the family and then with the government.
• Residency requirement as eligibility for services was established by the Law of Settlement.

50 maniacs at Bicetre Hospital in Paris (see Chapter 4). This period is often called the first revolution in mental health. For those in mental institutions, this period meant improved diets, regular exercise, religious observance, and the development of the mind. As you will read in the next section, in the United States these efforts were led by Amariah Brigham, Samuel B. Woodward, and Benjamin Rush. Unfortunately, the rise in moral treatment lasted only until the mid-19th century because of limited resources, overcrowding, and the passage of time (Macht, 1990).

Human Services in the United States: Colonial America

As we examine the history of human services in the United States, we see the influence of the English developments discussed in the preceding section. During the years of colonization, public relief was supported by individuals and groups, who donated resources and labor to institutions such as schools and hospitals or directly to needy people. Much assistance took the form of neighborly kindness or mutual aid. As the populations of the cities in the colonies grew, so did the number of indigents, idlers, criminals, orphans, and others who needed assistance. The colonists used the Elizabethan Poor Law as a model of how to meet the needs of those individuals.

The four principles that formed the basis of the local practice of poor relief in the colonies can be traced directly to the Elizabethan Poor Law of 1601. The first principle defined poor relief as a public responsibility. The second principle, the question of legal residence, therefore became a practical one, as services were provided at the local or parish level. The third principle spelled

1600s	Recognition of the needs of the poor
1600–1700s	Almshouses established
1773	State hospital opens in Williamsburg, VA
1792	Philippe Pinel advocates more humane treatment
1800s	Established district workhouses

Human Services in Colonial America Timeline

out the responsibility family members had to needy individuals; public aid was denied those who had parents, grandparents, adult children, or grandchildren. Finally, legislation combined concerns about children and work by declaring that the children of paupers were to be apprenticed to farmers and artisans who agreed to care for them.

Like England, the colonies responded to the needy by developing institutions. The first almshouse was built in Massachusetts in 1662 for dependents such as persons with mental illness, the elderly, children, the able-bodied poor, those with physical disabilities, and criminals. Almshouses were not developed systematically, but over the next 150 years they were established throughout the colonies as the need arose. The numbers of these houses made it increasingly obvious that there were large groups of needy individuals the towns could not support. With this realization began the trend for larger governmental units to accept the responsibility for the "state poor." By the early 1800s, a system of district workhouses had been developed. Besides the almshouses, there were very few specialized formal institutions. Criminals were held in jail until trial and, if found guilty, were fined, whipped, or executed. Poor strangers or vagrants were simply told to leave town. People with mental illness had no special facilities before the American Revolution; their care was the responsibility of their families. Those without relatives to care for them were placed in almshouses. Those with mental illness were often locked up by their families in an attic or cellar or left to wander about the countryside.

Benjamin Franklin was instrumental in establishing one of the few formal institutions for people with mental disturbances, a section of the Pennsylvania Hospital. Another facility devoted exclusively to those with mental disturbances was a state hospital at Williamsburg, Virginia, which opened in 1773. Little attention was given to the treatment of mental disease because it was viewed as an economic and social problem rather than a medical one. Determining insanity was the responsibility of officials, such as governors and church wardens, not members of the medical profession.

1800s Rapid industrialization
1813   Practice of probation begins
1810s Benjamin Rush influences mental health care
1820s Rise of the philosophy of individualism
1830s Orphanages begin, Poor Law Reform Bill of 1834
1840s Dorothea Dix teaches prisoners
1850s Rise of the philosophy of Social Darwinism
1854   Care of mentally ill becomes state responsibility
1880s Philanthropy emerges
1889   Opening of the Hull House

The 19th Century: A Time of Change Timeline

The 19th Century: A Time of Change

Large-scale immigration, rapid industrialization, and widespread urbanization led to many societal changes during the colonial years. These changes brought more poverty and more outlays for relief of the poor. During the Middle Ages, need was believed to arise from misfortune, for which society should assume responsibility. Belief in the right to public assistance was established and endorsed by the Elizabethan Poor Law, which placed the responsibility on the government. In the early years in the United States, colonists used the English system as a model for their philosophy toward and services for the poor and needy. By the early 1800s, however, the philosophy in the United States had changed.

Destitution was viewed as the fault of the individual, and public aid was thought to cause and encourage poverty. This punitive attitude toward the poor—the belief that to be poor was a crime—was manifested in the Poor Law Reform Bill of 1834. Its purpose was to limit the expansion of services provided to the poor or the have-nots. This bill introduced the concept of "less eligibility," stating that assistance to any person in need must be lower than the lowest working wage paid. The social philosophies of individualism, the work ethic, economic laissez-faire, and Social Darwinism promoted further changes in attitudes toward the poor and the needy.

Social Philosophies

During the 19th century, those espousing the philosophy of individualism viewed America as the land of opportunity. Hard work was the road to success, and that road could be traveled by anyone. The individual was held solely responsible for any failure. Similarly, proponents of the work ethic emphasized the importance of hard work and thrift for financial success and viewed poverty as a sign of spiritual weakness. Wealth was virtuous, and hard work represented the road to salvation.

Laissez-faire was an economic concept that focused on societal rather than individual responsibility. The original French phrase means "leave alone," and this concept encouraged a social attitude of "live and let live." The most desirable government, then, was the one that governed least—negating society's responsibility to help its less fortunate citizens. Those adhering to this philosophy opposed the provision of any human services as a right of the individual.

Social Darwinism, in combination with laissez-faire and the work ethic, created a climate for the reform that was to follow. An outgrowth of Charles Darwin's theory of evolution, it was used to explain social and economic phenomena. According to those who interpreted Darwin in social terms, the natural order of life was that the fittest would survive, creating a society of perfect people. Those who were unfit would not be able to meet their own needs

TABLE 2-3 ✦ SUMMARY POINTS: SOCIAL PHILOSOPHIES
OF THE 19TH CENTURY

- **Individualism**—hard work was the road to success and poverty was a sign of spiritual weakness.
- **Laissez-faire**—an economic concept that focused on societal rather than individual responsibility.
- **Social Darwinism**—any attempts to help the less fortunate would impede progress and facilitate the survival of the "unfit."

and would not survive. Supporters of Social Darwinism called for the repeal of poor laws and state-supported human services that facilitated the survival of the "unfit," as they believed that all change must be natural. Any attempt to help the less fortunate would be against progress, which depended on "natural selection."

This belief was especially popular between 1870 and 1880. In reality, it often served as a rationalization for unscrupulous business practices. Furthermore, it encouraged the belief that nothing could be done about the situation of the working class and the poor, who faced long work hours, low wages, child labor, and unhealthy working conditions.

These prevailing philosophies discouraged the provision of human services and limited services to those who desperately needed assistance. The private sector became very important in filling the need. Wealthy individuals were instrumental in organizing and reforming institutions. Mental hospitals, almshouses, workhouses, penitentiaries, and institutions for unwed mothers and delinquent youth appeared. Philanthropic societies were formed to support these institutions. By the middle of the 19th century, public and private sectors were working side by side. As welfare problems grew, the private sector was unable to meet increasing needs. In spite of the prevailing philosophies, there was growing demand for public agencies to assume more responsibility for the poor and needy. (See Table 2-3.)

By the 1850s, specialized institutions had been established for persons with mental illness, juvenile delinquents, the deaf and blind, and criminals. These institutions were established primarily in the belief that reform, rehabilitation, and education were possible. Institutions could improve society by protecting individuals from negative environmental influences.

In summary, the 19th century was a time of dramatic change in the way society viewed its responsibilities toward the poor and needy. Government relinquished some of its role in providing services, and the private sector assumed more responsibility. Unfortunately, the problems of those in need multiplied, and gradually the government began to increase its assistance again. Institutions also developed in response to the needs of specific populations. Probation, mental health, and child welfare provide examples of how 19th-century attitudes affected the delivery of human services to specific populations.

Probation

In the United States, the earliest practice similar to probation as we know it today occurred in 1813, when Judge Peter O. Thatcher of Boston began placing youthful offenders under the supervision of officials such as sheriffs and constables. In 1841, the concept of "friendly supervision" was introduced by John Augustus, a shoemaker. He helped drunks and other unfortunates by bailing them out, sometimes paying their fines, and then providing "friendly supervision" as the individuals adjusted to a new life.

The most well-known organization to provide assistance to ex-convicts was the Salvation Army, created in England in the late 19th century by William Booth. Its members believed in taking a more sympathetic approach to the problems and circumstances of those in need. For example, members of its Prison Gate Brigade met prisoners upon their release and provided whatever assistance they could, including a home, food, and employment (Collier, 1965).

Treatment of Persons with Mental Illness

Patients in the early asylums were mostly psychotic or severely retarded. Treatment was medically oriented, and many patients were treated as if they had a physical illness. The beginnings of reform in the late 1700s can be attributed to Dr. Benjamin Rush at the Pennsylvania Hospital in Philadelphia. Dr. Rush, who is considered the father of American psychiatry, fought the superstition and ignorance surrounding mental illness and elevated the study of mental illness to a scientific level. In 1812, he wrote *Medical Inquiries and Observations upon the Diseases of the Mind,* the first scientific treatise explaining the nature of mental illness. Before his writings, mental patients lived in atrocious conditions and were treated with brutality and cruelty; customary treatment methods were bleeding, restraint, and cold showers. Dr. Rush introduced occupational therapy, amusements, and exercise for patients.

Dorothea Dix was another pioneer who fought to improve conditions and services for people with mental illness during the 19th century. She became involved in social reform when, in 1841, she accepted an offer to teach a Sunday school class of 20 female prisoners in the jail at East Cambridge, Massachusetts. She was appalled at the conditions she found in the jail: overcrowding, filthy quarters, and little or no heat. What alarmed her most was the crowding together of criminals and the insane. She began a personal investigation of all the jails and almshouses in Massachusetts and made careful, systematic records of what she saw. Backed by a group of broad-minded, public-spirited citizens, Dix launched a whole new career as a moral reformer, calling for more enlightened treatment of those with mental illness. Controversy and outrage engulfed her, but those who checked her accounts found them to be factual. Her appeals were based on respect for Christian values and the advancement of civilization (Marshall, 1937).

Throughout the 1840s and 1850s, Dix campaigned before state legislatures to establish asylums for people with mental illness and the developmentally disabled who were housed in jails and almshouses. She encouraged the national government to assume additional responsibility for the care and treatment of people with mental illness. Using such methods as fact gathering, preparing memoranda and bills, and rallying public opinion, she began her campaign in Massachusetts, where the number of dependent insane was twice the total capacity of the state's three mental institutions (Trattner, 1999). She won her fight for enlarged facilities for indigent mental patients. The years between 1843 and 1853 are sometimes called her "decade of victory," because she was personally responsible for founding state hospitals in nine states.

Note the brief history of the East Tennessee Asylum for the Insane included here as it traces its founding and development. The asylum was built in a pastoral setting along a river, reflecting the belief of the times that a pastoral setting would have a calming influence on patients. More recent history illustrates the decline and deinstitutionalization experienced by so many mental hospitals.

In the *Providence Journal* on April 10, 1844, Dix published an article titled, "Astonishing Tenacity of Life." It is not signed by her but by Thomas G. Hazard. We know from a public document of her own, however, that she provided Hazard with the facts on which his article was based. The facts concerned her first visit to Little Compton, where she had discovered Abram Simmons, confined in complete darkness, in an unheated cell, seven feet square and six and one-half feet high, built entirely of stone. This dungeon stood in the courtyard of the poorhouse. Simmons had been imprisoned there for over three years. One of his legs was fastened by an ox-chain, shackled to an iron staple in the rock overhead. The article (Hazard, 1844, pp. 252–253) describes Simmons as follows:

> There he stood, near the door, motionless and silent; his tangled hair fell about his shoulders; his bare feet pressed the filthy wet stone floor; he was emaciated to a shadow and more resembled a disinterred corpse than any living creature. Never have I looked upon an object so pitiable, so woe-struck, so imaging despair. Notwithstanding the assertions of the Mistress that he would kill me I took his hands and endeavored to warm them by gentle friction. I spoke to him of release, of liberty, of care and kindness. A tear stole over the hollow cheek, but no words answered my importunities; no other movement indicated consciousness or perception of sensibility.

Dix is also recognized as the founder of St. Elizabeth's Hospital in Washington, D.C. Today we remember her for her tireless work in founding or enlarging 32 mental hospitals in the United States and abroad.

By 1854, the U.S. Congress had declared the financial care of persons with mental illness the responsibility of the states. This responsibility included paying for construction of proper facilities and needed treatment. In reality, however, the state systems were custodial warehouses, characterized by inadequate doctor–patient ratio, untrained personnel, overcrowding, and lack of public interest.

●●●●●●●●●

An Imprecise History of Lyons View

1873
The General Assembly appropriates $75,000 and appoints a board to oversee building a mental hospital near Knoxville, in order to ease overcrowding at the insane asylum near Nashville.

1874
The state buys 300 acres of farmland along the Tennessee River from Tom Lyons for $19,500. Construction begins on the new hospital.

1886
The East Tennessee Asylum for the Insane finally opens, after a lack of state funding delayed completion for several years. With a capacity of 250 patients, the hospital is heated by steam and lit by coal oil lamps. Families of the superintendent, physician, steward, and matron live on the top two floors. Treatment at that time consisted of tender loving care, says Lea Acuff, a former chaplain and historian of Lakeshore. "It involved getting people out of the stressful situations of their life and helping them work through the cycle of their illness."

1896
The Underhill Building for black patients is constructed. It remained the only building for black people until the hospital was integrated in the 1960s.

Early 1900s
Physicians began to be licensed and the philosophy toward treating mental illness became more clinical (clinical for its day, at least). Doctors learned how syphilis affected people, and would infect patients with malaria in order to produce a high fever in hopes of arresting the disease's progress (usually, though, the disease had progressed too far for the strategy to work). This period also marks a change in treatment philosophy. Acuff says, the families are encouraged to forget about their ill relatives. "When it became scientific, they begin to have inklings about the physical causes of mental illness. It wasn't long before people believed they just don't recover," he says. "There's no great optimism."

1915
Dr. Michael Campbell, the hospital's first and longest serving superintendent resigns. During his 30-year tenure, Campbell's attempts to make the hospital a "model institution for the treatment of the insane . . . were continually thwarted by a penny-pinching legislature," according to *Beyond the Asylum, The History of Mental Handicap Policy in Tennessee*. At

the time, the state spent 37.5 cents a day on each patient, less than it did on prisoners. "The Knoxville hospital . . . became a custodial institution, overcrowded with patients of all types housed together and subjected to the use of restraints and drugs."

1927
The hospital undertakes many building projects and changes its name to Eastern State Hospital.

1930s
The hospital begins using various hydrotherapy and shock treatments. With hydrotherapy, patients were doused or soaked several times alternately in hot and cold waters. "The trauma of it seemed to produce some changes, at least they thought it did," Acuff says. Later that decade, electric shock therapy—where convulsions were induced—came into use. Electrotherapy is still considered a viable treatment option, but doctors at the time often overused it. Psychoanalysis is also in vogue, but Eastern State (like most state hospitals) does not have the money, staff, or time for it.

1940
Newspaper articles accuse the Eastern State staff of alcoholism, abusing patients, and keeping inhumane conditions. The state investigates, then swaps superintendents of its Western and Eastern hospitals, bringing Dr. Bedford F. Peterson to Lyons View, where he served for 24 years. He constructs several new buildings (including the marble-interior treatment building, which included electro-, hydro- and hyper-term facilities), and started a patient newspaper, recreational and employee training programs, and community education efforts. "He had a deep attachment with the people. He knew them, knew their names, knew their families. He carried a lot of information in his head, which is why it didn't get written in charts," Acuff says.

1944
The Tennessee Valley Authority creates Fort Loudoun Lake, covering much of the hospital's farmland. The state gives the hospital farmland in another part of the county.

1953
The state creates a department of mental health, removing Eastern State from the prison system. This period also marked a philosophical

continued

An Imprecise History of Lyons View (continued)

change—one geared toward helping the mentally ill function in society. The discovery of thorazine and the effects it had on the mentally ill begins pharmaceutical-based treatments throughout the United States.

1960
Dr. Peterson opens the Therapeutic Village, a model community of 12 cottages, a chapel, and shops, designed to prepare ill patients to function in society. Unfortunately, it can accommodate only 240 of the hospital's 2,800 patients, so most of them remain locked in overcrowded wards. Today, many of the cottages are being rented out to Knox Youth Sports and Knox County, among others.

1965
The hospital is renamed Eastern State Psychiatric Hospital.

1971
The hospital's biggest scandal unfolds when the *Knoxville Journal* and State Representative Richard Krieg pay a midnight visit, reporting about the overcrowded, unsanitary, unsafe conditions there. The state holds formal hearings, and several hospital administrators either quit or are fired. The new superintendent, Dr. John Marshall, begins a more earnest effort to stabilize the mentally ill with drugs, and move them back into the community, using outpatient programs and halfway houses.

1972
The wings of the original hospital are demolished. It becomes the first state hospital to admit all minors to a unit separate from adults.

1973
Overlook Mental Health Center, stressing outpatient treatment, opens at Lyons View.

By the late 19th century, states began to separate persons with mental illness and those with developmental disabilities. There was an attempt to upgrade research, treatment, and physical facilities, and the hospitals eventually provided aftercare and outpatient clinics. The medically oriented approach continued to prevail in institutions, and mental disorders were defined and classified into two groups: those caused by organic brain disturbance and those with no apparent physical cause (psychogenetic).

1974
Eastern State becomes accredited. The lawsuit *Townsend v. Treadway* requires state institutions to pay patients for work they do there, thus bringing an end to Lakeshore patients doing farming, laundry, and other work.

1976
Name changes to Lakeshore Mental Health Institute.

1980s
As its budget continues to shrink, the institute releases more and more patients into the community, and cuts staff. In 1981, the state almost turns Lakeshore over to a private company. In 1983, lawmakers consider selling the land—appraised at the time between $6.6 and $8.4 million—and building another hospital elsewhere.

1992
The state announces plans to consolidate Lakeshore and Chattanooga's institute within five years, fueling employees' and mental health advocates' fears. So far, plans have not been utilized.

1994
Eighty acres of Lakeshore's property becomes a public park, owned and rented by the City of Knoxville, and managed by Knox Youth Sports.

1999
To date, the Lakeshore facility continues to serve adults, children, and youth. Many of the patients are diagnosed with severe mental illness and cannot successfully live in the community.

SOURCE: http://metro pulse.com/dir_zine/dir_1999/909/t_cover2.html. From "An Imprecise History of Lyons View," 1999. Copyright, 1999, MetroPulse, p. 95. Used with permission.

Child Welfare

Many approaches to child welfare were tried from the mid-19th century to the beginning of the 20th century. One was the removal of dependent, neglected, and delinquent children from almshouses and institutions. Another was the placement of those children in private homes. The first permanent orphanage, Bethesda, in Savannah, Georgia, is still in operation today as a modern child care center for emotionally disturbed children (Trattner, 1999). The

• • • • • • • • • •

INTERNATIONAL FOCUS
Mental Health in Developing Countries

All countries have systems of economics, religion, education, and law that have developed over time. Colonization by Western European countries interrupted the evolution of these systems in many developing countries, as Western traditions supplanted earlier systems, including mental health care systems.

Examples of developing countries using European systems of institutionalization or custodial care can be found in Southeast Asia in the early 1800s. In Singapore and Penang, lunatic asylums and hospitals for the insane were modeled after European facilities. No better than warehouses for persons with mental illness, these institutions also housed criminals, vagrants, and other social undesirables. With little hope of better care, many stayed for the remainder of their lives. By the end of the 19th century, the practice of institutionalization had expanded into India and Indonesia. Because such custodial care facilities did little to better the lives of persons with mental illness, a negative perception of institutionalization still influences the attitudes of people in Southeast Asia today.

Based on studies in several parts of the world, the World Health Organization (1975) concluded that there are no fundamental differences among nations with regard to the range or prevalence of mental disorders. In the predominantly rural populations and rapidly growing cities of developing countries, however, a combination of overcrowding, unemployment, limited and outdated health facilities, and rapid social change makes mental disorders a major problem. This problem is compounded when mental disorders take the form of physical complaints or criminal activity.

Mental disorders may be a source of fear, not only to family members and friends but also to administrators, health workers, and politicians. The belief that these conditions are caused by the supernatural continues to be widespread; it can lead to a person's rejection by or isolation from family members and community, skepticism among the public about treatment programs, and regressive attitudes regarding the development of mental health services. Institutionalization remains a dominant form of treatment.

first juvenile reformatory in America, the House of Refuge for Juvenile Delinquents in New York City, was supported by state funds. Massachusetts and Ohio quickly followed by establishing juvenile facilities. After the 1830s, the number of such institutions multiplied, as the public demanded the removal of children from almshouses. Unfortunately, juvenile institutions were not always an improvement, and overcrowded conditions and poor care prompted the establishment of a system that placed children in private homes.

Other forms of child welfare were the provision of mothers' or widows' pensions, the creation of juvenile courts and probation systems, the passage of compulsory school attendance laws, and crusades against child labor. These actions had several reasons. Many people believed that children are the most vulnerable and deserving group in society, and it was difficult to argue that the children were responsible for their own conditions. Children also constituted one of the largest groups of neglected and needy.

Reform Movements

By the latter half of the 19th century, two population shifts were affecting the provision of services to people in need: immigration from abroad and migration from rural to urban areas. In 1860, one-sixth of Americans lived in the cities; by 1900, this figure was one-third; and by 1920, one-half (Trattner, 1999). Between 1860 and 1900, approximately 14 million immigrants from abroad settled in cities, creating an urban population that consisted primarily of former farmers and immigrants. Most were unskilled or semiskilled workers in search of employment. This population explosion in the urban areas created many problems for the urban governments. Two responses to these problems were the organized charity movement and the settlement house movement.

THE ORGANIZED CHARITY MOVEMENT

The goal of the organized charity movement was to eliminate difficulties such as fraud or duplication in the provision of services (Trattner, 1999). According to the movement, the best way to deal with poverty was through personal contact or "friendly visiting" between the rich and the poor. Influenced by laissez-faire, individualism, and Puritanism, the movement soon shifted to reform, seeking better conditions in institutions, promoting better sanitation and health regulations, developing parks and recreation areas, and writing and enforcing housing codes.

The Charity Organization Society, a forerunner of the Community Chest and the United Way, is an example of society's response to the expanding urban population. Members of the Charity Organization Society believed that giving handouts of money and food actually encouraged people to remain poor and to beg for services. They supported the systematic distribution of alms only to the poor who needed them, thus helping the deserving poor while discouraging begging. They hoped to encourage thrift and independence among the poor. Eventually, this group evolved into a clearinghouse for all the city's charitable organizations, similar to the United Way of today.

THE SETTLEMENT HOUSE MOVEMENT

The development of the settlement house movement was in large part a reaction to the inability of the organized charity movement to improve the living

and working conditions of the poor. The leaders of the settlement house movement, unlike the leaders of the organized charity movement, did not support
the laissez-faire philosophy. They wanted reform that included adequate housing, better schools, the abolition of child labor, and an end to the sweatshops.
They thought that the best way to achieve this reform was not through alms
or "friendly visiting" but through "social engineering." Human service workers and reformers were "engineers"; they must participate in the system all the
time, not only when something was wrong. Individual workers and reformers
were perceived as members of an active and attentive movement that inter-
vened at the neighborhood level. The settlement house is an example of social
engineering in practice.

Typically, a settlement house was a large house in a slum area. It served as
a community center, sponsoring such activities as recreation; classes in English, cooking, and citizenship; vocational training; and child care. Different
settlement houses concentrated on different activities, depending on the needs
of the neighborhood. Key elements to the success of a settlement house were
the commitment of the workers and the location of the house. Social engineering could not be accomplished from afar; workers lived in the house or in
the community in which they served. The house was part of the community.
Perhaps the best example of a settlement house is Hull House in Chicago,
founded by Jane Addams in 1889. Addams was inspired by Toynbee Hall, a pioneer English settlement house she visited while in England in the 1880s.
Upon returning from Europe, she and her college friend, Ellen Starr, moved to
the poor section of Chicago and began raising money to support what was to
become Hull House. Because of her upper-middle-class background, she had
connections to the wealthy. Friends from college also supported the venture,
but the house gathered its greatest support from churches and missions. Hull
House was located in the middle of the immigrant section in Chicago. Addams
and Starr moved in and invited their immigrant neighbors to read Italian nov-
els and see slides of Italian art. The women came and brought their children;
the presence of children necessitated a nursery. Soon a boys' club was established, and then a men's club. Over the years, more than 50 services were available from Hull House.

Walter Lippmann describes the qualities and service of Jane Addams very
aptly (Tims, 1961, p. 150):

> Yet if that were all her life has meant, Jane Addams would only stand in
> a large company of men and women who in every land and under all
> conditions are persistently kind to their fellow beings. It is not all. There
> is something else, which was visible in the beauty of her countenance,
> was audible in her unaffected voice, is in the style of her writings, and
> was the special element in her influence. It was the quality within her
> which made it possible for her to descend into the pits of squalor and
> meanness and cruelty and evil, and yet never to lose, in fact always to
> hold clearly, the distinctions that are precious to a maturely civilized be-
> ing. She had compassion without condescension. She had pity without

retreat into vulgarity. She had infinite sympathy for common things without forgetfulness of those that are uncommon. That, I think, is why those who have known her say that she was not only good but great.

These movements are important because they illustrate the continual struggle during the 19th century to assist those in need. Generally, the assistance took two forms: provision of services and advocacy of reform. It was difficult to blame all the problems of urban poverty on the individual. The settlement house movement, in particular, introduced a new philosophy of helping that recognized the impact of societal forces on the lives of individuals. This new philosophy continued to develop in the 20th century.

 ## The 20th Century: New Directions

The early 1900s, sometimes called the *sociological era*, continued the period of social reform. During this time, two significant events or changes affected the history of helping and human services. The first was the development of a new profession. Settlement house and Charity Organization Society workers became known as *social workers*. The basis for the new profession was the belief that such people needed specific skills, knowledge, and understanding to work effectively with the poor. Good intentions were admirable but not sufficient to provide assistance. During this time, social diagnosis, or casework, evolved as the method of practice. Mary Richmond, the author of *Social Diagnosis* (1917), identified this process as one of investigation, diagnosis, prognosis, and treatment. Her book is regarded as the first treatise on social casework theory and method (Zimbalist, 1977). The development of the social work profession is significant; it represents the beginning of the professionalization of human services. Later in this century, the fields of welfare, mental health, child guidance, and probation also became professionalized.

Also during the early 20th century, a reexamination of the causes of poverty took place. A group of writers called muckrakers actively criticized the wealthy, accusing them of moral decay, cheating, and bribery. (The term was first used by President Theodore Roosevelt in criticizing sensationalist,

1900s	First social workers
1909	National Committee for Mental Hygiene founded
1910s	Muckrakers publicize social ills
1920–1930s	Free clinics for mentally ill open
1935	Social Security Act passed
1945	Beers published *A Mind that Found Itself*
1955	Joint Commission on Mental Illness and Health meets

Twentieth Century: New Directions Timeline

untruthful writers.) Muckrakers such as Lincoln Steffens and Upton Sinclair exposed unfair business, government, and labor practices. They supported the idea that poverty was caused by social and economic conditions, not by the individual, and proposed that poverty was a condition that prevented people from reaching their potential. They claimed that because poverty and need resulted from societal shortcomings, improvements in housing and working conditions could help eliminate poverty.

The Mental Health Movement

Clifford Beers, a victim of mental illness, was confined for three years in public and private mental institutions, where he experienced deprivation and cruelty. To publicize the plight of those with mental illness, he wrote about his collapse and treatment in A *Mind that Found Itself* (1945). In 1908, he founded the Connecticut Society for Mental Hygiene, considered by many to be the beginning of the organized mental health movement in America. By the following year, this pioneer state society had written a prospectus that included the following guidelines (Beers, 1945, p. 395):

I
"After all, what the insane most need is a friend!" By coordinating the friendly impulses of those who, if they but knew how, would gladly help the insane, the Society for Mental Hygiene can prove itself that friend.

II
It is the aim of the Society for Mental Hygiene to become a permanent agency for education and reform in the field of nervous and mental diseases; an agency for education always, for reform as long as radical changes may be needed.

III
The chief object of the Society for Mental Hygiene shall be the improvement of conditions among those actually insane and confined, and the protection of the mental health of the public at large.

Beers also proposed a national society, the National Committee for Mental Hygiene, which was formed in 1909. This group later changed its name to the National Association for Mental Health and is known today as the Mental Health Association. Its aim is to improve mental hospitals, arouse public concern, and prevent disease. By providing education on causes, diagnosis, prevention, and treatment, this organization furthered the development of the mental health movement.

Services for persons with mental illness continued to improve and expand. By the 1920s and 1930s, most large cities had free clinics for mental patients, where treatment and social services were provided. In fact, human services as we know it today began with the impact of World Wars I and II on the mental

• • • • • • • • • •

✦ *An Asylum in 1902*

After fifteen interminable hours the straitjacket was removed. Whereas just prior to its putting on I had been in a vigorous enough condition to offer stout resistance when wantonly assaulted, now, on coming out of it, I was helpless. When my arms were released from their constricted position, the pain was intense. Every joint had been racked. I had no control over the fingers of either hand, and could not have dressed myself had I been promised my freedom for doing so.

For more than the following week I suffered as already described, though of course with gradually decreasing intensity as my racked body became accustomed to the unnatural positions it was forced to take. This first experience occurred on the night of October 18th, 1902. I was subjected to the same unfair, unnecessary, and unscientific ordeal for twenty-one consecutive nights and parts of each of the corresponding twenty-one days. On more than one occasion, indeed, the attendant placed me in the straitjacket during the day for refusing to obey some trivial command. This, too, without an explicit order from the doctor in charge, though perhaps he acted under a general order.

During most of this time I was held also in seclusion in a padded cell. A padded cell is a vile hole. The side walls are padded as high as a man can reach, as is also the inside of the door. One of the worst features of such cells is the lack of ventilation, which deficiency of course aggravates their general unsanitary condition. The cell which I was forced to occupy was practically without heat, and as winter was coming on, I suffered intensely from the cold. Frequently it was so cold I could see my breath. Though my canvas jacket served to protect part of that body which it was at the same time racking, I was seldom comfortably warm; for, once uncovered, my arms being pinioned, I had no way of rearranging the blankets. What little sleep I managed to get I took lying on a hard mattress placed on the bare floor. The condition of the mattress I found in the cell was such that I objected to its further use, and the fact that another was supplied, at a time when few of my requests were being granted, proves its disgusting condition.

For this period of three weeks—from October 18th until November 8th, 1902, when I left this institution and was transferred to a state hospital—I was continuously either under lock and key (in the padded cell or some other room) or under the eye of an attendant. Over half the time I was in the snug, but cruel embrace of a straitjacket—about three hundred hours in all.

SOURCE: Excerpt from *A Mind that Found Itself*, by Clifford W. Beers, pp. 133–134, 395. Copyright; © 1907, 1917, 1921, 1923, 1931, 1932, 1934, 1935, 1937, 1939, 1940, 1942, 1944, 1948, 1953 by The American Foundation of Mental Hygiene, Inc. Reprinted by permission of Doubleday, a division of Random House, Inc.

health field By the end of World War II, the profession of clinical psychology
was created, in part because the number of veterans who were hospitalized in
Veterans Administration (VA) facilities for psychiatric evaluation had reached
more than 40,000 (Cranston, 1986).

Until the 1930s, individual leaders such as Jane Addams, Clifford Beers,
and the muckrakers spearheaded the development of services and the reform
of conditions for the impoverished. As described above, the development of
professions that trained workers in social services also began. As important as
these contributions were, they had little impact on poverty, mental illness, or
other human service concerns on a large scale or at a national level. As a result, the federal government increased its financial commitment to those in
need. Presidents of the United States assumed a leadership role in providing
services.

Increased Federal Involvement

The Great Depression was marked by vast unemployment, failing business
ventures, and the collapse of banks. The economic situation created a wave of
panic and long-term psychological and economic depression for individuals
who could see no end to financial hardship. President Franklin D. Roosevelt
introduced New Deal legislation that fundamentally changed the federal government's role in providing human services, focusing on two goals. The first
was to provide short-term aid to those who were unemployed. The Works
Progress Administration (WPA) and the Civilian Conservation Corps (CCC)
were but two of the work relief programs he initiated. The second focus was

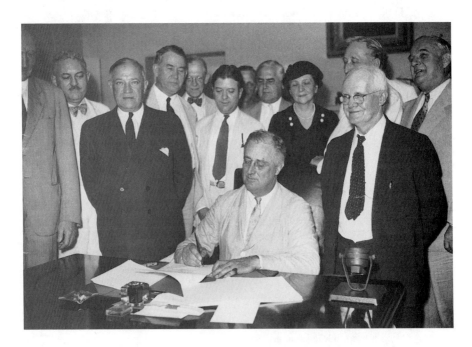

the enactment of the Social Security Act of 1935 as protection against future economic hardships.

The Social Security Act of 1935, the cornerstone of the present American social welfare system, was passed in response to the need for human services. This landmark piece of legislation was significant for several reasons. First, it translated into action the belief that Americans had the right to protection from economic instability. The federal government assumed responsibility for the economic security of all citizens, and thus began the American welfare state. Second, it expanded welfare activities and improved their standards by establishing a new alignment of responsibility in public welfare. The policy of federal aid or grants to states began, thus closing the door on three centuries of the "poor law" principle of local responsibility.

What the act actually did was to provide assistance in three areas: social insurance, public assistance, and health and welfare services. Social insurance programs included old-age, survivors, disability, and unemployment insurance, all of which supported an individual's right to benefits regardless of need. Public assistance provided federal funds to states to establish programs such as Aid to the Permanently and Totally Disabled (APTD), Aid to Families with Dependent Children (AFDC), Aid to the Blind, and Old Age Assistance (OAA). Also available under this category were programs of general assistance to needy people who were not eligible under any other program. The third area, health and welfare services, focused on child welfare, vocational rehabilitation, public health, children with disabilities, and maternal and child health. (See Table 2-4.)

Of course, some pieces were missing from these new social welfare efforts. The Social Security Act did not provide for long-term hardships. Unemployment benefits were available for only a limited amount of time, and neither health insurance nor permanent physical disability insurance was provided (Ehrenreich, 1985). In spite of these limitations, the initiatives of the Social Security Act became well-established components of the social welfare system. Few new programs would be developed during the next 20 years.

Under the administration of Harry Truman, the New Deal expanded into the Fair Deal. Most noteworthy were an enlarged Social Security program and public power projects on the Arkansas, Columbia, and Missouri rivers, bringing electricity and employment to these rural areas.

An important step in the provision of services to those with mental illness was the passage of the National Mental Health Act of 1946 (Public Law 79-487).

TABLE 2-4 ✦ SUMMARY POINTS: THE SOCIAL SECURITY ACT (1935)

- Social insurance programs (old-age, survivors, disability, and unemployment insurance) supported an individual's rights to benefits regardless of need.
- Public assistance helped states establish programs for the needy (e.g., Aid to Families with Dependent Children, Old Age Assistance, and Aid to the Blind).
- Health and welfare services provided programs for public health, vocational rehabilitation, and child welfare among others.

This act created a Mental Hygiene Division within the U.S. Public Health Service and a center for information and research, which later became the National Institute for Mental Health (NIMH). The Mental Hygiene Division emphasized preventive health measures. Its functions were to assist in the development of state and community health services; to study the causes, prevention, and treatment of mental illness; and to support training of psychiatrists, psychologists, social workers, and nurses. This agency played a critical role in the developing human service movement.

A second piece of legislation that helped set the stage for the emergence of human services was the Mental Health Study Act of 1955 (Public Law 84-182), which provided funding for a Joint Commission on Mental Illness and Health. The charge to the commission was "to analyze and evaluate the needs and resources of the mentally ill in the United States and make recommendations for a national mental health program." The commission included representatives of 36 organizations chosen by the NIMH. *Action for Mental Health,* by George Albee (1961a), was the final volume of the commission's report, containing recommendations for personnel needs, facilities, and costs. The commission then made recommendations for training, research, facilities, and programs.

Two of the commission's recommendations directly affected the human service movement. First, the commission concluded that the professional sector alone could not meet the health care needs of the majority of people if only traditional mental health professionals were used. According to the commission,

> [a]ll mental health professions should recognize that nonmedical mental health workers with aptitude, sound training, practical experience, and demonstrable competence should be permitted to do general, short-term psychotherapy—namely, treating persons by objective, permissive, nondirective techniques of listening to their troubles and helping them resolve these troubles in an individually insightful and socially useful way. Such therapy, combining some elements of psychiatric treatment, client counseling, 'someone to tell one's troubles to,' and love for one's fellow man, obviously can be carried out in a variety of settings by institutions, groups, and individuals, but in all cases should be undertaken under the auspices of recognized mental health agencies. (Albee, 1961b, p. x)

The commission also recommended that "a national mental health program should set as an objective one fully staffed, full-time mental health clinic available to each 50,000 of population" (Albee, 1961b, p. xiv). A major impact of the Mental Health Study Act on the human service movement was that it acknowledged the personnel shortage that existed, suggested a new type of mental health worker who could be trained in less time, and recommended a setting in which such new workers could be utilized effectively.

The commission's recommendations were well received and quickly became law. The conditions that encouraged this immediate action were an awareness of the increasing numbers of people with mental health problems, the rising costs of institutional care, and the need for more effective use of personnel, treatment facilities, and treatment (James, 1981).

Presidential Leadership

Presidential leadership also created a climate in which attention to social services and the needs of the have-nots flourished. In 1960, John F. Kennedy was elected president by a slim margin. He ran on a Democratic platform that emphasized the development of social policies to assist the unemployed, persons with mental illness, and persons with mental retardation. During his administration, the Manpower Development and Training Act was passed, funding programs that taught new skills to the unemployed so they could work. Kennedy sponsored aid to underdeveloped rural areas of the country, such as Appalachia, in redevelopment legislation that established special programs in locales with high poverty and unemployment rates. He also responded to the need for changes in the Social Security system. An amendment to the act provided casework to families that were chronically unemployed.

Kennedy renewed the government's commitment to mental health and the treatment of mental illness. He chose to focus on the problems of mental health and mental retardation, "because they are of such actual size and tragic impact and because their susceptibility to public action is so much greater than the attention they have received" (Kennedy, 1964b). He called for a national plan to investigate causes, strengthen resources, and improve training and facilities. Comprehensive community care, commonplace in the 1980s, was also a part of Kennedy's vision for addressing these problems.

In a speech on proposed measures to combat mental illness and mental retardation, he stated:

> I have sent to the Congress today a series of proposals to help fight mental illness and mental retardation. These two afflictions have been long neglected. They occur more frequently, affect more people, require more prolonged treatment, cause more individual and family suffering than any other condition in American life.
>
> It has been tolerated too long. It has troubled our national conscience, but only as a problem unpleasant to mention, easy to postpone, and despairing of solution. (Kennedy, 1964b, p. 51)

Funding for the recommendations of the commission was provided by the Community Mental Health Centers Act of 1963, which directed NIMH to set up requirements and regulations for the establishment of community mental health centers. Additionally, grants were to be made available for activities such as staffing, planning, initial operations, consultation, and education services. The idea behind this act was to provide diverse services to the population, including inpatient and outpatient care, emergency services, assistance to the courts, and services for the mental health of children and the elderly. By 1975, Congress had authorized over 609 multiservice centers (James, 1981).

Another response to the personnel shortage was the Scheuer Subprofessional Career Act of 1966, administered by the Department of Labor. The philosophical basis for the act was that poor people and minority group members, if trained appropriately, could provide effective mental health services. Programs were developed to train such people to be teacher aides, child care workers, corrections officers, and mental health workers. Most of the education was essentially in-service training, but some programs had links to vocational schools or community colleges. (See Table 2-5.)

Kennedy viewed human services as a comprehensive set of services to assist the needy. In the text of the speech he was to deliver in Austin, Texas, on the day of his assassination, he provided an overall definition of human services that encompasses the range of problems and service activity that characterizes human services today. "From public works to public health, wherever Government programs operate, the past three years we have seen a new burst of action and progress" (Kennedy, 1964a, p. 897). Specifically, he included crime, slums, poverty, pollution, and unemployment. He cited as evidence of his administration's concern and action the hospitals, clinics, and nursing homes being built; the new attack on mental health and mental retardation; the training of more dentists and doctors; and increases in Social Security benefits.

During Kennedy's years as president, he set the tone for increased emphasis on the eradication of poverty in the United States. His vision brought much hope to populations that had despaired of changing their situations without assistance. Kennedy ignited the support of the nation to help the less fortunate.

Following the assassination of Kennedy in 1963, Lyndon B. Johnson took the oath of office as president. Johnson assumed the legacy of Kennedy's commitment to the impoverished, but this was not a new role for him. Before his election to the vice presidency, he had spent 23 years as an advocate for those who had little hope for the future and no one to represent them.

Varying estimates are made of the number of poor people in America during the Johnson era. John K. Galbraith's (1976) well-known book, *The Affluent Society,* described a country in which people continuously improved their standard of living and the quality of their lives. Michael Harrington (1962) depicted the country very differently in *The Other America.* According to his research, 50 to 60 million Americans lived in poverty, a good many of them in isolated rural regions of the country, especially in the South and the Southeast,

---

TABLE 2-5 ✦ SUMMARY POINTS: MENTAL HEALTH LEGISLATION

- National Mental Health Act of 1946 created the National Institute of Mental Health (NIMH), a center for information and research.
- The Mental Health Study Act of 1955 provided funding for a Joint Commission on Mental Illness and Health to evaluate the mental health needs and recommend a national mental health program.
- The Community Mental Health Centers Act of 1963 provided funding for community mental health centers.
- Scheuer Subprofessional Career Act of 1966 supported the development of programs to train poor and minority group members to provide effective mental health services.

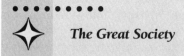

The Great Society

The following excerpts are from President Lyndon Johnson's speech at the University of Michigan's commencement on May 22, 1964. The Great Society, a name used in this speech, was to become a watchword for the social programs of the 1960s and early 1970s. Johnson eloquently paints a picture of his dream of eradicating poverty. The social legislation passed during his term to ensure "equality" to every individual was heralded as a step toward the Great Society.

... For in your time we have the opportunity to move not only toward the rich society and the powerful society, but upward to the Great Society. The Great Society rests on abundance and liberty for all. It demands an end to poverty and racial injustice, to which we are totally committed in our time. But that is just the beginning.

The Great Society is a place where every child can find knowledge to enrich his mind and to enlarge his talents. It is a place where leisure is a welcome chance to build and reflects not a feared cause of boredom and restlessness. It is a place where the city of man serves not only the needs of the body and the demands of commerce, but the desire for beauty and the hunger for community.

It is a place where man can renew contact with nature. It is a place which honors creation for its own sake and for what it adds to the understanding of the race. It is a place where men are more concerned with the quality of their goals than the quantity of their goods. But most of all, the Great Society is not a safe harbor, a resting place, a final objective, a finished work. It is a challenge constantly renewed, beckoning us toward a destiny where the meaning of our lives matches the marvelous products of our labor. . . .

For better or for worse, your generation has been appointed by history to deal with those problems and to lead America toward a new age. . . .

So will you join in the battle to give every citizen the full equality which God enjoins and the law requires, whatever his belief, or race, or the color of his skin? Will you join in the battle to give every citizen an escape from the crushing weight of poverty? Will you join in the battle to make it possible for all nations to live in enduring peace as neighbors and not as mortal enemies? Will you join in the battle to build the Great Society, to prove that our material progress is only the foundation on which we will build a richer life of mind and Spirit?

SOURCE: Excerpts from "President's Michigan Speech on the 'Great Society,' " by Lyndon Baines Johnson, in *Congressional Quarterly,* 20 (1964), p. 874. Reprinted by permission.

and others in large cities on the West and East coasts. These poor people had few skills for employment, lived in substandard housing, and were malnourished and illiterate.

In 1964, Johnson ran for president on a platform addressing the social problems described by Harrington. He proposed a comprehensive network of social policies and program initiatives. His opponent, Republican Senator Barry Goldwater, advocated reducing the government's role in addressing social problems. The public response to positive government social intervention was overwhelming, and Johnson was reelected by a large majority.

In his 1965 State of the Union address, he declared an "unconditional war on poverty" in order to create a "Great Society." Johnson believed the roots of poverty had to be attacked. Programs developed in the War on Poverty and Great Society initiatives included VISTA, the Neighborhood Youth Corps, the Job Corps, College Work Study, and Head Start. Their objective was to eradicate poverty by providing ways for the poor to improve their economic conditions. Many community action programs encouraged client participation in planning, delivering, and evaluating services.

Johnson also promoted the rights of the poor. For example, the Voting Rights Act of 1965 abolished the literacy tests that had been used to deny uneducated people the vote, and the Affirmative Action Order of 1968 and the Office of Economic Opportunity improved employment opportunities for minorities. Further evidence of the president's commitment were Medicare and Medicaid, amendments to the Social Security Act approved by President Johnson on July 30, 1965. Medicare (Title XVIII) provides health insurance for people over 65. Medicaid (Title XVIX) gives grants to the states to assist them in helping medically indigent citizens receive medical and hospital care.

Growth of the Human Service Movement

Since the 1960s, the human service movement has experienced unprecedented growth, evidenced by the increase in the number of training programs, the increased size of the mental health delivery system, and the development of the human service administration at the federal level. In 1966, the first human service program was established at Purdue University, a two-year associate degree program that focused on the training of entry-level mental health workers.

Originally, a new type of human service worker was envisioned that was a cross between the professional with an advanced degree and the volunteer. A major assumption about the new workers was that their firsthand work experiences, coupled with education and training, would enable them to establish greater rapport and credibility with their clients. In addition, their firsthand knowledge of the problems would give them greater understanding of clients and their difficulties. The initial intent was for these workers to perform innovative roles such as client advocacy and client–community liaison, but in reality they came to perform more traditional roles such as direct caregiving (Southern Regional Education Board, 1979).

NIMH continued its involvement with the movement during the 1970s. The New Careers branch of NIMH was established to provide leadership in the development of entry-level programs for disadvantaged persons. In 1975, this became the Paraprofessional Manpower Branch, which led the way in defining and developing the training for all levels of paraprofessional workers. There was much concern in the existing mental health system about who the new paraprofessionals would be, what jobs they would perform, and whether they would perform adequately. It was the responsibility of the Manpower Branch to address these questions.

In spite of the concern voiced by the other professionals in the mental health system, many of these newly trained human service workers were welcomed. During the 1970s, the number of clients served by the mental health system increased dramatically. New workers were needed, and the traditional ways of providing mental health services were not efficient or effective in meeting the changing needs. Highly skilled professionals with advanced degrees had been serving small numbers of clients. Human service workers could now provide the simpler direct-care services to greater numbers of clients while the highly skilled professionals worked with the more difficult problems and supervised the human service workers. Deinstitutionalization, a movement that began in the 1950s, called for transferring many institutionalized patients to the community for outpatient care. By the 1970s, a major segment of mental health treatment had shifted from the isolation of the institution to the complex environment of the community. As the concept of community mental health developed, different types of professional services were needed.

During this same time period, organizations emerged that signaled a move toward professionalism. Such organizations serve many purposes. They may regulate a profession or its workers, facilitate communication among its members, or foster excellence in research or service within the profession. Two organizations in particular were instrumental in the move toward a human service profession. These two influential organizations, the National Organization for Human Service Education (NOHSE) and the Council for Standards in Human Service Education (CSHSE), are still active today. Their websites are at http://www.nohse.com and http://www.cshse.com.

The Decline in Federal Involvement

The election of Richard Nixon as president in 1968 marked two important changes in the federal government's involvement in social reform: a decline in federal spending and a different way of managing human service programs. Both represented a return to more traditional values and a much more conservative approach to human services. Nixon's New Federalism called for individuals to assume responsibility for their own situations. It started power, resources, and influence flowing back to the states and local communities. The emphasis was on the development of self-help programs and provision of services by the private sector.

President Nixon introduced a new management system, management by objective (MBO), in a memo sent to 23 departments in 1973 (Gruber, 1981). The intent of this management system was to correct the problems associated with the vague goals of human service programs and organizations. MBO required specific steps in the administration of programs. First, managers were to establish goals; then each goal was to be translated into specific objectives, with a plan for their achievement; finally, the program would be evaluated, with both the goals and the results assessed.

With regard to human services, Nixon focused on a commitment to the family and a commitment to eradicating poverty. He believed that families were able to determine their own needs and should use aid as they determined best (Bowler, 1974). The Supplemental Security Income (SSI) program, which provided additional financial support for people needing assistance, translated this theory into practice.

President Gerald Ford's major impact on the human service delivery system was to continue the reduction of the federal government's involvement in human services. Ford supported an increased commitment by the private sector to support assistance to the needy. He had a major impact on human services through his 60 vetoes, which cut more than $9.5 billion that had been appropriated by Congress. Among the programs he vetoed were proposed improvements in federal aid to education, the school lunch program, and health care.

Focus on Mental Health

During his campaign for the presidency, Jimmy Carter discussed reorganizing the federal executive branch. After his election in 1976, he appointed a reorganization team directed by Bert Lance, the director of the Office of Management and Budget. The Human Resource group directed the study of the human services areas.

Five departments (Health, Education, and Welfare; Agriculture; Justice; Labor; and Interior) were involved in the reorganization. Initially, the services had been divided into categories of federal funding rather than sets of human problems. One-third of these programs either overlapped with each other or with programs in other departments. The major problem was in the Department of Health, Education, and Welfare; more than 300 of its programs crossed over into other departments. Another impetus for the reorganization was to fulfill a campaign promise by separating education programs from health and welfare services. The result was the creation of separate departments: the Department of Health and Human Services and the Department of Education. The use of the term *human services* denoted the wide variety of program services addressing human needs. The choice of the term clearly marks the point when human services became associated with a wide range of services, not restricted to those associated with mental health.

Carter also attempted to address a problem that had received attention from Kennedy and Johnson: unemployment. He proposed a Better Jobs and Income

Program that would have employed 1.4 million people in service positions developed by the government. In addition, more than 32 million people would have received payment for health, Social Security, welfare, and educational services. The program could not generate the political support that was needed because it was too complex to understand and too complicated to administer.

During the Carter administration, the President's Commission on Mental Health, chaired by Rosalyn Carter, found that between 10 and 15% of the population (20 to 32 million people) needed some form of mental health services at any one time. Unfortunately, the commission also discovered that many people did not have access to good, affordable mental health care. Further, there was a lack of support services for persons with chronic mental illness, which included approximately 1.5 million people in mental hospitals, nursing homes, and other residential facilities. On May 15, 1979, President Carter proposed the Mental Health Systems Act, which promised comprehensiveness, flexibility, and innovation by emphasizing services for persons with chronic mental illness and by emphasizing prevention. It also attempted to address the shortage of mental health personnel in underserved areas, requiring people who received federal money for their training to work in an area with a personnel shortage for a period as long as the time they received financial support. Congress passed the Mental Health Systems Act and authorized funding through 1984.

Dismantling the Welfare System

From the 1930s to the 1980s, the government's social policy was to assume responsibility for citizens who could not provide a reasonable quality of life for themselves. Voters in the 1980s and 1990s elected presidents who advocated substantial reduction of the federal budget and decreased federal government involvement in human services—a stark contrast to the policies of the previous administrations.

One of the first signs of retrenchment came from California. On June 7, 1978, California voters passed Proposition 13, an amendment to the state constitution (Pilisuk, 1980). The goal of the legislation was to amend the property tax structure. One result was that less money became available to fund a variety of services, including social services. People were beginning to question the effectiveness and efficiency of the government; they did not want to pay for so much government intervention. When the proposition passed, its supporters predicted that there would be substantial reductions in the services offered by government, and an increase in resources available from private sources.

What actually happened was that fewer professionals were employed, but the number of people in need did not decrease. Human service workers, serving larger caseloads, felt overworked, ineffective, and devalued. Their jobs seemed to have lost what little status they had; voters had sent a clear message that the services they provided were not supported. Existing programs were cut back, and fewer new programs were funded, but the needs were as great as ever. Self-care, community support systems, and natural helping networks had to take up the slack. More people in need began to turn to neighborhood groups, churches, friends, and families for assistance.

The passage of Proposition 13 was an early sign of the changing attitude of the American public toward government spending for human services. In 1980, Ronald Reagan was elected president on a platform that called for establishing new priorities in human services, slashing government spending, and reducing the government's involvement in human services. One of Reagan's priorities was to return the administration of human services to the individual states, communities, and private sources. His reasoning was that it is not the government's function to provide such services and that government delivery of such services is not effective or efficient. He terminated a number of social programs and drastically cut spending on others. Those affected included "AFDC, childcare, school lunch and other nutrition programs, food stamps, subsidized housing, energy assistance, family planning, public and mental health services, alcohol and drug abuse counseling, legal aid, the Job Corps, and the like" (Trattner, 1999, p. 365).

Reagan's reelection in 1984 was another overwhelming victory. His second term continued to emphasize the economy, defense, and foreign policy (Ginsberg, 1987). The plight of the poor worsened during this period and one result was a welfare reform bill designed to help single parents, particularly women, enter the job market. The Family Support Act was signed into law in 1988. Among the programs authorized was the JOBS program, which required single parents on welfare with children older than 3 years to work or be in training in order to receive assistance. The act also mandated new procedures for collecting child support payments and one year of support for child care and transportation so that single parents could work or participate in training. For the most part, though, both Reagan administrations largely ignored the plight of the poor and disenfranchised, focusing instead on defense spending and tax cuts.

As a result of Reagan's policy, there was a shift in service delivery. The number of nonprofit and private agencies in human services expanded, and human service institutions and agencies contracted out for services (Ginsberg, 1987). Reagan also advocated transferring federally owned housing and prisons to the private sector.

Just as the labor market tends to respond to economic demands, the human service labor market reflects human service demands (Austin, 1983). During the 1960s and 1970s, the human service market was growing, and the number of opportunities for employment and for advancement increased. During the 1980s that growth slowed. Opportunities did develop in the private sector with, for example, the privatization of correctional facilities and the development of employee assistance programs in private industry.

George Bush, Reagan's vice president, won the 1988 presidential election and claimed a mandate to continue many of the policies of the Reagan administrations. Generally, Bush's administration is noted for its emphasis on foreign policy and its lack of attention to domestic issues. In fact, because of the pressure of deficit spending, Bush and legislators agreed to slowly cut military spending. In 1990, military expenditures were cut, with the understanding that

Highlights of the New Law

The welfare reform bill signed into law by President Clinton makes the most dramatic changes in federal anti-poverty programs in six decades. Following are highlights:

Ends a 61-year guarantee of federal aid for poor children. Instead, Aid to Families with Dependent Children, the main federal cash welfare program, and smaller programs are folded into block grants that states will use to operate their own programs.

Reduces spending by about $55 billion over six years, mainly by cutting food stamps and aid to legal immigrants.

Imposes a five-year lifetime limit on welfare benefits. States can exempt up to 20% of their caseload for hardship reasons and set shorter time limits.

Requires recipients to begin working two years after receiving welfare and mandates that 50% of single-parent families work 30 hours a week by 2002. States already running welfare work programs under federally approved waivers can continue the programs until the waivers expire.

Reduces spending on food stamps, the federal coupons redeemed for food at supermarkets, by $28 billion over six years and allows able-bodied individuals without children to receive food stamps for only three months in any three-year period, unless they are working part time. Individuals can get another three months if they are laid off from work.

Bars most federal aid, including Medicaid and cash welfare, to future legal immigrants for five years.

Current immigrants cannot receive disability and food stamps during their first five years in the USA, and states have the option to deny other aid. Exceptions include refugees and immigrants who have generally worked for 10 years.

Makes it more difficult for children to receive federal disability payments due to mental problems—a program that has been widely abused, critics say.

SOURCE: From "Highlights of the New Law," *USA Today,* August 23, 1996, p. 3A. Copyright © 1996, *USA Today.* Reprinted with permission.

the money would not be shifted to support social programs. The most significant legislation of his four years was the Americans with Disabilities Act (ADA), which was passed in 1990. With little cost to the federal government, ADA was designed to get people into the workforce who otherwise would not be able to enter or who were kept out for other reasons, such as discrimination.

Bill Clinton and Welfare Reform

A declining economy, the growing gap between rich and poor, and the need for welfare reform all contributed to the election in 1992 of Democrat Bill Clinton, governor of Arkansas. One of his campaign pledges was to "end welfare as we know it."

In 1996, The Personal Responsibility and Work Opportunity Reconciliation Act replaced the Aid to Families with Dependent Children, which was the primary welfare law sponsored by the federal government to provide aid to eligible mothers with children. This legislation ended the federal government's six-decade guarantee of aid to the poor. Under the former welfare program, eligibility for support was based on income and was regulated by the federal government. The key components in the reformed welfare system are state control, work requirements, time limits, and penalties (Survey: New rules leading cause of decline in welfare rolls, 1999). The states receive federal funds in a block grant program called Temporary Assistance to Needy Families (TANF) and there is flexibility concerning how the states spend their money. Each state receives a fixed amount of money each year until 2001. If states are to receive their allotted amount, they must also contribute to the welfare program. The state contribution is called the mandated maintenance of effort (MOE). The funds are spent on eligible families (Reichert, 1998a). Many states have used their TANF and MOE dollars to provide traditional welfare services such as cash assistance, employment services, child care, and emergency assistance; however, some states have expanded their services. For example, Virginia provides a state-earned tax credit for eligible working families. New Mexico is using MOE funding to provide nonmedical substance abuse services to Native Americans. Illinois is using MOE support to provide services to homeless and at-risk families through the homeless shelter system. New Jersey is supporting legal immigrants who lost food stamps by providing nutritional programs (Reichert, 1998b).

The initial report on the success of the welfare reform is mixed. In 1999, President Clinton announced that the number of welfare recipients is at a 30-year low, down 44% from 1994 ("Welfare rolls hit a 30-year low," 1999). A positive report comes in from many states, and by 1999, Wisconsin was able to document that 83% of those surveyed had worked at least part of the time since leaving the rolls (Study: Most former Wisconsin welfare recipients now working, 1999). Unfortunately there are still many problems facing these poor families. Many clients are working, but for $7 or $8 per hour (Tweedie, 1999). They went straight to work, receiving little training and no education; and once the state support is discontinued, they will join the growing ranks of the working poor. According to welfare program administrators, "To ease these hard-core adult recipients into jobs . . . it will take much more—more skills, more services, more money and more patience—than was needed to nudge the first . . . (clients) off the rolls" (Healy, 1998).

The following quotes from welfare mothers voice their concerns within the program.

• • • • • • • • • •

WEB SOURCES
Find Out More About Welfare Reform

http://www.nasulgc.org/clinton_welfare_announcement.htm

This site is a record of the announcement that President Clinton made to announce the changes in the welfare-to-work programs, focusing on helping fathers support their children and families.

http://www.sfgate.com/cgi-bin/article/archive/1998/12/02/MN45270.DTL

This article describes welfare reform success and its difficulties.

http://www.ncsl.org/statefed/welfare/8quest.htm

This site is provided by the National Conference of State Legislatures. It answers eight questions that are asked about welfare reform, including the following: Are effective programs in place to help hard-to-serve recipients? Does the state plan deal with recipients keeping jobs and getting better jobs and finding work in rural areas and city centers? Will it survive an economic downturn?

http://www.welfare-policy.org/impact.htm

This site addresses many questions about welfare reform such as the following: Why are caseloads declining? What types of jobs are welfare recipients getting? Are families better off? Included are very current questions and responses.

http://www.childrensdefense.org/fairstart-welfare2what.html

This site is a joint report released by the Children's Defense Fund and the National Coalition for the Homeless documenting the results of the welfare-to-work program. The report compiles more than 30 state and local studies and presents national and local findings, cataloguing both current questions and responses.

http://aspe.os.dhhs.gov/hsp/isp/reform.htm

This site compares the prior law with the Personal Responsibility and Work Opportunity Reconciliation Act of 1996 (P.L. 104-193).

Of California's welfare-to-work program, Jewell Bibs, age 21, says, "They made it sound so good . . . they help you with child care. They help you with bus fare. But they tell you, you can find a good job. And to them, a good job is any job. You can get one of them and you're still going to be poor" (Golden, 1996, p. 9).

Phyllis Martin in Boston has been on a continuous welfare-to-work cycle since 1987. She has twice trained for jobs, worked, and then been part of a large company layoff. She has this to say about her current job as a filing clerk in an architectural firm: "I hope this is it. I mean, I hope this is it" (Nifong, 1996, p. 10).

Manda Seefield of Coal Valley, Illinois, mother of two young children, has been on welfare for the past six years. She says of her ability to

1996 Welfare into Law Speech

What we are trying to do today is to overcome the flaws of the welfare system for the people who are trapped in it. We all know that the typical family on welfare today is very different from the one that welfare was designed to deal with 60 years ago. We all know that there are a lot of good people on welfare who just get off of it in the ordinary course of business, but that a significant number of people are trapped on welfare for a very long time, exiling them from the entire community of work that gives structure to our lives.

Nearly 30 years ago Robert Kennedy said, "Work is the meaning of what this country is all about. We need it as individuals. We need to sense it in our fellow citizens. And we need it as a society and as a people." He was right then, and it's right now. From now on our nation's answer to this great social challenge will no longer be a never-ending cycle of welfare: it will be the dignity, the power, and the ethic of work. Today we are taking an historic chance to make welfare what it was meant to be: a second chance, not a way of life. The bill I am about to sign, as I have said many times, is far from perfect. But it has come a very long way.

Congress sent me two previous bills that I strongly believe failed to protect our children and did too little to move people from welfare to work. I vetoed both of them. This bill had broad bipartisan support and is much, much better on both counts.

The new bill restores America's basic bargain of providing opportunity and demanding in return responsibility. It provides $14 billion for child care, $4 billion more than the present law does. It is good because without the assurance of child care it's all but impossible for a mother with young children to go to work.

It requires states to maintain their own spending on welfare reform, and gives them powerful performance incentives to place more people on welfare in jobs. It gives states the capacity to create jobs by taking money now used for welfare checks and giving it to employers as subsidies, as incentives to hire people. This bill will help people that go to work so they can stop drawing a welfare check and start drawing a paycheck.

It's also better for children. It preserves the national safety net of food stamps and school lunches. It drops the deep cuts and the devastating changes in child protection, adoption and help for disabled children. It preserves the national guaranty of health care for poor children, the disabled, the elderly and people on welfare—the most important preservation of all.

It includes the tough child support enforcement measures that as far as I know every member of Congress and everybody in the administration and

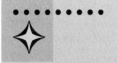

every thinking person in the country has supported for more than two years now. It's the most sweeping crackdown on deadbeat parents in history. We have succeeded in increasing child support collection 40 percent. But over a third of the cases where there are delinquencies involve people who cross state lines. For a lot of women and children, the only reason they're on welfare today, the only reason, is that the father up and walked away when he could have made a contribution to the welfare of the children. That is wrong. If every parent paid the child support that he or she owes legally today, we could move 800,000 women and children off welfare immediately.

With this bill, we say, if you don't pay the child support you owe, we'll garnish your wages, take away your driver's license, track you across state lines, if necessary make you work off what you owe. It is a good thing, and it will help dramatically to reduce welfare, increase independence and reinforce parental responsibility.

SOURCE: Office of the Press Secretary, The White House, August 22, 1996. Remarks by the president at the signing of the Personal Responsibility and Work Opportunity Reconciliation Act (http://www.pub.whitehouse.gov/white-house-publications/1996/08/1996-08-22-president-remarks).

find work, "They don't want you unless you have experience . . . but how do you get experience, unless somebody is going to give you a job?" (Johnson, 1996, p. A7).

These mothers express only a few of the problems they see with the new welfare reform. Teena Briton, a welfare mother who attends North Shore Community College in Salem, Massachusetts, summarizes their concerns: "I feel [the state's] going to keep chipping away, chipping away at us until finally it's going to be, like, 'Hey, you've got to get off welfare and that's it.' And that's OK. But let me stay on it long enough to get some hope" (Nifong, 1997, p. 10).

The debate will continue over the impact of the welfare reform legislation, but today there are three major concerns. One is the sufficiency of resources to help people get education, training, and other necessities. A second concern is the lack of ongoing social services such as substance abuse treatment, domestic violence shelters, and homelessness retreats for those who are now off the welfare rolls but still have multiple problems. A third concern is that the $56 billion cuts in AFDC, food stamps, and other programs might throw 1.1 million children into poverty. However these concerns are addressed, this legislation is a significant historical event in the move to dismantle the welfare system in the United States.

TABLE 2-6 ✦ SUMMARY POINTS: PRESIDENTIAL LEADERSHIP IN HUMAN SERVICES

Franklin D. Roosevelt
- Short-term aid in the form of Works Progress Administration and the Civilian Conservation Corps to the unemployed
- Social Security Act of 1935 as protection against future economic hardships

Harry Truman
- An enlarged Social Security program
- Public power projects
- National Mental Health Act of 1946

Dwight D. Eisenhower
- Mental Health Study Act of 1955

John F. Kennedy
- Manpower Development and Training Act to teach new skills to unemployed
- Aid to underdeveloped areas nationally and internationally
- Changes in Social Security Act to provide casework to families chronically unemployed
- Community Mental Health Centers Act of 1963

Lyndon B. Johnson
- Older Americans Act of 1965 that funded support programs for senior citizens
- Scheurer Subprofessional Career Act of 1966
- War on Poverty and Great Society initiatives including Neighborhood Youth Corps, Job Corps, College Work Study, and Head Start
- Voting Rights Act of 1965
- Affirmative Action Order of 1968
- Medicare and Medicaid Amendments to the Social Security Act

Richard Nixon
- Decline in federal spending and provision of services by private sector
- Management by objective (MBO), a new management system
- Supplemental Security Income (SSI) program that provided additional financial support to those needing assistance

Gerald Ford
- Continued reduction of federal involvement in human services
- Vetoed improvements in federal aid to education, the school lunch program, and health care

Jimmy Carter
- Department of Health, Education, and Welfare becomes the Department of Health and Human Services and the Department of Education.
- Appointed the President's Commission on Mental Health
- Proposed the Mental Health Systems Act, which was passed and funded through 1984

Ronald Reagan
- Terminated and reduced a number of human service programs.
- Family Support Act (1988) authorized the JOBS program.

George Bush
- Lack of attention to domestic issues
- Americans with Disabilities Act (1990)

Bill Clinton
- Personal Responsibility and Work Opportunity Reconciliation Act (1996) replaced Aid to Families with Dependent Children (AFDC).

During the Clinton years, attention was also focused on developing support for family caregivers. This effort was in direct response to the growing number of elderly in the United States. Today one in four households are providing care to these older citizens. Three-fourths of the caregivers are women, many of whom are older themselves. A predominant number of these women are also employed full time, run their own households, and have children of their own (Administration on Aging, 1999). Currently the Older Americans Act of 1965 includes several support programs for older Americans such as meals-on-wheels programs, rides to the doctor or pharmacy for visits, protection against elder abuse, and counseling. The proposed reauthorization of the Older Americans Act would add the creation of the National Family Caregiver Support Program. Through this program, families who care for the elderly would receive support to improve the quality of long-term care. In addition, counseling and training would be available for these caregivers to help them understand both their new responsibilities and the needs of their elderly charges. In addition, the reauthorization would include a tax credit for caring for the elderly, housing for the elderly, and Medicaid support for home and community-based care (Administration on Aging, 1999). (See Table 2-6.)

New challenges face human service professionals as we enter the 21st century. Managed care, technological advances, nontraditional service settings, and a shrinking global community are only a few of the changes with which service providers must cope. These challenges will be explored in the next chapter as you begin thinking about human services today.

Things to Remember

1. Before the Middle Ages, people believed that mental illness was caused by evil spirits, and early forms of treatment focused on ridding the body of these spirits.
2. Until the 1500s, the Catholic Church was chiefly responsible for providing human services. Under the Church's guidance, many institutions were founded for the poor, orphans, the elderly, and the handicapped.
3. The decline of feudalism, the growth of commerce, and the beginning of industrialization made it necessary to find new ways of assisting those in need.
4. Pressures caused by the increasing number of poor in the cities created the need for a large-scale attack on poverty and prompted the passage of the Elizabethan Poor Law of 1601, critical legislation that guided social welfare practices in England and the United States for the next 350 years.
5. In the early years, the colonists used the English system as a model for their philosophy toward and services for the poor and needy. By the early 1800s, however, other philosophies prevailed, ones that discouraged and limited the provision of human services.

6. Major reforms during the late 1800s concentrated on improving the treatment of the institutionalized mentally ill and children.
7. The Charity Organization Society, a forerunner of the Community Chest and the United Way, is an example of society's response to the needs of an expanding urban population.
8. A settlement house was a large house in a slum area that served as a community center, sponsoring such activities as recreation; classes in English, cooking, and citizenship; vocational training; and child care.
9. President Franklin D. Roosevelt introduced the Social Security Act of 1935, which fundamentally changed the federal government's role in providing human services.
10. During the years John F. Kennedy served as president, he set the tone for increased emphasis on the eradication of poverty in the United States, bringing hope to populations that had despaired of changing their situations without assistance.
11. The emergence of human service training programs and the development of a human service philosophy mirror the historical events and presidential leadership from the 1960s to the present.
12. In his 1965 State of the Union address, President Lyndon Johnson declared an "unconditional war on poverty." He developed programs that attacked the roots of poverty in order to create a "Great Society."
13. The National Organization for Human Service Education and the Council for Standards in Human Service Education have been instrumental in the development of the human service profession.
14. The election of Richard Nixon as president marked two important changes in the federal government's involvement in social reform: a decline in federal spending and a different way of managing human service programs.
15. During the presidency of Ronald Reagan, commitment to human services passed from the federal government to state and local governments, the private sector, and needy individuals themselves.
16. The Bush administration supported the passage of the Americans with Disabilities Act which provided guidelines to reduce the discrimination of individuals with disabilities.
17. Bill Clinton reformed the welfare system by proposing a new law that emphasized training, education, short-term support, and personal responsibility.

Additional Readings: Focus on History

Beers, Clifford W. (1945). *A mind that found itself: An autobiography.* Garden City, NY: Doubleday, Doran.
Clifford Beers writes of his experiences as a three-time patient in mental institutions around the turn of the century.

Butterfield, F. (1996). *All God's children: The Bosket family and the American tradition of violence.* New York: Avon Books.

This chronicle of the history of a black family through five generations shows how early struggles in the antebellum South finally led to lives of rage and violence on the streets of New York City.

Johnson, A. B. (1990). *Out of bedlam: The truth about deinstitutionalization.* New York: Basic Books.

The author reviews the history of deinstitutionalization by focusing on the fiscal pressures faced by states and the opportunities to shift costs to the federal government. As a mental health professional herself, Johnson illustrates how bureaucratic complexity and confusion have given deinstitutionalization a bum rap.

Marshall, Helen E. (1937). *The forgotten samaritan.* Chapel Hill, NC: University of North Carolina Press.

Marshall has produced a well-written biography of Dorothea Dix, humanitarian and reformer.

Trattner, Walter I. (1999). *From poor law to welfare state: A history of social welfare in America.* New York: Free Press.

Trattner gives an overview of social welfare in the United States from the colonial era to the present. He includes highlights of the mental health, child welfare, and public health movements, as well as beginnings of social welfare as a profession.

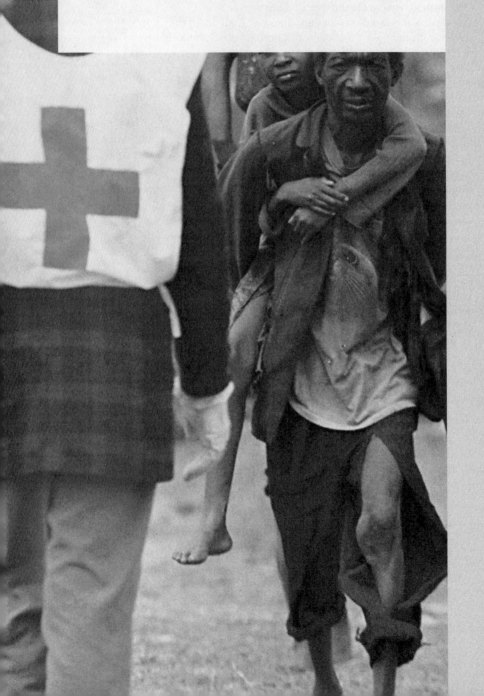

 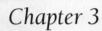

One facet of the definition of human services is how and where services are delivered today. This chapter examines new settings, new skills, and recent trends in human service delivery. As you read this chapter, you will see that human services today has a much broader scope than ever before. It takes place in a variety of settings, addresses global human needs, interfaces with the managed care system, and reflects recent advances in communication and technology. This chapter examines each of these dimensions in more detail to help expand your definition of human services.

New Settings for Human Service Delivery

One way to describe the broadening scope of human services today is to think about where services are delivered. In many instances, services continue to be delivered in agencies or institutional settings; but with a growing emphasis on making services accessible and comprehensive, service delivery in nontraditional settings has increased. Rural services, industrial and military settings, and schools are highlighted in this section.

Institutional and Community-Based Services

There has been a change in philosophy regarding the delivery of services in institutional settings and in the community. The difference in settings is an obvious factor. Earlier institutions were located in remote places because pastoral settings were believed to be peaceful and calming. These settings may also have been chosen because members of society did not like to be reminded of the existence of people with mental illness. Correctional facilities have been built in rural areas because the criminal population is considered dangerous to others. Again, people who were not incarcerated did not like to be reminded of this population. Now, however, in mental health, the trend is toward downsizing institutions and increasing the number of community-based services. In the past, many people who were institutionalized could have functioned in the community with some professional support. The goal of community-based mental health care is to enable clients to interact with their environments in the least restrictive setting in which they can function.

Community-based mental health has changed the nature of service delivery. The focus of treatment has become health and wellness instead of illness. The process involves other social institutions such as schools, recreation facilities, and churches. In addition, the psychological and medical treatment received by clients has been adapted for community-based care. Much of the human service work is in case management: The human service worker acts as planner, consultant, and liaison between the mental health agency, the client, and the other institutions. Human service professionals also provide support for the families of persons with mental illness.

Community-based care in corrections is designed to take individuals from prisons and local jails and place them in the community within supervised, planned programs. These programs link educational services, counseling, substance abuse treatment, and employment assistance. In these programs, much of the responsibility falls to the client to take the initiative in using available services.

Another area of community-based care has developed between human services professionals and families of children who have behavioral, emotional, and/or mental problems. In the earlier model, the family and the child were seen as clients; now the parents are considered part of the helping network. According to Cohen and Lavach (1995), in the parents-as-helpers model, parents are seen as

- Experts on and teachers of their own children
- Advocates for their children
- Change agents in improving the environment in which their children live

In this model, families are empowered to assume responsibility for their own care and the care of their children, but are still eligible for support when it is appropriate.

Since the 1970s, interest in providing services in rural areas has increased. Two factors account for this interest. First, historically those living in rural areas have been disadvantaged, experiencing a steady erosion in population and quality of life. They are more likely to be elderly, be members of disadvantaged minorities, lack the kinds of opportunities available to metropolitan counterparts, and need the help of human service agencies and professionals (Ginsberg, 1998). Evidence also suggests, however, a growing pattern of relocation to rural areas and small towns, which is a reversal of 20th-century migrating trends from rural to urban areas. Small towns and rural areas are attracting those who see advantages in living where there are lower crime rates, opportunities for professional advancement, and larger labor pools with lower wage expectations. Thus, an increased number of people live in rural areas who are not disadvantaged, but rather may have significant wealth. They include property owners, professionals, and business people. Those who are living in rural poverty, and those who are not disadvantaged, may experience similar problems that require the help of social service agencies and helping professionals, such as mental illness, family conflicts, and physical limitations.

A second reason for the interest in human services in rural areas is the number of difficulties or barriers in providing accessible and adequate services. Shortages of trained health care and helping professionals, the large geographic distances between clients and providers, the cost of services, the maintenance of confidentiality, and the coordination of care are all problematic in rural areas. Another significant barrier is the community stigma attached to having problems and receiving services (Hook & Ford, 1998). Often this negative perception prevents individuals and families from getting the help they need. One helpful model of service is the home visit, which is necessary when clients will not come to an agency:

> They believe it is a place for crazy people and fear that anyone seeing them going in or coming out will think they are crazy. On the other hand, a case manager and two other people (therapist, physician) seen going into their house could be taken for relatives. (Garrett, 1998, p. 10)

The provision of mental health services is particularly problematic in rural areas. In addition to the problems mentioned, mental health problems often remain undiagnosed (Rost, Humphrey, & Kelleher, 1994). Rural primary care providers such as physicians and nurse practitioners are likely to care for those with mental health problems and will encounter difficulties in referring them for specialized care. Here again, distance, stigma, and costs are among the barriers that prevent successful referrals.

Recognition that significant challenges exist in human service provision in rural areas has prompted federal support for improved services. Unfortunately, the support has waxed and waned over the years. From 1978 to 1981, federal policies encouraged collaborative community efforts. By 1981, however, federal policy began to decrease support for linkages between mental health and other community services. Additional legislation that has narrowed the focus of mental health has also curtailed rural mental health funding (U.S. Congress, 1990). The last significant effort to address these problems occurred during the farm crisis of the 1980s when the National Institute of Mental Health (NIMH) encouraged collaborative efforts to respond to the needs of economically troubled rural families.

Linkage arrangements among existing area agencies and organizations have been particularly effective when they have been employed. Their benefits include improved access to mental health services, facilitation of appropriate use of mental and primary health services, a reduction in the burden of primary care providers to meet mental health needs, and better continuity of care (Burns, Burke, & Ozarin, 1983). But there are also problems with linkages. Turf issues, ineffective communication, and organizational differences with procedures, policies, and philosophies make the establishment and operation of linkages difficult. Workers in effective linkage arrangements are those who have excellent skills to engender the respect of medical staff, understand the culture and policies of the general health sector, and practice good communication skills (Hook & Ford, 1998).

In recent years many efforts have been developed to improve rural service delivery (Ginsberg, 1998). *Human Services in Rural Environment,* a professional journal, is published by the School of Social Work and Human Services at Eastern Washington University. Articles on the same topic now appear with some regularity in other more general professional journals. Books have also been published recently that focus on rural issues, and several federal and state government agencies such as the National Institute of Mental Health, the Public

Health Service, and the Department of Housing and Urban Development have established special programs to deal with rural areas and concerns.

Human Services in Industry and the Military

Traditionally, human services has been associated with people in financial need, particularly those who are unemployed or who are labeled as poor. Today's employers recognize that workers who are physically and psychologically well are more productive employees. Industry has learned to identify signals that indicate when an employee needs assistance, such as tardiness, absenteeism, ineffective job performance, and inability to cooperate or communicate with others. Many companies now encourage their workers to seek help.

Industry's initial interest in human services began when drug and alcohol abuse among employees showed alarming increases. The federal government was instrumental in establishing guidelines for treating this problem. The Federal Comprehensive Alcohol Abuse and Alcohol Prevention, Treatment and Rehabilitation Act (the Hughes Act) was passed in 1970 and created the National Institute on Alcohol Abuse and Alcoholism. The act was significant for the field of human services because it established an approach that was different from the treatment for persons with mental illness. The act required federal agencies to have alcohol abuse and prevention programs available to employees—programs now well known as employee assistance programs (EAPs). EAP services are offered to employees of most major corporations. Some address broad needs of workers such as counseling for abuse, personal issues, and marital problems; encouraging wellness with diet counseling, exercise, stress management, and personal awareness education; and developing work-related skills through such programs as employee orientation, management development, human relations training, team building, organizational development, and preparation for retirement. Most professionals who provide this support have baccalaureate and master's level training. The scope of human services has once again expanded beyond the fundamental provision of basic assistance.

Passage of the Americans with Disabilities Act (ADA) has also had a significant impact on business, industry, and other employers. Signed into law by President George Bush on July 26, 1990, ADA was patterned after the 1964 Civil Rights Act. The intent and spirit of ADA was, and continues to be, to enable people with disabilities to have access to goods and services—including employment—that is equal to the access available to citizens without disabilities. ADA is nondiscriminatory legislation, not affirmative action legislation. This act makes it unlawful for employers to discriminate against people with disabilities in regard to hiring, firing, compensation, training, and advancement. The act affects almost 50 million Americans with disabilities. The five titles in the act delineate the areas it addresses:

- Employment
- Public Services, including transportation systems (federal, state, and local government)

- Access to Goods and Services in the Public Sector
- Telecommunications
- Miscellaneous Provisions (e.g., insurance issues, limits regarding modifications to historical buildings and other structures)

The overwhelming majority of the nation's employers openly embrace ADA's equal access and reasonable accommodation tenets. If a candidate is qualified for a particular job and can perform the essential job functions, that person has the same opportunities as anyone else. The employer must make alterations to the work setting to account for the disability. Through mediation, alternative dispute resolution, arbitration, and litigation, case law is further defining and clarifying ADA's parameters. The integration and acceptance of people with disabilities has increased greatly in the short period since passage of the act, but more remains to be done.

Another nontraditional setting for human service delivery is the military. Meeting basic human needs in the military is different from accomplishing the same in a civilian setting, partly because of the atmosphere of discipline and commitment to the organization. In 1881, the American Red Cross began providing social services to the military out of a concern for the health and welfare of the individuals in uniform. A medical orientation characterized military social service until 1976, when the Service to Armed Forces (SAF) was developed to help the military better serve the families of military personnel. Field offices were established in military hospitals and military installations to assist communication between service personnel and families. The field offices provide a team of professionals, including a human service worker, to counsel military personnel (Masi, 1982). In January 1999, the Navy also announced a new program that would link personnel and families by e-mail. The new Navy site, LIFElines Web, is part of a $3.4 million Quality of Life program that promotes "a national model leading the way in human resources support services. Interactive family support, counseling and training is available on-line" (Brewin, 1999).

Schools as Part of the Human Service Delivery System

Schools are now a site for human service delivery in many communities. The following observations by public school teachers illustrate the challenges they encounter in schools today and the need for expanded services in educational settings.

> *Donna Viveiros, a teacher from Fall River, Massachusetts:* "Children come to school with all kinds of problems from home. Students can't sit still; they're hungry; their home life is just upside down." (Vreeland, 1991, p. B1)

> *Joy G. Dryfoos, an elementary education teacher:* "Schools are being called on to be those 'surrogate parents' that can increase the 'teachability' of children who arrive on their doorsteps in poor shape." (Hornblower, 1996, p. 37)

Russell Yeany, dean of the College of Education, University of Georgia:
"We are asking teachers to do a lot, but we don't have any choice. We don't have the luxury of focusing just on academic issues. The classroom has become the last safety net." (Anderson, 1998, A1)

Teachers such as these encounter the problems of children and youth each time they enter the classroom. They ask: "Can learning occur in an environment characterized by gangs, dropouts, teenage pregnancy, substance abuse, AIDS, and violence?" Predictions for the future do not offer much hope.

The challenge to human service professionals is to build on the commonalities they share with professional educators to coordinate comprehensive services that assist the whole person. Because human service and educational professionals share the same clients, a team approach ensures that those clients receive services with little duplication but much reinforcement. Another role they have in common is that of service delivery. Whether interacting with clients in a school classroom, an agency office, or an institutional setting, every helping professional plays many roles: teacher/educator, caregiver, advocate, and broker.

A partnership between human services and education is essential to meet the complex needs of children and families. School-based services or full-service schools are popular terms that describe the creation of an array of integrated support services in schools that children, youth, and families need to be successful (Dryfoos, 1994). This movement melds quality education and support services.

What services are provided in full-service schools? The answer depends on several factors such as the needs of students and their families, the viability of school reform, and the cooperative efforts of local agencies. Dryfoos (1994) suggests that the result may actually be a combination of the settlement house (see Chapter 2) with the school, where educational, health, and social welfare services are integrated. One example of a successful collaboration effort is Roosevelt Healthy Start, an initiative in Los Angeles that strives to increase the number of physically and mentally healthy children and families, to improve the resiliency of families and adolescents, and to increase the number of students who stay in school and graduate. (See Table 3-1.) Read about this program in the accompanying box.

As described, human services occur in an increasing diversity of settings; the challenge for the generalist helper is to use skills, knowledge, and values to serve clients effectively across these varied settings. One of those skills is using technology.

 # The Impact of Technology

Recent advances in technology continue to change the delivery of human services, although not without cost. Many organizations find the initial investment in equipment, software, and training to be quite expensive. Even so,

••••••••••

 Roosevelt Healthy Start

The Roosevelt Healthy Start is part of the California Healthy Start initiative which was launched in 1991 in response to Senate Bill 620. The main purpose of Senate Bill 620 is "to restructure the state's fragmented systems of education, health, mental health, and social services for children and families" (Wagner, 1994, p. 1). In 1993, the Boyle Heights area of Los Angeles administrators, teachers, students, parents, and community agencies organized to address the mental and physical health needs of their students. Their purpose was to identify human and material resources within the collaborative or from other interested agencies, which could be reorganized into a continuum of services most needed by the families in the Boyle Heights community. The collaborative now brings services to Roosevelt High School, Hollenbeck Middle School, and Sheridan Elementary School. All three schools are located in East Los Angeles (which includes the Boyle Heights community), a highly urbanized, densely populated, economically depressed residential area comprised of first-, second-, and third-generation Hispanic families of primarily Mexican-American descent. The community is fraught with poverty, social and political decay, high crime rates, low levels of school success, limited-English-speaking residents, limited transportation, and high unemployment rates.

The services provided by Roosevelt Healthy Start include coordinated case management for families and/or adolescents experiencing significant health, mental health, and social problems that interfere with family functioning and school success. They have served 9,100 students and their offsprings include one or more of the following services:

TABLE 3-1   ✦   SUMMARY POINTS: SERVICE DELIVERY SETTINGS

- Human service delivery continues in traditional settings such as social service agencies and institutions.
- Mental health, corrections, and families are examples of community-based service delivery.
- Rural human service delivery faces many barriers including distance, cost, confidentiality, and shortages of professionals.
- The Federal Comprehensive Alcohol Abuse and Alcohol Prevention, Treatment and Rehabilitation Act prompted the establishment of employee assistance programs in the workplace.
- The Americans with Disabilities Act ensures equal access to goods and services for persons with disabilities.
- Full-service schools integrate educational, health, and social welfare services.

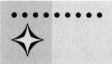

- Mental health counseling services for suicide prevention, physical and sexual abuse, family-interaction difficulties, behavior problems, gender identifying, and students in grief
- Medical services including physical exams, diagnosis/treatment of minor illnesses, immunizations, health promotion and preventive care, health education/counseling, reproductive health services, and medical/mental health referrals
- Health education to provide workshops, classes, and one-on-one counseling in health-related issues to students
- Adolescent and family life program to provide case management for students identified as "at risk" for dropping out, and pregnant and/or parenting teens
- Medi-Cal eligibility worker on site to screen and accept applications for MediCal
- Immediate Needs Transportation Program Distributing Agency to serve families and children who have an urgent transportation need
- Free legal consultation to students and families regarding emancipation, home evictions, immigration, and other legal matters

An evaluation of Roosevelt Healthy Start found that it has made a significant impact in areas such as increased immunization of kindergarten students, reduced absences due to illness, decreased teen pregnancy, increased family access to mental and physical health care, increased family use of appropriate private and public support systems, increased participation of parents and adolescents in activities, and increased attendance rates for all schools.

new technologies have been introduced into the human service delivery system in the areas of communication, information management, service delivery, and professional development. Many of these areas have experienced great changes; and continued change is predicted. Administrators of services, direct service providers, and clients are all "customers" of the new computer systems that have emerged during the technology revolution. We expect growth in the creative use of technology to continue occurring at a rapid pace.

The primary goal for using technology in the human service delivery system is to provide services more effectively and efficiently. For many human service professionals, use of technology has already helped them provide better quality services in a more cost-effective manner. As these technologies become more interwoven in our lives, they also will be used simply because they represent the standard way of doing business. Next we examine several areas where computers and other new technologies have been integrated into human service practice and delivery. One ethical concern about the increased use of technology is the protection of confidentiality. With the shift from paper or face-to-face communication to technology-driven methods, protection of the client and the helping activity must continue to be ensured.

Communication

Computer technologies and the advances in satellite communications have changed the ways many interactions occur in human service settings. One innovation is electronic mail (e-mail) which human service professionals use for daily interactions with colleagues, whether they are in the same building or across the state, nation, or sometimes the globe. The advantage of e-mail is convenience. When a computer is linked to an e-mail service, users can write messages on the computer and send them immediately, any time of day or night. Recipients can open messages and read them at their convenience, often at a different computer from their own by signing on as a guest or gaining access from the World Wide Web. Any message—incoming and outgoing—can also be printed if a paper copy of the message is desired. Within the human services context, much of this communication focuses on understanding procedures to help clients, seeking services, acquiring information, and sharing ideas.

Human service professionals also use computer technologies in other ways to communicate. Distribution lists and listservs are used when individuals with a common interest wish to talk with one another and share ideas and concerns. One such listserv is the International Counselor Network (ICN). The members in this network are continually discussing issues such as ethics, treatment, managed care, and funding. When you belong to a listserv such as the ICN, you can read all messages sent between the members, but you are not committed to responding in any way. You can also actively join the dialogue at any time by writing a response to an issue being discussed or by raising a question. Each member receives your communication and is free to answer. The entire membership receives all communications among members. Figure 3-1 shows an example of a message similar to those sent in the ICN. More than 850 counselors received the message (Marino, 1996).

Another way human service professionals in distant locations can communicate with each other is by teleconferencing. Many large organizations find this technology a cost-effective way to conduct meetings and to talk with each other about service delivery, new programming for clients, and ways to learn new information and skills. Teleconferencing is used by many state agencies to stay in touch with their local branches. This technology is also being used to reach clients. For example, in Korea, conferencing is used in rural areas where clients have difficulty accessing services. Education, counseling, assessment, and therapy are being delivered in this manner from a central site to three distant communities (Freddolino & Han, 1998).

Date: Mon, 18 Sep 1995 20:02:57 -0500
Reply-To: XXXXXXXXXXXXXXXXXXXXXXXXXXXXXXXXXX
Sender: "International Counselor Network (ICN)"
<ICN@UTKVMl.BITNET>
From: XXXXXXXXXXXXXXXXXXXXXXXXXXXXXXXXXXXXX
Organization: XXXXXXXXXXXXXXXXXXXXXXXXXXXX
Subject: Sleepwalking
X-To: ICN <icn@utkvml.utk.edu>
To: Multiple recipients of list ICN
<ICN@UTKVM1.BITNET>

Hello, I have two students ages 8 and 9 who have come to me and said they are concerned about their sleepwalking. I do not know anything about sleepwalking, so I am asking for your help. Any information about the causes or what contributes to it would be helpful. I would also like to know the counseling issues behind sleepwalking. Do you feel a school counselor should try to help the student or should they be referred to outside sources? I work in a school where most parents could not afford outside treatment. I will appreciate any information you might have.

Figure 3-1 ✦ Example of a Listserv Message

SOURCE: Reprinted from "Counselors in Cyberspace Debate Whether Client Discussions Are Ethical," by T. W. Marino, January, 1996, *Counseling Today,* p. 18.; © ACA. Reprinted with permission. No further reproduction authorized without permission of the American Counseling Association.

Cellular phones and pagers are becoming increasingly popular communication tools for administrators and those providing direct services to clients. These devices also allow professionals to be available at all times. A case manager working with adult substance abusers says, "I carry my beeper with me 24 hours a day. In this work, I need to be available for my clients anytime they need me. They can call me anytime, day or night, and I can help them through their critical times. Many of them tell me that just knowing that I am there for them and easily accessible (even though they do not call) makes the difficult times easier" (Bill Draney, personal communication, August 13, 1999). These devices also provide security to many workers when they are in dangerous or isolated situations.

Another method of expanding communications is through the World Wide Web. Through individualized web pages, many individuals and organizations can provide information to those online. Today with access to the Web increasing, it is used as both an outreach and educational tool. For example, note the online human service directory for San Francisco, called the San Francisco Connection: City and County Online Human Service Directory (http://www.gii.com/nicampgnJ2f2e.htm). This site was created with the cooperation of city agencies and community-based organizations. Professionals use the San Francisco Public Library platform so that users can access a single source as an information and referral database. There is also a neighborhood database, a nonprofit organization, and government agency database. Each of these sites allows users to make suggestions for improvement and to post comments.

Agencies are also using the Web to advertise services that they provide. For example, Planned Parenthood Corporation of Columbia/Willamette (Oregon) (http://www.ppcw.org/welcome.htm) maintains an extensive website that details patient services such as contraception, abortion, services for men, and services for sexually transmitted diseases, screening, and treatment. They also include clinic sites and patient stories while maintaining patient confidentiality. Another example is the site provided by Family Services of El Paso (http://www.utep.edu/socwork/Student/Fs.htm). This site is simply a web presence which provides a list of services offered by the agency and contact information such as location, telephone and fax numbers, and the current director. Teencentral.net (http://www.teencentral.net) is a national site where teens have discussions with counselors and read about solutions other teens have found.

Not only are agencies advertising their services, but they are also providing the public with information about topics of concern and interest such as mental health, adolescent difficulties, parenting, eldercare, and health. The Planned Parenthood of Willamette site offers users a reference list of topics that includes contraception and abortion, as well as policy issues, women's health, and many others. Other sites focus primarily on education. For example, Mental Health Net (http://mentalhelp.net) is an index of worldwide mental health services and organizations, with 9,300 resources and links listed. This site offers links to the National Mental Health Association, Brazelton Center for Mental Health Law, Australian International Mental Health Strategy, California Coalition for Ethical Mental Health Care, Canadian Mental Health Association, and many others. The site also provides articles published from a variety of sources that focus on mental health issues, reference books, an Internet forum for discussions concerning mental health, updates on mental health issues, and self-help resources. This site is just one example of the literally thousands of websites provided as educational tools.

Organizations are also using the Web to reach their members and to recruit potential new members. As an example, the web page for the National Organization for Human Service Education (http://www.nohse.com) offers information about the organization, including links to its role and mission, the board of directors, the regional organization, and membership.

Unfortunately, access to the Web is not uniform across the country. According to Yovovick (1997), users of the Web are divided into either the elite and experts who are web and computer savvy or others for whom the computer and its offerings are much less accessible. Minorities and women are less likely to use the computer or achieve a comfort level with its use (Hoffman & Novak, 1998; "NCAAP targets minority gap," 1999; "Study shows minorities less likely," 1999). Community initiatives are widening the access as state-funded computer centers in neighborhoods, public libraries, and schools develop across the country (http://www.civicaction.org).

In spite of the disparity in utilization of the World Wide Web, this communication medium can also be a powerful multicultural tool used to connect people to other people (Karger & Levine, 1999). As you will read later in this chapter, the need to increase one's understanding of cultures and human diversity is necessary given the rapidly changing demographics of the United States and the world and the ethical implications of a multicultural society (Chapter 9). The Web allows the sharing of stories, histories, choices, reflections, and interactions that reach beyond what has been traditionally available in books, periodicals, or classrooms. For example, many books provide information on ethnic gangs in the United States, their cultures, and behaviors, but the Web allows a student or a human service professional to communicate and interact with a former Puerto Rican gang member.

Just as technology supports better communication, it also offers an improved way of managing information. There are many ways in which computers and their software help manage this information within the human service delivery system.

Information Management

Using computer technology, managers can coordinate information from a variety of sources and then organize the data to facilitate planning, decision making, and reporting. Information can also be managed to support evaluation and help tie service delivery to outcomes and cost. The information entered into a human service database can include a client's name and other relevant demographic data (age, gender, race, marital status), prior use of the human service delivery system, intake information and assessment results, problem identification, treatment plans, treatment records of services provided, and evaluation of those services according to outcomes reached and client satisfaction.

In addition, in this environment of managed care, the information system may also include service costs, payment, the cost of each service delivered, and a record of the interaction with the managed care organization. The interaction record may show the kinds of services authorized by frequency, duration, and definition of the service provider (Webb, 1996). Table 3-2 shows the types of information in an information management system that can be used for foster care (Webb, 1996).

Another example of an information system supporting the delivery of services is an information care network established for use with determining appropriate treatment for substance abuse patients. This system collects and maintains a database of patient information and treatment paths. In addition to maintaining a database, this system also analyzes the treatment decisions made and the outcomes, and assists in determining the appropriate treatment for these patients (Linn, McCreery, Kasab, & Schneider, 1998).

One advantage of a management information system is its ability to transfer information electronically across organizations and among workers. This feature benefits both human service professionals and clients in several ways.

TABLE 3-2   ♦   FOSTER CARE DATA ELEMENTS

Data elements	Categories
1. State	
2. Report period ending date	
3. Local agency FIPS code	
4. Record number	
5. Most recent periodic review date	Child's demographic information 5–17
6. Date of birth	
7. Sex	
8. Race	
9. Hispanic origin	
10. Child diagnosed with disabilities	
11. Mental retardation	
12. Visually or hearing impaired	
13. Physically disabled	
14. Emotionally disturbed	
15. Other diagnosed conditions	
16. Has child ever been adopted	
17. Age of child when adopted	
18. Date of first removal from home	Removal/placement setting indicators 18–24
19. Total number of removals	
20. Discharge date from last episode	
21. Date of latest removal	
22. Computer-generated date	
23. Placement date in current setting	
24. # of previous settings in episode	
25. Manner of removal for episode	Circumstances associated with removal 25–40
26. Physical abuse	
27. Sexual abuse	
28. Neglect	
29. Parent alcohol abuse	
30. Parent drug abuse	
31. Child alcohol abuse	
32. Child drug abuse	
33. Child disability	
34. Child's behavior problem	
35. Death of parent	

TABLE 3-2   ✦   *continued*

Data elements	Categories
36. Incarceration of parent	
37. Caretaker inability to cope	
38. Abandonment	
39. Relinquishment	
40. Inadequate housing	
41. Current placement setting	Current placement setting 41–42
42. Out of state placement	
43. Most recent case plan goal	Most recent case plan goal 43
44. Caretaker family structure	Principal caretaker information 44–46
45. 1st principal caretaker birth year	
46. 2nd principal caretaker birth year	
47. Date of mother's TPR	Parental rights termination 47–56
48. Date of father's TPR	
49. Foster family structure	
50. 1st foster caretaker's year of birth	
51. 2nd foster caretaker's year of birth	
52. 1st foster caretaker's race	
53. 1st foster caretaker's Hispanic origin	
54. 2nd foster caretaker's race	
55. 2nd foster caretaker's Hispanic origin	
56. Date of discharge from foster care	
57. Computer-generated date	Discharge date 57–58
58. Reasons for discharge	
59. Title IV-E (foster care)	Sources of federal financial support/assistance for child 59–65
60. Title IV-E (adoption assistance)	
61. Title IV-a (AFDC)	
62. Title IV-D (Child Support)	
63. Title XIX (Medicaid)	
64. SSI or other social security	
65. None of the above	

SOURCE: From "The Management of Information," by Bruce Webb (1996), presentation conducted at the Managed Care Institute—Futurecare: Preparing for Managed Care and Children's Services, Nashville, Tennessee. Reprinted by permission.

First, the client and the professional save the time and energy required to generate the data for a second or a third time. If the data represent intake or initial assessment information, the professional can review it with the client and request additional information to ensure accuracy. Second, work can begin with the client much earlier because, in some cases, much of the information-gathering is complete. Access to broad information gives the human service professional a more comprehensive review of a client's experience within the service delivery system. Human service professionals are also able to provide better service because they can coordinate their care of the client with any other current services the client is receiving.

Telemedicine has been extremely useful in rural emergency rooms, correctional facilities, home health care, and psychiatry. This method of communication uses electronic signals to transfer medical data, including patient records, videoconferencing, and high-resolution photographs. For example, one state has contracted with a psychiatrist to serve individuals who are deaf and mentally ill throughout the state by means of videoconferencing.

Just as technology is becoming an effective way to support human service work using management information systems, it is also being developed to provide services to clients.

Providing Services to Clients

The services available through new models of service delivery range from computer programs which assess client knowledge or skill and recommend a plan of action to actual counseling online in real time. A telecommunications system was developed to assess adolescents who are at risk in terms of their health (Alemangno, Frank, Mosavel, & Butts, 1998). Using this program, the clients listen to a standard set of questions and then answer by touch tone. Once they have completed the questionnaire, they receive a report that is faxed from a health professional. This report describes the at-risk status of the client and makes recommendations for positive interventions.

Many software programs and tools are available to teach clients specific knowledge or skills to enhance their daily living or increase their vocational potential. Many of the programs are designed for clients who are experiencing difficulties. One such program, BUSTED, was developed to reduce antisocial behavior of youth involved in the criminal justice system. The computer game SMACK was developed for at-risk teens to help them learn the consequences of bad decisions and drug use (Oalcley, 1994; Resnick, 1994). Some programs are proactive and promote good health and wellness. One example is BARN, a health education game designed to teach adolescents about issues ranging from AIDS to sexual and body awareness (Bosworth, 1994). HealthWorks is an AIDS education program for early-adolescent middle schoolers (Cahill, 1994). Both SMACK and BARN are educational tools that can be used in the schools and in child, youth, and family programs.

Technology has also influenced the delivery of counseling services. In many programs, the client uses an interactive computer program, followed by a discussion with a human service professional of the client's responses. One such in-

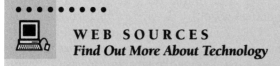

● ● ● ● ● ● ● ● ● ●

WEB SOURCES
Find Out More About Technology

The following websites illustrate the wide range of ways that school counselor professionals are using technology. Many of these were provided by Marino (1999).

SCHOOL VIOLENCE SITES

http://www.ncsu.edu/cpsv

This site provided by The Center for the Prevention of School Violence lists schools involved in support of positive climate, describes the current issues that surround violence, describes special projects that schools are proposing and providing to counter school violence, and provides access to newsletter, research, and briefs on the issues.

http://edc.org/HHD/csn

This site is the Children's Safety Network (CSN) home page. It provides the CSN, which is supported by the National Injury and Violence Prevention Resource Center. Its purpose is to collect and develop resources for agencies whose purpose is to reduce injuries and violence to children. Examples of materials are publications relating to violence and children, effective strategies for evaluating community-based interventions, and descriptions of building safe community programs. The site also combines efforts and resources with traffic safety and public health and provides links to other injury prevention resources on the World Wide Web.

http://www.counseling.org/schoolviolence

This site was prepared by the American Counseling Association (ACA) to provide resources for professionals who are addressing the issues that surround school violence. It includes articles and editorials prepared by ACA staff, and links to other sites.

http://www.educ.sfu.ca/cnps/cscrp.html

This site was developed by a Canadian counselor, David Paterson. It links with professional organizations, the counseling professional, resources, and a discussion page used by counselors to talk about professional issues.

LISTSERVS

Listserv@utkvml.utk.edu

This e-mail address enables users to subscribe to the International Counselor's Network (ICN). The listserv discusses counseling issues, of which the dialogue includes professionals worldwide.

http://www.plattsburgh.edu/projects/cnet/listservs/listserv.html

This website provides information about many listservs that focus on counseling issues.

teractive multimedia system, developed by the Beck Institute for Cognitive Therapy and Research, computerizes cognitive therapy and is used at the Norton Psychiatric Clinic in Louisville, Kentucky ("New Interactive Multimedia System," 1995). "The program instructs patients on how to recognize maladaptive thoughts and behavior thereby reinforcing the positive aspects of therapy, such as modifying 'automatic thoughts,' generating alternative thoughts and activity scheduling. Each time the patient uses the video, a printed progress report is generated to help therapists focus on key areas of concern" (p. 44).

Counseling services and other support services are also provided online. This allows human service professionals to be available via e-mail or the WWW to work with individuals who are experiencing specific difficulties, thereby increasing access to services. Proponents of online counseling believe that without this venue, many people would not be able to benefit from the knowledge and care of helpers (Karger & Levine, 1999). Others, however, believe that the use of online counseling is controversial because of concerns about confidentiality, informed consent, and competence. Nevertheless, the number of participants continues to grow. Certain sites also provide medical consultation and child care advice. Thus, the phrase, "the doctor is always in," reflects the constancy of the Internet and its easy accessibility.

Because of the prevalence of "e-therapy"—online or internet therapy—and the accompanying concerns of members of the professional community, guidelines are emerging for those clients who wish to use such therapy. These guidelines address the following types of questions (Ainsworth, 1999): Are you a good candidate for online therapy? How do you find a credentialed professional? How do you make an appropriate choice among professionals? How do you locate online counseling websites and compare? How do you ensure confidentiality? As e-therapy becomes more integrated into professional practice, even more attention will be given to issues of confidentiality and competence.

Online chat forums also help to provide support to those in need. They address a range of topics and are accessible on many networks. One example is a "chat group" for law enforcement officers and their families, who invite those with problems to share them electronically. A second example is the discussion network developed by the Nebraska Network for Children and Families to focus on eldercare (Nebraska Network for Children and Families, 1999). The discussion page, CARETALK, "is a special discussion group designed for caregivers of adults with special needs." Those who use this discussion group can read past questions and subsequent dialogue. They may be silent participants who only read what others have submitted or they may be active participants who use the discussion page to gather information and opinions and help other discussants.

Another type of client support provided by technology involves assistive technology. This support is available for clients with disabilities. Its purpose is to help individuals with handicaps to "increase, maintain, or improve their functional capacities" (Ray & Warden, 1995, p. 4). See the accompanying box for a detailed description of assistive technology as defined and mandated by Public Law 101-476. These assistive devices are being developed or upgraded continually and the list includes devices that support individuals in their learning and in their daily living.

Assistive technology addresses needs in the areas of vision, hearing, learning, speech and language, and mobility. One example of assistive technology is that which supports the functioning of individuals with visual impairments. Many individuals cannot read regular print and need assistive devices to help them input data into the computer. One such device is Braille to print, with six keys of the standard keyboard used to input Braille with full access to the function keys. Special software such as BRLkeys for the IBM makes this adaptation possible. Additional assistive technologies translate Braille to print and Braille to voice. Software allows the input to produce a printed copy and a Braille copy.

• • • • • • • • • •

 ### Assistive Technology Defined

- Defines assistive technology device to mean any item, piece of equipment, or product, whether acquired commercially off the shelf, modified, or customized, which is used to increase, maintain, or improve functional capabilities of individuals with disabilities (same definition as is used in PL 100-407, Technology-Related Assistance for Individuals with Disabilities Act [1988]).
- Defines assistive technology service to mean any service that directly assists an individual with a disability in the selection, acquisition, or use of an assistive technology device. Such term includes
  A. The evaluation of the needs of an individual with a disability, including a functional evaluation of the individual in the individual's customary environment
  B. Purchasing, leasing, or otherwise providing for the acquisition of assistive technology devices by individuals with disabilities
  C. Selecting, designing, fitting, customizing, adapting, applying, maintaining, repairing, or replacing of assistive technology devices
  D. Coordinating and using other therapies, interventions, or services with assistive technology devices, such as those associated with existing education and rehabilitation places and programs
  E. Training or technical assistance for an individual with disabilities, or, where appropriate, the family of an individual with disabilities
  F. Training or technical assistance for professionals (including individuals providing education and rehabilitation service), employers, or other individuals who provide services to, employ, or are otherwise substantially involved in the major life functions of individuals with disabilities.

SOURCE: From *Technology, Computers, and the Special Needs Learner,* by J. Ray and M. K. Warden, ©1995. Reprinted with permission of Wadsworth, a division of Thomson Learning. Fax 800-730-2215..

A portable note-taking device, the BrailleMate (TeleSensory), combines the note-taking device with a Braille keypad, voice output, and a single refreshable Braille cell output. This device has the capability of sorting information within the device itself or transferring the information to external disk drives, Braille and print devices, or other computers (Ray & Warden, 1995).

These are only a few of the many assistive technologies available to facilitate the functioning of the visually impaired. Technology not only facilitates the education and training of clients but is also used for the education and training of human service professionals who desire new knowledge, information, and skills to support their work with clients. Computers are also used in this area.

Professional Development

Professional development is an important aspect of lifelong learning, and technology has made it easier for human service professionals to take advantage of the latest information about populations being served as well as the knowledge and skills of emerging best practice. One way this information is available is by CD-ROM. Most compact discs of interest to the human service professional may be found in a local university or city library. One advantage of using these CDs for research is the easy access to current information.

Another advancement in professional development is the availability of software that facilitates skill development. Programs are available to teach interviewing, problem solving, rehabilitation counseling, decision making, counseling, crisis counseling, organizational assessment, case management, and many other skills. Much of the software is interactive and uses simulation as the primary instructional tool. In teaching problem solving in case management, many programs use simulated cases of individuals with severe problems and difficulties. Students and practitioners are asked to identify and prioritize needs, and to choose alternatives and outcomes. Most programs provide the client's current status and other, more detailed information about client history.

In addition, offering professional development on the World Wide Web is beginning to emerge as a teaching tool. For example, the American Association on Aging has developed a series of workshops delivered on the Web (www.asa.org). The workshops include instructions, activities, and dialogue focused on problems in aging and allow professionals worldwide to participate in seminars with experts in the field. (See Table 3-3.)

In summary, human service professionals are currently using technologies to improve the ways they communicate with each other, to expand the ways information is managed, to provide services to clients, and to engage in professional development. We predict that technology will continue to have an impact on the profession during the 21st century.

TABLE 3-3   ✦   SUMMARY POINTS: USES OF TECHNOLOGY

- Communication in human services is enhanced by e-mail, listservs, teleconferencing, and the World Wide Web (WWW).
- Telemedicine, management systems, and care networks are examples of information management systems.
- Direct services to clients by means of technology include assessment, counseling, information, and education.
- Technology allows human service professionals to utilize the latest information about practice, client groups, and skill development.

Managed Care

In the past decade, managed care has had a profound effect on the delivery of human services. Its influence is felt by both the client and the human service professional as they work together to plan and provide services. Today, managed care organizations administer a large percentage of the group health insurance, and the movement of managed care into mental health care, child care, corrections, and other social services is on the rise (Dewan, 1999; Lyons, Libman-Minzer, & Kisiel, 1998; Tuckfelt, Fink, Warren, & Travis, 1999; Villani & Sharfstein, 1999). We now look at managed care and how it has affected the delivery of health, mental health, and other services.

Managed care is a term used to describe a set of tools or methods designed to manage resources and deliver human services, especially in the areas of health care and mental health. It developed from the public's demand for accountability of service delivery and from the rising costs in health and mental health care. Although the American public was seriously concerned about the cost of health care in the 1980s, today there is growing concern about managed care and its responsibility to deterioration of care (Kilborn, 1997). Prior to the use of managed care to allocate resources and services, most care was provided on a fee-for-service basis. In other words, a health or human service professional would provide a specific service and charge a standard rate. The payment for these services would come from the client, an insurance provider, or the agency or organization supporting the client care.

The Influence of Managed Care

A broad definition of managed care is that it involves "any patient care that is not determined solely by the provider" (Goodman, Brown, & Dietz, 1992, p. 5). In the case of human services, a provider is a professional who delivers services to a client or clients. Managed care influences the process of service delivery by *using external reviews, developing standards of good practice, and emphasizing a continuum of care.*

Managed care organizations provide several types of external reviews. One review authorizes the expense of needed services for a client. For the human service professional, this means that before a service can be provided and before the professional can be reimbursed or paid, the managed care organization reviews the requested service. According to Goodman et al. (1992), those conducting this external review ask the following questions:

- What is the problem?
- What is the proposed treatment?
- Why is the proposed treatment recommended?
- What evidence supports the proposed treatment?

A guiding principle for managed care review is to approve the lowest level of care that will meet the client's needs. In other words, if hospitalization has been recommended, the managed care reviewer asks, "Could the client also be treated in the home?" If ten weeks of therapy is recommended, the question is, "Will four weeks be adequate?" If the client needs a vocational assessment, psychological assessment, physical assessment, and a social history, managed care reviewers may recommend conducting the physical and the psychological assessment first and then determining whether the others are needed.

Another component of the external review is related to the provision of good quality services. The previous set of questions is asked prior to service provision; questions are also asked *after* service delivery. Goodman et al. (1992, p. 21) listed the questions that guide the managed care organization as it determines whether good quality care was provided to the client.

- Is the care appropriate (i.e., clinically necessary for the condition)?
- Is the provider competent to provide that care?
- Is the care effective?
- Is the care cost-effective?
- Is the care accessible?
- Is the care safe?
- Is the patient satisfied?

Other considerations surround quality of care and many of those focus on fair treatment of the client, such as the ease with which the client can access the services, the meeting of client expectations, the attention to and fair disposition of client appeals and grievances, and client satisfaction. Satisfaction within the service delivery system extends beyond the client to families of clients and to the human service professional. One issue to surface within the professional, client/patient, and political context is "patient rights" within the managed care context.

The Joint Initiative of Mental Health Professional Organizations has published the *Mental Health Patient's Bill of Rights: Principles for the Provisions of Mental Health and Substance Abuse Treatment Services,* which lists the rights that patients should expect when receiving mental health services. The rights are explained in detail with an emphasis both on the rights and the appropriate questions the client can ask the managed care professional when discussing benefits and services. The bill of rights covers issues such as the right to know, confidentiality, choice, determination of treatment, nondiscrimination, and treatment review. Similar material has been published by the National Clearing House on Managed Care and Long-Term Support and Services for People with Developmental Disabilities and Their Families. Each is concerned with client empowerment, fair treatment, quality of care, and satisfaction within the managed care environment (National Coalition of Mental Health, 1999; National Clearing House on Managed Care, 1999).

Continuous review is another way managed care interfaces with service delivery. In continuous review, there is periodic dialogue between human service providers and the managed care personnel about the status of the client and the effectiveness of the services. The purpose of this review is to identify any problems with the assessment, the treatment plan, or its implementation. Another purpose of the review is to remind those providing services of the guideline that says to provide "the right services at the right time in the right amounts, no more, no less" (Schafer, 1996, p. 2). Many professionals believe that both quality of care and reasonable cost should guide decisions about services (Indritz, 1997). The following case illustrates what one client experienced:

Jimmy Jones, a 14-year-old, single, white male, has recently been truant from school and was caught fighting with other students. His difficult behavior began about the time his father, with whom he has a close relationship, was diagnosed with cancer. Jimmy's doctor recommended that he see a counselor who specializes in working with adolescents to help him cope with his father's illness. After an initial visit with the counselor, ten visits are authorized by the Jones' insurance company. Part of the authorization requires the counselor to file periodic progress reports. After the tenth visit, a review of the case will determine whether additional visits will be authorized.

Managed care also affects the way we think about and deliver services to specific client populations. Because managed care emphasizes appropriate services for clients and matching services to specific outcomes, both managed care personnel and human service professionals are working to develop standards of best practice for meeting specific client needs. In the past, human service professionals have had great difficulty stating clearly the appropriate services for addressing the needs of their clients—needs that stem from poverty, unemployment, illiteracy, juvenile delinquency, child abuse, and other difficulties. Further complicating the task of developing standards is the complexity and large number of problems that many clients face.

Examples of standards of best practice are provided by Barker (1996), referring to best practices in child welfare. For issues of access, he suggests that the current system is based on voluntary access and that the system does not always reach those who need care. The best practice would be good preventive and crisis services with access to all who are in need. The way managed care would be responsive to best practice would be to have a single point of entry to all who have needs and to provide services immediately after access. As you can see from this example, the standard of best practice is high, and in many cases, it is different from what is available for clients now.

Within the framework of standards of best practice and managed care, professionals are now being asked to specify their outcomes, relate those outcomes to services, and provide the services as efficiently and effectively as possible. Because resources are limited, managed care organizations suggest that only a few outcomes should be attempted and all services should be tied to outcomes. This limitation means that helpers may not be able to address all the needs of their clients. They must set and then focus on priorities. An example of the specific standard of practice is described in the following box, which describes a short-term, computer-based therapy, *Therapeutic Learning Program,* by explaining the focus of each session and the session's goals.

This therapy meets specific needs and was developed to help "patients define a specific problem, propose an active solution and resolve their conflicts about taking action" (Gould, 1992, p. 351). The program focuses on three questions:

- What is hurting you and how can you help yourself?
- Would the action you propose be a smart and safe one?
- What serious concerns do you have that keep you from acting?

At the conclusion of the ten sessions, clients are asked whether they can answer the three preceding questions. This process is one example of focusing the service and then linking the service received to specific outcomes.

Another important concept for delivering human services within the managed care environment is *continuum of care.* Continuum of care describes an integrated system of settings, services, professionals, and levels of care and services. The client moves from site to site as the needs dictate and receives appropriate care as needed. There are many examples of continuum of care. For the elderly, this continuum may include physician services, emergency services, acute care, skilled nursing facilities, outpatient centers, home care programs, day treatment programs, mental health services, and family/community support (American Dietetic Association, 1999). Continuum of care was the focus of grants to assist the homeless to "get housing, job training, child care, mental health services and substance abuse" (Boland, 1998). The goal was to move 330,000 American homeless from the streets to self-sufficiency. The programs approved were those that stressed efforts to address the complexities of homelessness and to provide long-term support as needed by the clients served. During the assessment phase of the helping process, human service professionals and clients work together to identify the problems, assess their severity or seriousness, and decide on the type of treatment that is needed. Type of treatment includes a decision about the level or continuum of care. In the philosophy of managed care, an assessment should determine the intensity of care to be delivered to the client, and clients should not be given more treatment than they need. The level of care needed should also be continually reviewed, and client treatment should be moved along a continuum from more intense to less intense when appropriate. Of course, at times clients will require more elaborate interventions and will move from less intense to more intense care.

An abbreviated continuum of care for children and adolescents is presented in Table 3-4. Note in the left column that there is intensive treatment, inpatient/acute psychiatric care. This level of treatment is appropriate when children and youth need constant supervision, medical intervention, and therapy. Many times clients receive these services when there is a probable threat of violence to self or others. At the other end of the continuum is home-based therapy, which is appropriate when children and youth are in troubled situations that can be addressed with brief, short-term interventions.

As you can see, managed care is influencing the way all human services are delivered by introducing or emphasizing such concepts as external review, standards of best practice, and continuum of care. These in turn affect the way human service professionals do their work. (See Table 3-5.)

Managed Care and the Human Service Professional

Managed care has affected the daily work of the human service professional, especially in providing direct service. This interaction has required a shift in the roles and responsibilities of the professional in five ways: an emphasis on case management responsibilities, increasing demands for documentation, growing use of gatekeepers, expansion of resolution-focused helping strategies, and continuing importance of confidentiality and providing high-quality services.

Today, more human service professionals than ever are using case management in providing services to their clients. With an emphasis on cost-effective service delivery, coordination of care through a case manager has emerged as a method to better ensure efficiency and high-quality service. The purpose of case management, as discussed in Chapter 1, is to oversee the comprehensive care of a client. It can include (1) assessment, (2) planning, coordinating, and monitoring of treatment, and (3) evaluation. Human service literature describes two types of case managers. One is a case manager in a human service organization who assumes many of the responsibilities described above; the other works for a managed care organization. The following examples illustrate their different responsibilities.

Chris Bachman, a rehabilitation counselor, has a caseload of 70 clients. Chris works with each client to develop a plan of services, some delivered by Chris himself, but most provided by professionals at other agencies. Chris monitors the delivery of services, authorizes payment on behalf of his agency, and evaluates with the client the services received. (Continued on p. 115.)

• • • • • • • • • •

 Therapeutic Learning Program (TLP) Session Goals

Session 1: Identifying stress-related problems, conflicts, and symptoms
  a. to identify sources of stress and ineffective responses
  b. to sort out stressful issues from developmental stress problems
  c. to prioritize one clearly stated stress problem that calls for some action

Session 2: Clarifying goals and focusing on action
  a. to identify the developmental goal that addresses the adaptational demand
  b. to clarify and define the action or behavior change that is necessary
  c. to build an action intention that represents the recovery of the underdeveloped function

Session 3: Thinking through the consequences of taking action
  a. to distinguish realistic dangers from exaggerated dangers
  b. to isolate and expose the fears as predictions confused with memories
  c. to reach a conscious cost-benefit positive decision about the intended action

Session 4: Uncovering hidden motives and fears of failure and success
  a. to clarify that certain strongly felt fears are not objective dangers
  b. to weaken the hold of irrational fears
  c. to learn to identify thinking errors as a useful concept
  d. to distinguish between healthy and unhealthy motives
  e. to demonstrate that fears of failure and success rarely point to real dangers

Session 5: Exploring anger and guilt as obstacles to action
  a. to clarify that certain strong anxiety feelings are not indicative of external dangers
  b. to demonstrate that angry feelings are controllable by rational considerations
  c. to demonstrate that the feeling of guilt is information that can be processed to clarify value
  d. to continue to confirm that the intended action is safe and doable

Session 6: Confronting issues of self-esteem
  a. to identify and acknowledge self-esteem sensitivities
  b. to begin to accept the universality and mystery of these sensitivities

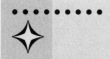

   c. to entertain the thought that this powerful inner voice represents a historical fiction

   d. to understand that the self-esteem sensitivity is the biggest block to resolving the developmental conflict

Session 7: Examining old and detrimental patterns of behavior

   a. to identify the deepest vulnerability that is being challenged by the action intention

   b. to see how the self-doubt triggers the ineffective protective behavior

   c. to examine and demonstrate how the self-doubt system feeds itself

   d. to begin to challenge the automatic response

Session 8: Understanding the history of self-doubts

   a. to expose the illusion of permanent damage

   b. to see that responses to early events were limited and naturally protective

   c. to see that these early protective behaviors were automatic responses to feeling inadequate

   d. to view the self-doubt as an initial response to events by the immature mind

Session 9: Analyzing a current incident involving the self-doubt

   a. to demonstrate and diminish self-fulfilling prophecies

   b. to identify the erroneous thinking that currently feeds the powerful self-doubt

   c. to understand that feeding the doubt by misinterpretation is a choice, not a necessity

   d. to recognize that to continue to do this is to avoid growth

Session 10: Evaluating the changes experienced during the course

   a. to see that fears are to be overcome and not submitted to

   b. to see the action intention as part of ongoing recovery of function

   c. to understand that recovery of function and individuation are necessary

   d. to consolidate new views of reality

SOURCE: From "Adult Developmental Brief Computer-Assisted Therapy," by P. L. Gould, 1992, in J. L. Feldman and R. J. Fitzpatrick (Eds.), *Managed Mental Healthcare* (pp. 347–358). Washington, DC: American Psychiatric Press. Reprinted by permission.

TABLE 3-4 ♦ CONTINUUM OF CARE

Inpatient/acute psychiatric care	Residential treatment	Partial hospitalization	Therapeutic respite care emergency shelter	Therapeutic foster care	Outpatient treatment
• Suicidal attempts, or ideation, with a plan and the likelihood of carrying out the threat, need for continued observation to prevent any at-risk behaviors.	• Client requires full 24-hour daily supervision care and treatment; not functioning adequately enough to benefit from treatment while living at home or alternative living situation.	• Client has symptoms and/or behavioral manifestations of such severity that there is a significant interference with social, family, and/or educational functions.	• Client required supervision and out-of-home placement due to an emergency situation or crisis in the family.	• Client is in need of services more intensive than outpatient treatment, but less intensive than the level of care provided by partial hospitalization, or 24-hour residential or hospital treatment.	• Diagnostic evaluation establishes the presence of behavioral/emotional problems amenable to outpatient problem-focused psychotherapy.
• Assaultive, aggressive, or self-destructive behavior, with the likelihood of harm to self or others. Need for continued observation to limit behavior and protect self or others.	• Significant dysfunction in family or interpersonal relationships and/or in the school or community setting.	• Client does not present significant danger to self or others, such as imminent suicidal risk, assaultive or homicidal behaviors, severe disorganization or disorientation, extreme impulsivity, severe uncontrolled substance abuse or acting-out behavior.	• Client has history of physical, emotional, and/or sexual abuse.	• Client has DSM Axis I diagnosis, with a history of neglect and abuse.	• Client's symptoms warrant a DMS Axis I diagnosis.
• Crisis stabilization with intensive individual, family, group therapy, and/or appropriate medication therapy.	• Not an imminent suicide risk, not physically abusive to self or others.	• Client is not a high-elopement risk.	• Client is experiencing mild or moderate emotional problems.	• Client requires 24-hour supervision and support which the family is unable to provide.	• Client does not demonstrate problems of sufficient severity to warrant more intensive treatment.
	• Not destructive toward other people or propriety.		• Client may be aggressive and oppositional but is able to respond to external control and structure of 24-hour program.	• Client presents mild to moderate risk of harm to self or others, with the need for observation and monitoring.	• Degree of danger to self or others is judged to be manageable.
	• Not a high-elopement risk (for unlocked programs).		• Client has not been successful with previous out-of-home placements.		• Family is willing to participate in child's treatment plan.

SOURCE: From "The Management of information," by B. Barker, 1(996), presentation conducted at the Managed Care Institute—Futurecare: Preparing for Managed Care and Children's Services, Nashville, Tennessee. Reprinted by permission.

TABLE 3-5   ✦   SUMMARY POINTS: MANAGED CARE TERMS

- **External reviews**—evaluation of a request for services prior to service delivery
- **Standards of good practice**—specification of outcomes, relationship of outcomes to services, and efficient and effective service delivery
- **Continuum of care**—integrated system of settings, services, professionals, and levels of care

(Continued from p. 111.)

Tasha Jones is a case manager who works for Healthcare, Inc., a managed care organization that has clients in five counties. Her major responsibilities include external utilization review and resource allocation. Her contact with human service professionals like Chris Bachman is through applications, forms, or phone calls. She has never met a client or a human service professional in person.

As more services are regulated and directed by managed care organizations, the need for the services of both types of case managers will grow.

Another influence of managed care is the increased documentation associated with service delivery. The workload for many human service professionals has doubled as they use the managed care external review process. A request for services can include an initial assessment, a detailed description of the client's problem, a service plan, a periodic assessment of the implementation of the plan and status of outcomes, requests for reimbursement, and termination of clients. Often the documentation required for the managed care process is different from that required by the agency. Thus, unless the managed care organization has established the same information system as the organization, the professional may have two systems of documentation to maintain.

Another change that has emerged is an elaborate gatekeeping function for initial screening of clients. Gatekeeping in the managed care system, especially in the area of mental health, is a method used to control access to services. Often, to receive mental health services, clients must have a referral from a physician. The purpose of this physician referral is to decrease the utilization of mental health services, but the result has been to increase the client load of the physician who must sign the referrals. Gatekeeping also occurs when a special service, not considered part of the standard of good practice, is needed or recommended. The client is not free to take the initiative to seek that service but must have the permission of and referral from the primary caretaker—in most cases, the physician. The introduction of the gatekeeper to mental health services places hardships on both the client and the human service professional. Clients see this visit to the physician as a barrier to getting services, and they often encounter physicians who are not sympathetic to their nonmedical problems. Sometimes they must wait to see the physician, and this wait delays their receiving the mental health services they need. For human service professionals, the gatekeeper is another layer of bureaucracy between them and their clients. On a positive note, however, many of these professionals are working with the gatekeeper physicians to help them understand the mental health needs of their clients.

Resolution-Focused Helping

Another influence of managed care is the need to develop resolution-focused helping strategies that are limited in time and in scope. This brief counseling type of intervention focuses on reaching specific outcomes in a relatively short time by making an immediate difference in the client's life, targeting behaviors that need to be changed and facilitating that change, and helping clients make new choices about thinking and behaving. Action is central to resolution-focused helping but takes place rather quickly. It now appears in treatment for chemical dependency, in children and youth services, and in mental health services.

Several legal and ethical issues, such as confidentiality, have emerged from the interface of managed care and human service delivery. Much of the information that is transferred to managed care organizations is sensitive and provided in confidence by the client. Human service professionals worry about who will see the information on clients that is transmitted to the managed care organization. They are also concerned about how the information will be used and how it will be stored. There is also an increased concern for information stored using technology. Human service professionals urge consideration of security practices such as logon procedures, firewalls, and encryption (Rock & Congress, 1999). Most human service professionals understand well the importance of confidentiality of information, but they know little about the commitment to confidentiality of staff in managed care organizations.

Another concern that human service professionals have about the managed care system and its influence on service delivery is the impact on quality. One purpose of managed care is to contain costs, and professionals believe that this focus can lead managed care organizations to sacrifice quality in their services to clients. Those outside the managed care organization worry that these for-profit companies have financial gain as their primary goal. Human service professionals have expressed specific complaints about quality that include insufficient mental health treatment, insufficient reimbursement, rejection of justifications for services, and a resistance to approve treatment. They are concerned that specific populations, such as the elderly and the poor, receive less than acceptable care. They also have doubts about the professional qualifications of case managers in the managed care setting, especially when these professionals are conducting the external review and approving service delivery.

Many in the human service sector recognize the problems with managed care but also concede that it is now part of service delivery. If the problems are to be addressed to improve the quality of client care, human service professionals need to create a partnership with managed care organizations. The following strategies may help accomplish this goal:

- Human service organizations can hire consultants to help them work with managed care organizations.
- Human service professionals can contract directly with case management organizations to provide services.
- Human service professionals can work with managed care organizations to document client problems and possible options of treatment to help them define standards of best practice.
- Human service workers can learn more about the world of managed care, its language, and business practices.

The International Dimension

Any discussion about human services today without considering its international dimension would be difficult. Everyone on the planet is drawing closer as a result of technological advances in transportation and communication. Today, people travel the world in a matter of hours rather than days or weeks. Advances in communication keep us instantly informed about developments throughout the world by satellite, electronic mail, and faxes. The internet, the world's largest computer network, had over 25 million users in 1995. The number of users who access the net at least once a week is projected to reach 720 million by 2005 (DeWitt, 1994; Paquet, 1999). It is also predicted that the majority of worldwide internet users will be non-English speaking by 2004 (Dillon, 1999). The "information superhighway" has no borders, with users in most countries on the globe. The world is becoming a smaller place when we consider factors other than physical distance; thus, we need to know what is happening internationally in terms of human services—the recent changes that have occurred and the challenges that remain.

Challenges in International Human Services

During 1995, the world's population grew by 100 million people to 5.75 billion, the largest increase ever. Ninety percent of the growth is in poor countries "already terribly torn by civil strife and social unrest and where all too many people live in brutal poverty," according to Werner Fornos of the Population Institute ("Poor Nations," 1995, p. A1). Although this information may seem discouraging, positive changes do occur. Since the devastation of World War II, vast improvements have come about in worldwide health care and living conditions. Average life expectancy—even in low-income nations such as Zaire, Egypt, and India—has risen from 40 years to 66 years (Desjarlais, Eisenberg, Good, & Kleinman, 1995). Diseases such as smallpox have been eradicated and others such as leprosy and epilepsy have been lessened by medical interventions. Infant mortality rates have fallen and literacy rates have risen.

Thoughts about the future trigger a global alarm, however. Calculations by the world's biggest super computer at the Hadley Center in England project the following:

- Thirty million people will be hungry in 50 years because it will be too dry to grow crops in large parts of Africa.
- An additional 170 million people will live in countries with extreme water shortages.
- Malaria, one of the world's most feared diseases, will threaten larger areas of the world—including Europe—by 2050. (*The Guardian,* 1998, p. A5)

A closer look at poverty and its related problems can help us understand their very serious nature at the present time as well as provide insights about future problems.

Urbanization, a long-term global trend, is most pronounced in poor countries that are least able to cope with its pressures. Today, a third of the world's population—about 600 million people—do not have the means to meet their basic needs such as clean water and sewage disposal. Mumbai (Bombay), the largest city in India, has a population of 15.1 million. By 2015, it will be the second largest metropolis in the world, with 27.4 million people. In Mumbai, between 200 and 250 families arrive each day, hoping for a better life in the city. Many begin their lives there as pavement dwellers because there is no other place to live. Land is scarce, and rooms and apartments are full. The newcomers may remain on the sidewalks for the rest of their lives, or they may move to a slum dwelling. In either case, clean water, electricity, paved paths/roads, and working community toilets are often nonexistent. Although

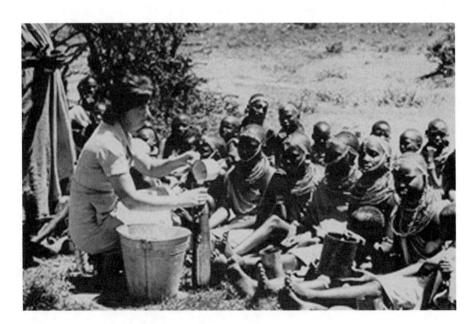

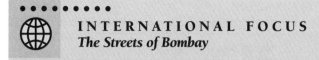

INTERNATIONAL FOCUS
The Streets of Bombay

Vikki, 17, has lived on Bombay's streets for a decade, since he ran away from his impoverished village and alcoholic father. He joined a population of homeless children that is larger than many cities.

Most of the estimated 100,000 street children in Bombay live in tarpaper shanties, at railway stations, or on the pavement. Most are doomed to lives of menial labor or petty crime.

But Vikki may have found an escape. He is one of 400 youths who have attended workshops run by a humanitarian group to teach street children the basics of good business.

Called Project Mainstream, the two-day workshops began in February to train teenagers how to be good salespeople; run profitable vegetable, betel nut, or snack stands; make incense sticks; or become florists.

Taking a pragmatic approach to the problems of small-time business, the courses also teach how to handle municipal officials who demand bribes, varying from 20 rupees (75 cents) to 200 rupees ($7.50), to overlook violations such as selling without a license. That usually means paying them.

Helped by a loan of $45, Vikki sells toasted vegetable sandwiches from his stand outside Crawford Market, the city's wholesale fruit market. At 5 rupees a serving, he's been turning a profit of about 100 rupees ($1.80), enough to buy two flimsy T-shirts or a meager meal for two at a roadside kiosk.

The pressure of life on the street is enormous. At least five street children attempt suicide every month in Bombay, says the Coordinating Committee for Vulnerable Children, a volunteer group.

About three-fourths of the street youngsters are substance abusers, usually of hashish or an adulterated form of heroin known as brown sugar, the committee says.

Project Mainstream is financed mainly by Indian and Canadian Rotary Clubs. "Any honest, money-making endeavor must be supported by the community," said Mahendra Mehta, of the Bombay Rotary Club.

In Bombay, as in many of India's megacities, the government cannot provide basic services such as health care and education to the influx of rural poor. Community and volunteer organizations take up some of that slack.

The Coordinating Committee directs 22 grass-roots organizations that reach an estimated 4,000 children. They run centers where children can bathe and receive counseling. They also conduct informal schools and try to reunite children with families and select children for Project Mainstream.

SOURCE: From "Bombay Street Kids Become Entrepreneurs," by Naresh Fernandes, October 15, 1995, *Seattle Times*, p. A4. Reprinted by permission of Associated Press.

TABLE 3-6 ✦ MATERNAL DEATHS
(Women who die each year in pregnancy or childbirth)

Area	Number of deaths
Europe	3,000
Central Asia	14,000
Americas	23,000
Mideast and North Africa	35,000
Sub-Saharan Africa	219,000
Asia and Pacific	291,000
World Total	585,000

SOURCE: From "A World in Need," Copyright, June 24, 1996, *U.S. News & World Report,* p. 20.

slum living represents upward mobility in many developing countries, slum dwellers complain about the gangs, high rent, drugs, violence, sewage, and floods.

Another widespread problem is the abuse and neglect suffered by women and children throughout the world. Over 18 million suffer debilitating illnesses or injuries that often disable them. A 1996 UNICEF report estimates that 585,000 women die each year in pregnancy and childbirth (Crossette, 1996). (See Table 3-6.) To get a perspective on the problem, consider these figures: Roughly 1 in 13 women in sub-Saharan Africa and 1 in 35 in South Asia dies of causes related to pregnancy and childbirth whereas the numbers are 1 in 3,200 in Europe, 1 in 3,300 in the United States, and 1 in 7,300 in Canada.

Child labor remains a reality today in many countries. The United Nations' (UN) International Labor Organization (ILO) estimates that there are at least 100 million child workers in the world (Hecht, 1996). In Africa, for example, the problem affects a minimum of 25% of all children between the ages of 10 and 14. In Senegal, the figure is as high as 40%. Child labor is a fact of life in third-world countries. Children work to supplement the family income, and many rural families send children to work rather than to school. Child labor means work; it does not mean learning to read and write, playing, or resting when ill.

Child prostitution is a reality in Cambodia, India, China, Thailand, the Philippines, Taiwan, and other countries. Social workers and governments estimate that more than 1 million girls and boys, age 17 and younger, are engaged in prostitution (Kristof, 1996). Many enter the sex trade unwillingly, sold by parents to brothel owners, drugged, or kidnapped off the street. The fear of AIDS is one of several factors driving customers to younger girls and boys who are regarded as more likely to be free of disease.

Education, particularly for girls, is by no means universal. Girls are far less likely than boys to attend primary school. Half of all girls in sub-Saharan Africa and 22% in North Africa, Asia, and the Middle East are not in school, compared with 14% of boys ("A World in Need," 1996). Girls are kept home to cook, clean, and mind younger children, or they work outside the home to bring in extra income.

The challenges in international human services continue to be great. The plights of refugees, those with AIDS, the homeless, drug users, and the displaced in the aftermath of natural disasters—in addition to the problems discussed here—are some of those challenges. Ishrat Husain, director of the Poverty and Social Policy Department at the World Bank in Washington, cites our improved understanding of poverty, the participation of the poor in the design and implementation of projects, and awareness of the damage done by discriminating against women and ethnic minorities as the keys to successful programs (Husain, 1996). He states:

> But all these strategies would serve no purpose if the poor cannot make a living. They can only do that if they have the health, strength, and education that will enable them to live and work productively. One of the most efficient ways to reduce poverty is to invest in the human capital of the poor. . . . No investment in education has a higher return than investment in educating girls. It has a powerful effect on almost every aspect of development. It lowers fertility rates, raises productivity, and helps the environment. Increasing female literacy in Africa could help lower infant mortality. (p. 19)

Influences on the United States

How does the international dimension of human services affect the United States? Although most information in this book concerns human services in this country, we must also be aware of its international dimension. Immigrants to the United States increase our awareness of those nationalities that have become or are becoming part of our population. In the early history of the country, immigration was limited primarily to Europeans; 100 years ago, 90% of the immigrants to the United States came from European countries. By 1985, however, nearly half of all immigrants to this country were Asians. In addition to Chinese and Japanese, there are substantial numbers of Filipino, Korean, Vietnamese, and Indian immigrants. Today, people born in another country comprise 9% of the American population, the highest figure since World War II. Latinos are the largest immigrant group, accounting for 46% of those born elsewhere (Grier, 1996).

We can continue to explore diversity in the United States by thinking about some population figures. America's population in the next century will experience profound shifts, making it more ethnically diverse than ever before. By 2050, about half the population will be non-Latino whites, making the United States a "majority minority" nation (Friedman, 1996). This

● ● ● ● ● ● ● ● ●

INTERNATIONAL FOCUS
Kevin Burns—A Peace Corps Experience

Namaste. This common Nepali greeting is derived from the literal meaning, "I salute the god within you." I am working in Nepal as a Peace Corps volunteer. I have been here about 18 months. It has been quite an experience for me. My first experience in Nepal was a week in Kathmandu, the capital of Nepal. We left for Tansen, a beautiful town in the mid-hills of Nepal, to begin our training. In Tansen during training, I lived with a host family that did not speak much English. They were very nice. Days were spent studying about the culture, learning the language, and learning the technical aspects of my upcoming job. Here I learned how to eat the typical way of the country: lentils and rice with vegetables (*dal-blaat*) for lunch and a big plate of rice for supper.

After our training we returned to Kathmandu for a week, and then I traveled to my post of two years—Mechinagar Municipality. It is located in the Teria on the Eastern border with India. I work in the new community development branch of the municipality. My job description says I will be working with programs in health, sanitation, education, income generation, and local organization coordination. While I have been doing my work, I have not always felt productive, but I have learned an enormous amount about living in another culture.

The community development section is brand new. I work with the community development coordinator. I have learned that in the work it is important to "drink tea." I also began to understand the importance of understanding how things work here, the culture, and even the importance of drinking tea—milk tea with sugar. Whatever you do, wherever you go, whether you visit a friend or an office, tea is served.

Our office is implementing a UNICEF urban out-of-school program with nonformal education and skill training for local youth who are not in school. We also have been working on improving local health care services. Other activities include women's literacy classes, an expanded local saving and credit program, and programs involving the local marginalized ethnic groups.

I live in three rooms of a family's house. I now have a Nepali mother, Ama, and father, Buwa. I am their new youngest son. They are a nice family. Ama doesn't speak any English and her Nepali is too fast. It has been

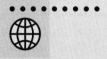

only recently that I have begun to understand her (sometimes). The house is located on the main road between the two bazaars. My rooms are downstairs in a two-story cement building. The family has a garden out front and chickens in the back. The housing here is usually either brick and cement, wooden with bamboo walls and tin roofs, or all bamboo huts with thatch roofs. In my neighborhood there is a mixture of all three. Away from the area is farmland, although 40 years ago this was a dense, malaria-infested jungle.

The cow is the most sacred animal in Nepal. It is a crime to kill one here. In early India the sacredness of cows helped during a famine because, if people ate the cattle, then the farm productivity would drop and only make the famine recovery worse. I think most Americans think of Buddhism in Nepal, but that is because most people know little about the mountain culture, which is more Buddhist. Nepal is the birthplace of Buddha. Over 85% of Nepalis are Hindu, with about 10% Buddhists and 2% Moslem. Hindus here also incorporate Buddhism in their worship, so it is an interesting mix. Hindus do not believe in one all-powerful God, but there are over 330,000 different gods and goddesses.

I am slowly learning to speak and read Nepali, which has a different alphabet from our Western one. Actually there are over 20 separate languages spoken in Nepal (maybe up to 100 dialects). The national language—Nepali—is spoken by most everyone.

One of the first things I learned when I arrived was that I know very little about how to help here. Nepal is poor; it ranks in the bottom ten of the lowest per capita income in the world. According to UNICEF, about 50% of the children in my area are malnourished. The literacy rate here is about 40%, which is up from 2% in 1945. In my district, which is the country's largest agricultural producer, 80% of the land is owned by 20 families. Looking at Nepal through the eyes of the United States can be depressing. Don't forget we spent many years dealing with the same issues that Nepal is beginning to tackle such as child labor, equal rights, and others.

SOURCE: Kevin Burns, Peace Corps Volunteer, 2000. Reprinted with permission.

proportion is down from three-quarters today and is accounted for by high immigration rates and high birth rates among Latino women. The Latino and Asian portion of the population will grow fastest, while blacks will nearly double in number by 2050. The population in the United States as a whole will grow from 262 million to 394 million, an increase of 50% (U.S. Census Bureau, 1996). This projection represents some of the slowest population growth in the country's history, but the Census Bureau notes that the United States is experiencing one of the most dramatic shifts in its racial and ethnic makeup since those brought on by slave trading in the 17th and 18th centuries and the immigration from Eastern and Southern Europe in the late 19th and early 20th centuries.

Projections of population in the future are only that—projections. They are subject to change because of several factors, including changes in legislation that regulates immigration and in fertility rates, and breakthroughs in medical care that impact life expectancy (Holmes, 1996). Nevertheless, the United States is the fastest growing country in the industrialized world today. After 2025, however, population growth will slow to an all-time low brought about by declining birth rates and increased deaths as the population ages. These changes will present new economic and social issues.

Today and in the foreseeable future, the United States must grapple with numerous issues related to diversity. Should changes in immigration laws reduce legal immigration rates? What efforts should be employed against illegal immigration? Do immigrants take jobs from unemployed citizens? Are immigrants entitled to public education and other benefits? Should English be the official language of the United States? What impact will these ethnic shifts have on Medicare and Social Security? While these questions are debated throughout the United States, we continue to be part of the global community and play a role in the international human services discussed earlier.

A direct way this is occurring is through the choice of some human service professionals to work as service providers or volunteers in other countries, particularly developing countries. Some are employed by UN agencies, the World Bank, or the Peace Corps, while others volunteer for shorter periods with religious groups such as the Missionaries of Charity or nonprofit organizations such as Cross-Cultural Solutions or the Red Cross.

Many other human service professionals elect to remain in the United States. Given the population projections, it is increasingly likely that these helpers will work with people of very different backgrounds from them. The Latino population presents an example of the complexity of the situation. In the United States this group is growing almost five times faster than that of non-Latinos and by 2010 is expected to be the nation's largest minority (U.S. Census Population Survey, 1994). Although ethnic groups from Spanish-speaking countries such as Mexico, Nicaragua, and Argentina are referred to as Latino or Hispanic, those cultures and customs are as diverse as English-speaking populations. It would be a mistake to assume that they are a uniform, cohesive group that is culturally homogenous. Hispanics or Latino communities are found in Miami, Spanish Harlem, and migrant labor camps, and each is culturally, ethnically, and geographically diverse, making an awareness and appreciation of each group's uniqueness necessary for effective human service delivery.

Trends in Human Services

Human services will be different in this century. We know that change occurs rapidly. In this chapter you have read about changes already taken place that impact service delivery today. The utilization of technology, managed care, and the diverse and nontraditional settings for helping activities will continue to impact human services, but other trends will influence what and how services will be delivered and to whom. It is appropriate that as part of our discussion of human services today, we devote some thought to the future. It will come quickly. To trigger your thinking about the future, we discuss four major trends as we conclude this chapter.

Aging in America

Growth and change of the elderly population in America rank among the most important demographic developments of the 20th century (Treas, 1995). This development has serious implications for the next 50 years. The population age 65 and older quadrupled during the first half of the 20th century. The pace of growth is slowing, but after the first baby boomers turn 65 in 2011, the older population will swell once again. In 1995, nearly 34 million Americans were age 65 or older. By 2030 that number will double as the last of the baby-boom generation passes age 65. It is not just the numbers that cause concern, however; some current trends among the elderly will be accentuated—and will impact human service delivery.

This larger group will have increasing educational levels, include more minority elderly, and include more women than men. Many will be reasonably healthy and live independent and active lives, although there will still be a great disparity in terms of income and health status in certain segments of the population (Clubok, 2001). These include older single women with low incomes, baby boomers with less education, and minority groups who have not benefited from economic prosperity (Friedland & Summer, 1999). Most interestingly, though, is that this older population is growing older. Gains in life expectancy, medical advances, and improved health and lifestyles contribute to the fact that the population age 85 and older is the fastest growing age group in the United States. As the 21st century begins, the oldest old constitute nearly 24% of the elderly population (age 65 and over). By 2050, the elderly population is projected to more than double; the proportion of the oldest old will increase 225% (Friedland & Summer, 1999).

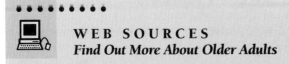

The following sites will help professionals who are working with older adults or children of older adults.

www.aarp.org

This website has articles of interest relevant for keeping up with the issues of today such as computer tips and technology updates, volunteering, and recent survey information on attitudes about death and dying. It also introduces travel and education opportunities, legislative issues related to seniors, and other informative articles and links.

www.agingwithdignity.org

This is the site of Aging with Dignity. Founded in 1996 by Jim Towey, Aging with Dignity is a privately funded, nonprofit organization that advocates for the needs of elders and their caregivers, with a particular emphasis on improving care for those who face the end of life. This organization has developed a document called Five Wishes, which allows people to communicate their preferences in terms of care and treatment should they become seriously ill.

www.elderweb.com

This website provides information about long-term care for older adults, with excellent links for legal, financial, medical, and housing issues.

www.estateplanninglinks.com

This website contains links to other sites on estate planning, elder law, and tax-related issues for both the layperson and the professional.

The expected changes in numbers, ethnicity, sex ratio, and other factors present challenges for human services in the next 50 years. While many people will enter their older years with the health and resources to pursue full and independent lives, there will also be a significant number who are troubled by poor health, dependency, and the inability to do simple tasks (Treas, 1995). Additionally, those who are in good health will not escape the transition from active and independent living to a time when greater assistance is necessary. Addressing these needs will present challenges for human services and society at large during the 21st century, particularly in the areas of income assistance, health care, housing alternatives, employment issues, leisure opportunities, and environmental modification.

An Emphasis on Diversity

Typically, when we think about diversity, it is the ethnic makeup of our country that comes to mind. In fact, earlier in this chapter you read about the changing demographics of both the United States and the world, and how those changes will impact human services. It is accepted today that as you enter the human service profession you will encounter clients who are different from you. You will also be working with other helping professionals who are different from you. For example, at an agency in Miami, a team of human service professionals represent a variety of countries: Spain, Cuba, El Salvador, Romania, and the Dominican Republic. Not only do they differ in the countries where they were raised, but they also speak different languages, come from different economic backgrounds, are different ages and genders, and they also have entered the United States under various circumstances. You prepare for working relationships such as these by learning about multicultural counseling, reading the plethora of books that address ethnic diversity, and increasing your awareness of other cultures through travel, interaction with other students, and television, books, and movies. Diversity, however, has a much broader connotation than ethnic diversity and it is an understanding of this more sweeping concept that will help us address the challenges of 21st-century problems.

As a human service professional, you will encounter diversity across disciplines and systems and among professionals and clients. You know that clients and coworkers will differ in ethnicity, gender, lifestyle, race, religion, and culture. You have also read in this chapter about the growing emphasis on managed care, schools as sites for human service delivery, and the competition for limited resources that require us to facilitate partnerships with other agencies, organizations, and professionals. We will best serve our clients if we can work collaboratively in teams across agencies and disciplines to increase our flexibility and resources, to serve the client, and to meet the needs of an increasingly diverse population.

How do we work with those who are ethnically different from us? All people are shaped by the culture in which they were raised, including those who consider themselves the dominant culture in the United States (Okun, Fried, & Okun, 1999). What do you know about your own culture and how it is perceived by others? Are you open to learning about others whose worlds are different? The ability to work effectively with diverse groups means establishing relationships based on the trust and respect for others, increasing our awareness and knowledge of other ways, listening without judgments, and appreciating the world view of others. The challenge to human service professionals in the 21st century is to take the lead to work effectively with others, whether that is a client, a neighborhood, a regional population, or other professionals.

Client Responsibility

As the 20th century ended, one well-accepted change that occurred over its last half was the role of the client in the helping process. For many years, the client was a passive recipient of services—accepting the decisions, following the direction of a helper, and generally assuming little responsibility for what occurred With the recognition of clients' rights, the emphasis on consumer satisfaction, and the advent of welfare reform, the participation of the client in human service delivery has increased greatly; in many instances, the client becomes actively involved in the helping process.

This change has necessitated efforts on the part of human service professionals to engage the client as a partner in the helping process. Establishing a collaborative relationship calls for skills that promote a climate of trust and a sense of partnership. Taking time to get to know the client, considering the client's point of view, and exploring client expectations are part of this process. Once a relationship exists, the client becomes an active participant in assessing the problem and the situation, collecting information, determining a course of action, and evaluating the process. As a result of these actions, the client shares responsibility for the success or failure of the endeavor.

An example of the current status of the client's role is welfare reform— legislation passed in 1996 that ended federal assistance to the poor. After the reform, each state was charged with developing its own welfare program. In practice, many of these state programs now require the active participation of the client. Some require client input in developing a plan for service delivery, determining problems, and deciding the services that are necessary to solve these problems. Part of the plan is the client's signature, which indicates the client's participation and commitment to the process. Other states use contracts that identify client responsibility and the consequences of failing to fulfill the contract. In some situations, clients actually become case managers of their own cases. These examples illustrate how client involvement has changed through the years.

For human service professionals this shift in the client's role has some benefits. First, the client shares the responsibility with the helper for the effectiveness of the helping process. Being actively engaged in the process increases the likelihood that the client will follow through on whatever tasks are necessary and will be more satisfied with the results. Second, the establishment of a relationship with the client also impacts the client's satisfaction. Having a good relationship with the helper means that clients believe that the helper listened, spent time with them, and provided follow-up services. Finally, clients have much to teach the human service professional about themselves, their problems, and the services they need. Ignoring these aspects of service delivery leads to ineffective and inefficient services. These are important lessons for helpers that will carry over to their work with other clients.

Changing Skills

This chapter presents the fact that human service delivery is changing rapidly. The problems people experience, societal conditions, resources, and many other factors are fluid and influence service delivery. Attending to these changes calls for different helping skills. Some, like advocacy, are recognized, accepted, and taught as human service skills and will continue to be emphasized in the future. Other skills may be more nontraditional, such as selling. Both advocacy and selling are discussed here as examples that will be critical for successful service delivery in the future.

As human services changes, there may be both positive and negative reactions. It is possible that services will become more streamlined yet less available, and cost containment will save money but become an overriding factor in limiting treatment and other services. It is even possible that legislation will become law that may be unfair to some groups or individuals. These possibilities make vigilance on the part of human service providers particularly important as they look out for the interests of their clients.

Advocacy means speaking out on behalf of clients or those who cannot speak for themselves. It frequently involves clients, their families, the community, and other professionals. Direct advocacy efforts may take many forms: empowering clients to act; improving environments; acting on behalf of a client by writing letters, filing forms, and so forth; informing clients about programs, services, and policies; and guiding a client through choices and changes. There are also situations that require advocacy on a larger scale. Are needed services provided? Are they available and accessible? Is the public policy fair and equitable? In these instances, a human service professional may act as a spokesperson to inform the public and legislators about what exists or what is needed. It may also be necessary to act as part of a collaborative effort for common agreement or support about an issue.

Kelly and Empson (1999) present the case of incarcerated women as an example of a client group that needs advocacy efforts both individually and societally. Nearly six times as many women are incarcerated in prison today as there were in 1930, an increase of 460%. They face numerous barriers that require the attention of an advocate: "limited access to outpatient treatment, acceptance into jail without evaluation for drug abuse, or unavailability of prison-based programs" (Kelly & Empson, 1999, p. 32). On a larger scale, collaborative efforts ensure a healthy environment for incarcerated women and empowerment to become their own advocates to speak to legislators and committees through client testimony and experiences that inform public opinion.

The advocacy role of the human service professional is discussed more completely in Chapter 6, but as you think about the future and the skills you will need to be an effective service provider, you also will want to think about how to prepare for this role. An effective advocate needs a variety of information and skills, but chief among them is the knowledge and awareness of the cultural values that influence communication, relationships, and a sense of self-determination. This further emphasizes the importance of diversity as discussed in this section.

A more nontraditional skill that is receiving attention is selling. Initial responses to this skill may be objections to sales as pushy, competitive, aggressive, manipulative, and fast-talking, whereas in reality many salespeople are professional, respectable people who do a good job selling because they believe it is a helping profession (Bartlett, 1994; Nirenberg, 1984). According to recent sales literature, a new model of selling has emerged, one that is compatible with human service values and easily integrated with such practice (Cathcart, 1990).

The new model of sales emphasizes a relationship approach to selling that focuses on the "we" in the relationship and the development of a partnership that is characterized by flexibility, two-way communication, and the resolution of concerns. The following quote illustrates how selling occurs in human services:

> We interview them, talk about our program a bit, and talk about why they were referred to us. So you think our program has something to offer you? Do you think there would be any benefit to us helping you? Could we work together? And 90% say yes. We are pretty good at selling our program. It is a sales job that is a part of health care that isn't discussed too often. It is selling that needs to go on, particularly with getting people into a program.

This quote is from the director/case manager of an intensive case management program in Los Angeles, which assists patients with severe mental illness who are living in this community that provides "cradle to grave" comprehensive services. The clients served by this program comprise the "revolving door" clientele at residential mental health centers and hospitals in the Los Angeles area. The agency's goal is to improve the quality of life for these clients by helping them live independently in the community and to reduce their stay in institutional settings. For many of these clients, residential mental health facilities are their residence of choice and their safety nets. They have never maintained a stable living arrangement in the community. During the initial phase of contact with clients, case managers in this program provide a "vision" to their potential clients for a new way of living in the community. They must have the client "buy in" for two reasons. First, without client commitment to

---

TABLE 3-7 ✦ SUMMARY POINTS: TRENDS

- The effect of urbanization in poor countries will continue to create difficulties in meeting the basic needs of people.
- Demographic shifts in the United States raise questions about immigration policies, language, employment, and entitlement programs.
- One important shift is the growth and change of the elderly population which projects an increase in the number of elderly as well as changes in their characteristics.
- Clients will remain active participants in human service delivery.
- Advocacy and selling are examples of helping skills that are becoming increasingly important.

the goals of the program and the services it offers, helping the client becomes very difficult. Second, because it is a voluntary program, clients must agree to participate, so the agency can receive the funding necessary to provide these intensive services. The focus of the selling in this setting is to successfully initiate client service.

Human service educators recognize that their field continues to change rapidly and innovative approaches to traditional helping may be needed to meet the demand of service delivery in the 21st century. It is also important to retain those traditional skills that are effective. As human service professionals, the challenge is to stay abreast of both societal trends and new developments in order to provide quality services to those who need assistance. (See Table 3-7.)

 ## Things to Remember

1. Human services are delivered to populations in a variety of settings, including rural areas, industry, the military, schools, and other community-based settings, all of which increase the number of clients who can be reached.

2. Schools have become a site for service delivery as teachers and human service professionals share the same clients.

3. The trend toward providing more services in community-based settings and less in institutional ones is helping to serve clients in the least restrictive environment.

4. Community-based services were first used with clients with mental illness who were deinstitutionalized; now, populations receiving community-based services include those in the criminal justice system, the developmentally disabled, and the elderly.

5. The barriers to service delivery in rural areas include shortages of workers, the large geographic distances between clients and providers, the cost of services, confidentiality issues, and coordination of care.

6. Technology has begun to change the way human service professionals meet their responsibilities, particularly in the areas of communication, information management, service provision, and professional development.

7. Communication avenues used by human service professionals include electronic mail, listservs, the World Wide Web, cellular phones, and teleconferencing.

8. Computer technology is available to help human service professionals manage information and use data to make decisions about planning programs, establishing costs, and reporting.

9. Technology is being effectively used to provide services to clients, including diagnosing and assessing, teaching new skills, and assisting those with disabilities or impairments.

10. The increased use managed care organizations is dramatically changing the delivery of human services through the use of external reviews, the demand to develop standards of best practice, the need for better information management, and an emphasis on a continuum of care.

11. Managed care standards, developed for accountability in health and human services, can be summarized as "providing the right services at the right time in the right amounts, no more, no less" (Schafer, 1996, p. 2).

12. Resolution-focused intervention has emerged as a way to help clients change in a brief period of time.

13. As technological advances draw the world closer, we become more aware of the human service challenges in an international context, including individuals and families in war-torn areas who are living in disruptive and life-threatening environments.

14. In the international context, many individuals live in large cities in poor countries where they struggle to meet basic needs and have little access to housing, sanitation, and nutritious food.

15. Among the trends in the United States that will influence future human service delivery are the growth and change of its elderly population, the increasing diversity of clients and professionals, the increasingly active participation of clients, and the development of new and in some cases nontraditional skills.

Additional Readings: New Trends

Anders, G. (1996). *Health against wealth: HMOs and the breakdown of medical trust.* Boston: Houghton Mifflin Company.
   Author George Anders, a reporter for *The Wall Street Journal,* documents the backlash against managed care by arguing that cost-driven managed care companies are systematically degrading the quality of medicine.

Desjarlais, R., Eisenberg, L., Good, B., & Kleinman, A. (1995). *World mental health: Problems and priorities in low-income countries.* New York: Oxford University Press.
   This report issues a call to action for individuals, communities, governments, and international agencies to take steps to stem the growing personal and social burdens due to mental illness and behavioral problems worldwide.

Dryfoos, J. (1994). *Full-service schools: A revolution in health and social services for children, youth, and families.* San Francisco: Jossey-Bass.
   This book describes the movement to create an array of integrated support services in schools that will help students and their families be successful.

Ginsberg, Leon H. (Ed.). (1998). *Social work in rural communities.* (3rd ed.). Alexandria, VA: Council on Social Work Education.
   This collection of readings addresses a number of concerns in rural service delivery, including concepts, special populations, problems, and social programs.

Skolnick, J. H., & Currie, E. (1997). *Crisis in American institutions.* New York: Longman.

This book of readings by well-known social scientists addresses a number of critical issues that face our society today, including racial segregation, poverty, ghetto joblessness, and corporate power among others.

Suro, R. (1998). *Strangers among us: How Latino immigration is transforming America.* New York: Alfred A. Knopf.

A former correspondent for *The New York Times,* the author documents how Latinos have become central to America's struggle with poverty and race.

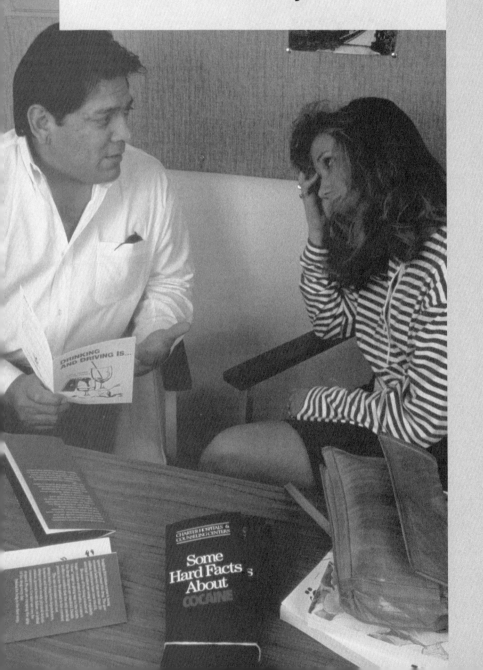

Chapter 4

Models of Human Service Delivery

In developing a definition of human services, we have discussed its various characterizations, briefly traced the history of service provision, and explored recent developments, emphasizing human services today. Another approach to defining human services is to examine the way it benefits service recipients. This chapter describes three models that represent different orientations in service delivery: the medical model, the public health model, and the human service model.

In this chapter you will meet clients who have received services delivered in the context of these three models. The cases of Robert Smith and Ralph Jones illustrate services provided by the medical model. Sean O'Reilley was a recipient of services provided by the public health model. Susan, her husband, Ted, and children, Matthew and Justin, illustrate the complexities of client needs and require multifaceted, long-term intervention.

All three models are used to deliver services today; some agencies may prefer one over the others, and one model may be more effective than the other two in some situations. Workers may be skilled in following one particular model, but you are likely to be working closely with practitioners who follow the other models. Therefore, you should know the characteristics of each model, its historical development, and how it is used. To help translate this information into human service practice, we examine a relevant social problem from the perspective of each model.

Each of the three models of service delivery has certain philosophical assumptions that guide its practice. These assumptions reflect beliefs about the causes of problems, their treatment, and the role of the professional in the model. To illustrate, we consider the nature of mental disorders from the perspectives of each of the three models.

The medical model is based on an orientation developed by the medical profession; it assumes that mental disorders are diseases or illnesses that impair an individual's ability to function. The disease or illness, in this case the mental disorder, has an organic basis and responds to medical interventions such as medication, laboratory studies, and physical therapies. Often the individual, or *patient*, receives treatment from a physician in a hospital or medical clinic.

The public health model resembles the medical model in its diagnosis and treatment process, but the models differ in recipients of services and methodologies of treatment. Whereas the medical model emphasizes individuals, the public health model focuses on *groups* in the population who may be identified by geography (community, country, region, or state), types of problems (abuse, poverty, specific illnesses), or specific characteristics such as age (children, the elderly). This model views mental disorders as the result of malfunctions or pressures created by the environment or by society. The mental disorder is evaluated for its impact not only on the individual but also on society at large. In addition to treating the individual, this model emphasizes preventing the problem through supporting activities such as use of films, speakers, school programs, and pamphlets, all aimed at educating the population about the problem.

The human service model is concerned with the interaction between the individual and the environment, stressing the need for balance between the two. Although recognizing both the medical and the public health perspectives, this model focuses on the interpersonal and environmental conflicts that may result from the problem (in this case, a mental disorder). Perhaps the individual (or *client* or *consumer*) has problems resulting from genetic predispositions, biochemical imbalances, faulty learning, lack of insight into behavior that may be inappropriate, a physical or mental disability, and/or influences from the social environment. Whatever the situation, the client is experiencing interpersonal and emotional difficulties that affect behavior. Treatment in this model encompasses services to both the individual and the environment through work with the client as well as the people and the institutions with which the client is involved. Each model provides a different perspective on the same problem. We now look at the development of each one.

 ## The Medical Model

Definition

The medical model sees the person coming for help as an individual whose problem is a disease or a sickness. The individual is "sick" or "ill," not healthy. Often called *patients,* these individuals depend on the physician or service provider to prescribe a treatment or cure for the "disease." This model can be summarized as a system that involves the following elements: symptom–diagnosis–treatment–cure (Reinhard, 1986).

The medical model, with a history that includes shamans, medicine men and women, and witch doctors, is perhaps the oldest of all treatment models. In fact, other models used it as they were developing. For example, in Chapter 2 we discussed the beginning of the new profession of social work at the turn of the 20th century. Mary Richmond, author of *Social Diagnosis* (1917), used the medical model to describe social casework. Believing that the presenting problem was rooted in the individual, she suggested that pauperism was a disease. The friendly visitor, therefore, became a social physician whose duty was to heal the complex conditions of poverty (Zimbalist, 1977).

The corrections field also adopted the medical model during the 1930s when its emphasis shifted from punishment to treatment. The change was based on the assumption that "criminal behavior is caused by biological or social conditions that require treatment" (Clear & Cole, 1997, p. 87). Theoretically, prisons were to become therapeutic communities, where inmates would be rehabilitated to reenter society. Unfortunately, budget constraints limited this change to one of name only; departments of prisons became "departments of corrections," but punishment continued to be the reality. Structurally, the system already included parole, probation, and the indeterminate sentence. All that remained to complete the incorporation of the medical model was the addition of a classification system to aid in diagnosis and treatment (Clear & Cole, 1997).

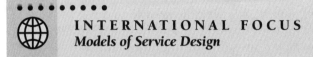

• • • • • • • • •

INTERNATIONAL FOCUS
Models of Service Design

Howard N. Higginbotham (1979) suggests three basic models of service design today: traditional psychiatry, the public health approach, and the village system.

The first model, traditional psychiatry, is similar to North American or European psychiatry, which has not been modified for use in non-Western settings. This model emphasizes residential facilities; the individuals who need these services must therefore leave their homes to get treatment. Unfortunately, long-term confinement often results. Treatment within such facilities varies from custodial management to programs of work "therapy," which may take the form of farming, sewing, or daily chores around the hospital. Programs of psychotropic medication and electroconvulsive shock (ECT) are often followed in the cases of new admissions and chronic patients. Less prevalent as a treatment modality is one-to-one psychotherapy.

The second model is a public health approach to services. In developing countries, this approach is characterized by its emphasis on primary prevention and the training of paraprofessionals. Consultation and educational activities are provided so as to maximize the utilization of resources. Maintaining the patient outside the hospital, by mobilizing and coordinating community resources, is also characteristic of this approach.

The third approach, the village system, developed as a response to frustrations in attempting to establish facilities based on Western models in such areas as Africa. In this system, patients live with relatives who reside near mental clinics. Treatment in the village system incorporates the use of native healers, therapeutic relationships, psychotropic drugs, and the natural therapeutic elements of the village, which include confession, dancing, and rituals.

SOURCE: Adapted from "Culture and Mental Services," by Howard N. Higginbotham. In Anthony J. Marsella, Roland G. Tharp, and Thomas Ciborowski (Eds.), *Perspectives on Cross-Cultural Psychology*, pp. 205–236. Copyright © 1979 by Academic Press, reprinted by permission of the publisher. All rights reserved.

History

As mentioned in Chapter 2, institutions developed as a way to meet the needs of some segments of society. Asylums were established primarily to care for persons with mental illness, shifting care from the local community to rural institutions and replacing local financing with state funding. Responsibility for the care of persons with mental illness rested with the medical profession.

Psychiatry emerged as a discipline at the end of the 18th century when Philippe Pinel became head of the Hospice de Bicetre and later of Salpetriere (mental institutions in France). Some mental disorders had been recognized as such early on, but Pinel's removal of chains from patients and other humane acts emphasized the belief that pathological behavioral disorders had organic origins and that their treatment belonged to medicine. Accordingly, those diagnosed as mentally ill were to be treated as patients by physicians in hospital settings, just like other patients with medical problems. Pinel, hoping to create a science of mental disease, is credited with introducing the medical model into psychiatry by stressing the clinical diagnosis and appropriate medical treatment. (See box.)

Until the end of the 19th century, insanity was socially defined: "An insane was a person whose behavior for pathological reasons was so disturbed that he had to be segregated in special institutions" (Pichot, 1985, p. 10). With the emergence of psychiatry as a medical specialty, a body of knowledge was established to explain the nature and causes of insanity. The discovery and application of the most effective treatments became a priority. Insanity became medically defined, meaning that the institution of treatment had to be a hospital instead of a prison, and the care of the patient would be handled by a physician, not a warden.

After the middle of the 19th century, use of the medical model to treat mental illness dominated. By the end of the century, however, the medical model was changing. A new school of thought rejected medical treatment and advocated psychotherapy for treatment of persons with mental illness. The new philosophy was based on the assumption that diseases of the soul were completely separate from diseases of the body. Psychiatry concerned itself with the medicine of the soul; psychosis was the disease of the soul, and neurosis was the disease of the nerves (Pichot, 1985). Sigmund Freud's work reflected this orientation.

Early in his career, Freud was a researcher and clinician in biology and neurology; he made outstanding contributions to both fields. He used the scientific method, insisting that medical problems of mental illness be studied in the rigorous laboratory setting.

Later, Freud rejected his earlier training and revolutionized the study and treatment of mental illness. He developed a method of therapy commonly known today as the *psychoanalytic method*. In this method, the client shares all thoughts with the therapist. The therapist interprets this material to explain to patients the nature of their repressions and the influence of these repressions on their present problems. Freud also developed a theory of neurosis and one of the normal mind, based on the assumption that mental disorders were psychologically rooted. Although Freud's impact was profound, psychoanalytic theory did not completely change the medical model or become the preferred method of treatment, for several reasons. First, its success was difficult to evaluate and to document. Second, it required too much time and expense to be a viable treatment for large numbers of people.

The treatment of persons with mental illness continued to develop in the 1940s; however, more psychiatrists and improved treatment were needed. A

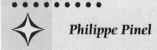

Philippe Pinel

Philippe Pinel (1745–1826) is famous in the history of medicine and mental health. In revolutionary France, Pinel courageously campaigned to secure a new status for persons with mental illness as people suffering from disease rather than being possessed by demons or manifesting the consequences of sin. Pinel argued, practiced, and taught that such persons require medical care rather than persecution or punishment, and that they are entitled to be treated with respect as persons and citizens. This was a revolutionary idea.

Pinel was born into a modest family of surgeons in southwestern France. Initially trained as a cleric and destined for service in the church, he decided to study science in Toulouse. By 1773, he had acquired a doctorate of medicine, but he continued his studies for four more years in Montpellier under Barthez. Sickness and health became his lifelong concern, and he systematically applied himself to learning all he could about medicine from ancient as well as contemporary sources. He acquired the education of a classicist and a humanist in addition to his extensive knowledge of the practice of medicine in his day. He moved to Paris in 1778 and supported himself by translating scientific and medical works and teaching mathematics. Though extremely shy, he became a member of an important group of reformers and medical thinkers called the Ideologues. Benjamin Franklin tried to convince Pinel to go to America. However, Pinel was a patriot and wished to help modernize medicine in his own country. His interest in insanity derived from the suicide of a seriously depressed friend and patient in 1783. In 1792, apparently because of his connections with the Ideologues, Pinel was appointed Physician of the Infirmaries to the Hospice de Bicetre, a huge Parisian custodial institution for indigent ailing men. In the same year, he wrote an essay on the subject of the clinical training of doctors. This essay remained unnoticed in the Archives of the National Academy of Medicine in Paris until 1935, when it was discovered by M. Gentry, curator of the academy. Translated and published in America in 1971, it gives a remarkable view of the attitudes, values, and practices of French medicine at the end of the 18th century.

Pinel's essay on the clinical training of doctors was written at the beginning of a period, 1794–1815, which medical historian E. H. Ackerknecht terms the "period of Pinel." During this time, Pinel managed two of the major hospitals in Paris and published three significant works: *Philosophical Nosography* (1798), *Treatise on Insanity* (1801), and *Clinical Medicine* (1802). The first book would serve for years as a text for the classification of diseases; the second would lay the foundation for mod-

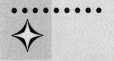

ern psychiatry; and the third, published in three successively enlarged editions, would spread his methodology and fame among the next generation.

In 1794, Pinel transferred to the Hospice de la Salpetriere, an institution that housed nearly 7,000 destitute women. He administered, practiced, and taught in this hospital for 30 years, applying the principles that gave him the reputation as a founder of modern psychiatry.

In medical practice, Pinel practically invented the role of the full-time resident physician who teaches and trains students, interns, and fellow researchers in a hospital ward. Along with other reformers, he argued for national curricula, standards, and diplomas for medical education. Pinel insisted that such education should be conducted in French and based on clinical practice and observations. He viewed the natural sciences as "accessories" to the practice of medicine.

With regard to mental health, Pinel is often given credit for what he learned from the uneducated but experienced and successful Keeper of the Insane at Bicetre, J. P. Pussin (1746–1811): namely, that the mental patients could be managed without cages, chains, or cruelty. Pinel brought Pussin to Salpetriere in 1802 to aid him in caring for the many unruly patients. Pinel combined Pussin's practical management principles with his own medical knowledge to develop his famous "moral method" for treating mental illness. This method assumes that mental illness is due to some imbalance in the patient, which the physician can treat and rectify. The crux of this method is extensive observation and knowledge about the patient. This knowledge makes possible detailed therapy, which the physician must carefully supervise. Pinel's approach is a far cry from bleeding, beating, purging, and imprisonment, which had been the usual methods of treating the insane.

Pinel's methods and publications made him well known, and students flocked to him. Among them were the future leaders of French medicine. Pinel's concern for humane treatment of persons with mental illness was realized in France and made that country a world leader in the enlightened treatment of mental illness. When Dorothea Dix traveled in Europe in the late 1850s, extending her great American crusade to reform in the treatment of the insane, she had only small changes to recommend to the French, and to the Turks in Constantinople who had been trained by the French.

SOURCE: Used by permission of H. Phillips Hamlin (1985).

common treatment during this decade was electroconvulsive or electroshock therapy. This treatment involved administering an electric shock of 70 to 130 volts to the brain, leaving the patient unconsciousness and/or in convulsions. On regaining consciousness, the patient sometimes experienced confusion and memory loss, but problem behaviors diminished after several weeks of treatments. Electroshock therapy was effective with depressed individuals, but it was used less successfully to treat other mental disorders. Its abuse during the 1960s resulted in negative perceptions of this treatment method, and these perceptions contributed to the growing popularity of psychotropic medications.

Psychotropic drugs, which act on the brain, are now among the most widely used treatments for mental disorders. Because of the prevalence of these medications, *psychopharmacology,* the study of the effects of drugs on mental health, is an area of interest to human service workers. Ponterotto (1985) suggested that familiarity with this information will help human service workers communicate with medical personnel and better understand the uses and limitations of these medications as they relate to client behavior.

Psychotropic medications can be divided into four major classes: antipsychotic drugs, antidepressant drugs, antianxiety drugs, and lithium salts. *Antipsychotic drugs* are effective in managing psychotic disorders such as bipolar disorder (colloquially known as manic depression) and schizophrenia. Although these drugs do not cure psychosis, they help to control certain psychotic behaviors such as suspiciousness, hallucinations, and impulsiveness. Haldol (haloperidol), Thorazine (chlorpromazine), Clozaril (clozapine), and Mellaril (thioridazine) are well-known examples of antipsychotic medication.

Antidepressant drugs, the second class, relieve depression. There are two kinds of antidepressant drugs: the tricyclic antidepressants and the monoamine oxidase inhibitors. Human service workers will most likely come in contact with widely used tricyclic antidepressants such as Elavil (amitriptyline) or Tofranil (imipramine); however, Prozac (fluoxetine), Paxil (paroxetine), Luvor (fluvoxamine), and Zoloft (sertraline)—antidepressants unrelated to tricyclic or monoamine oxidase inhibitors—have become increasingly popular in recent years because of fewer side effects. These drugs are selective seratonin reuptake inhibitors (SSRIs).

The most widely used psychotropic medications by far are the *antianxiety drugs, sedatives,* and *hypnotics.* Prescribed to relieve anxiety, fear, or tension, these medications may be classed as barbiturates, benzodiazepines, or antihistamines. Benzodiazepines such as Valium (diazepam), Xanax (alprazolam), Tranxene (clorazepate), and Librium (chlordiazepoxide) are especially popular, because they reduce anxiety without reducing overall performance.

The final class of psychotropic medication is *mood stabilizers.* They include lithium carbonate, calcium channel blockers (Calan, Isoptin), and anticonvulsants (Tegretol, Epitol). Used primarily in the treatment of bipolar disorder, these drugs are particularly effective in preventing the mania state, which is characterized by symptoms of extreme irritability, talkativeness, grandiose ideas, exaggerated self-esteem, and increased involvement in risky activities such as spending sprees or reckless driving.

• • • • • • • • • •

WEB SOURCES
Find Out More About Psychotropic Medications

http://www.cornerstonemh.com/psychotropic.html

This site provides basic information about psychotropic medications. It includes a summary description of each category and a discussion weighing the benefits of primary care treatment and psychiatric care treatment. In addition, there are links to other articles that focus on medication for treating mental illness.

http://www.psychnetworks.com/medic.html

Psychological Networks has prepared a rationale for administering and taking psychotropic medications. It is written for the layperson and makes a case for professional diagnosis prior to prescribing the drugs.

http://www.cqc.state.ny.us/cc26a.htm

New York State has prepared a summary of two cases in which the patient's right to refuse psychotropic medication is challenged. The legal and ethical dimensions are explored.

http://smhp.psych.ucla.edu/med/charta.htm

This site was prepared by the UCLA and was a school/mental health project. Psychotropic medications are categorized by child/adolescent diagnoses and are presented in chart format. The medications are listed with the diagnosis that leads to the prescription. The caveat is that continued monitoring of drug effects is essential.

http://www.applesforhealth.com/psymedchild1.html

This site describes the current information on the safety and efficacy of medications for children and adolescents with mental disorders. Data provide advanced knowledge of the effects of psychotropic drugs on children by the NIMH.

http://www.westerncarolinacenter.org/body_psychotropic_medications_mana.html

This site provides clinical guidelines for medicine management of psychotropic medicines. It includes guidelines for diagnosis, dosage, duration, duplication, evaluation, informed consent, and use of an interdisciplinary team.

http://php.iupui.edu/~flip/meds.html

This online booklet was prepared by the NIMH. It prepares the layperson to deal with mental illness of friends and family. Special emphasis is placed upon the use of psychotropic medications.

Psychotropic medications have revolutionized mental health by facilitating deinstitutionalization, but the effects have not always been positive. For example, critics say that antianxiety drugs mask symptoms so that individuals avoid dealing with the real problem. Clients who take major tranquilizers over a long period of time may suffer dangerous side effects, such as tardive dyskinesia, a neurological disorder characterized by abnormal, involuntary mouth or tongue movements. Table 4-1 lists other common side effects of the four major categories.

Today, those who deliver services in the medical model face several challenges. One is that the symptom–diagnosis–treatment–cure process more realistically leads to cure *or* control. Particularly with psychiatric illnesses, controlling the symptoms and making the patient functional are the guides for treatment. Complicating this issue are the numerous new drugs that appear with frequency. There are now many drugs that do not fit neatly into the four categories of psychotropic drugs just described. For example, the new seratonin drugs (Prozac, Paxil, and Zoloft), which do not fit one category, are broadly prescribed today to treat bulimia, obsessive-compulsive disorders, and anxiety disorders.

A second challenge is determining who controls medical services. Is it the physician, the patient, insurers or managed care organizations, employers, and/or the government? To varying degrees, all seem to have a role. For example, the intrusions of government become greater each year. Although it is sometimes difficult medically to separate the organic and psychiatric states, it has happened at some state government levels; that is, diagnosis and reimbursement guidelines have differentiated physical and mental conditions. A second example is the impact of managed care discussed in Chapter 3. Typi-

TABLE 4-1 ✦ POSSIBLE SIDE EFFECTS OF PSYCHOTROPIC MEDICATIONS

Antipsychotic drugs	Antidepressants	Antianxiety drugs	Mood stabilizers
Feelings of heaviness	Dry mouth	Drug tolerance	Toxic warning signs (nausea, tremors, muscle spasms)
Sluggishness	Blurred vision	Stumbling gait	
Weakness	Constipation	Slurred speech	Thyroid disorders
Faintness	Urinary retention	Drowsiness	Renal toxicity
Drowsiness	Lowered or raised	Conjunctivitis	Nausea
Dizziness	blood pressure	Dry mouth	Vomiting
Tremors	Agitation	Constipation	Diarrhea
Seizures	Raised temperature	Urinary problems	Sedation
Tardive dyskinesia	Hallucinations		Confusion
Loss of muscle tone	Convulsions		

cally, in a managed system, physicians receive a fixed amount per patient to take care of medical problems. A small part of the capitation fee is for behavioral health care. Once again, physicians are faced with an arbitrary separation between physical and psychiatric conditions. They also grapple daily with wanting to do the right thing but at the same time contain costs. Achieving this balance is difficult when physicians attend to the "whole" patient, which includes a consideration of the patient's environment and social circumstances. In some instances, physicians have lost their right to choose which drugs to prescribe because managed care staff overrule their recommendations with less expensive medicine.

The past 30 years have demystified psychiatric illness and made its acceptance widespread. The future may include new perspectives. One may be an awareness that we treat mild disease too aggressively. A second perspective is that in some cases it is society that is malfunctional, not the individual—that is, society places people in situations that are not normal but expects them not to behave abnormally. For example, think about the malfunctional mother who has a full-time job as well as responsibility for the home and the children. The problem may not be that she is malfunctional but that society's expectations are unrealistic. (See Table 4-2.)

Case Studies

One obvious example of the medical model's application to human service problems is its use in treating mental illness. Two illustrative case studies follow. The case of Robert Smith describes the mental illness and treatment of a man in the late 1870s. This narrative not only illustrates the orientation of the medical model but also expresses the attitudes of that time toward mental illness. The case of Ralph Jones represents the use of the medical model over 100 years later. The use of the medical model in the second case is especially reflected in the prescription of medication and other physical treatments for Ralph's illness. In both cases, note that the clients are considered ill and that their treatment reflects this diagnosis.

TABLE 4-2 ✦ SUMMARY POINTS: HISTORY OF THE MEDICAL
                    MODEL

- Individual is "sick."
- Recipient is called *patient.*
- 18th-century Philippe Pinel removed chains of mentally ill.
- Pinel stressed clinical diagnosis and treatment.
- Psychiatry emerges as a medical specialty.
- Mid-19th-century psychotherapy emerges as treatment.
- Freud develops psychoanalytic method.
- Electric shock was introduced in the 1940s.
- Today psychotropic drugs are the most widely used treatments.

ROBERT SMITH

Robert Smith was the fourth of six children and the third son. His family, third-generation immigrants from England, lived in Philadelphia. Robert was quiet and withdrawn as a child, and while he did the work the family found for him, he was never very energetic in seeking it out.

The Smith family was relatively poor. Their fortunes improved somewhat during the Civil War, when they were able to find employment in the war-related metal industry, but after the war they descended again into poverty.

In his late 20s, Robert began to have episodes of "mania," as a doctor later called it. While still usually quiet and withdrawn, Robert would become violent and aggressive if crossed by members of his family or neighbors or if frustrated by events. These episodes of mania cost him his job, and soon the family was having to watch him all the time. During an episode, he would sometimes attack anyone who tried to communicate with him; when the episode passed, he would again become withdrawn and listless.

When Robert's aggressiveness began to be expressed toward the neighbors as well as toward family members, the family began to seek help for him. They took him to physicians, who examined him but did not know what to do for him.

By the time he was 32, Robert Smith's behavior had become so distressing that his family was desperate. He had been arrested more than once for destroying property in the neighborhood and threatening neighbors. His family had only barely kept him out of prison. His father took him to the county commission, which, after hearing the testimony of the family and the local sheriff, agreed to send him to the Blockley Almshouse in the fall of 1875. Blockley Almshouse was a huge collection of buildings maintained by the city of Philadelphia for its insane poor. When it was time for Robert to go there, the combined efforts of several family members and neighbors were necessary to overcome his resistance and subdue him.

At first, Robert was kept in the general hospital to recover from the injuries he had received in resisting the move to Blockley. Then he was transferred to a crowded asylum building, where he was nominally under the care of Dr. Isaac Ray, whom he actually never saw except from a distance.

Robert had to sleep on a night bed put on the floor in a corridor. When his violent episodes occurred, he was put in a straight waistcoat, which reduced his ability to attack other patients or attendants. The ward was generally noisy and turbulent. There was little chance for a good night's sleep, nor was there anything much for the patients to do during the day except to excite each other, creating almost continual disturbances.

After a year in Blockley, and weeks in a straitjacket, Robert became less violent and more depressed. Cold-water treatments seemed to reduce his violent episodes while he was in Blockley. His family noticed that he had lost weight and they became worried about his physical health. They found the hospital dreary and depressing, but they were reluctant to have Robert discharged because they were afraid of what he would do outside. They were torn by their desire to get help for him and their concern that conditions at Blockley were unhealthy.

In the fall of 1876, the Smiths decided to move to Albany, New York. Because Robert seemed more manageable, if not better, they decided to take him with them. He made the journey all right, but the new environment seemed to bring on upsetting manic episodes such as he had had in Philadelphia. Within months, the family was again trying to decide what to do with him.

The business they had joined, begun by Mr. Smith's oldest brother, was modestly successful, so the family's financial resources were improved. When Robert's condition worsened, his family took him to a well-known local physician. After futile attempts to treat Robert, the doctor suggested that they take him to the Lunatic Asylum for the State of New York at Utica. The physician assured them that this asylum was a reputable one, much better than Blockley, and he signed a Certificate of Insanity, which helped them get Robert's admission to the asylum approved by a justice of the court.

In the early summer of 1877, Robert was taken to Utica by his father, uncle, and two older brothers. They traveled by boat, a short distance up the Hudson River, and then west on the Mohawk, a journey of some 150 miles.

The Smiths were impressed and encouraged by the asylum at Utica. They were shown the ward where Robert would stay; it was large, cheerful, and well furnished with large windows. None of the other patients were in straitjackets, and the Smiths were told that Dr. Gray, the superintendent, did not believe in mechanical restraints. Rather, he believed in an organized regimen of treatment that involved engaging the patients' minds and bodies in healthy activities, such as walking, bowling, gardening, and the mechanical arts.

Robert improved somewhat at Utica. The frequency and intensity of his manic episodes decreased, and within a year he was able to go home on a parole of about six months. However, he was never able to remain outside the asylum longer than that because his mania would return and intensify. He spent most of his remaining life in the asylum at Utica and died in 1890 from pneumonia, which he caught after a bout with influenza (Hamlin, 1985).

RALPH JONES

Ralph Jones has had a hard life. The third youngest of seven children, he apparently witnessed the suicide of his natural mother when he was 6. His natural father was either unable or unwilling to keep the family together, and all the children were sent to foster homes and orphanages.

Ralph was adopted at age 10 by a minister and a psychiatric social worker. He had a hard time getting along with them. He began dealing and using drugs when he was about 13 years old, abusing pot, phencyclidine (PCP), acid, and alcohol. He may have become an alcoholic by the age of 16. Ralph says that his adoptive parents were kind to him, but he just could not seem to do what they wanted, and after a while relations between them became very strained. At 16, Ralph was brought to the local youth program at the mental hospital because of his drug problems and violent acting out.

He did not complete high school but managed to get a GED while studying mechanics at a local vocational school while living in a group home. Ralph served 18 months in the Army. He was discharged with partial disability, caused by an injury to his left leg which he incurred playing football.

Ralph tends to be violent and lacks self-control when he has been drinking. Because of this behavior, he has lost many different jobs. Once, while drunk, he robbed and assaulted an elderly man in Florida—a crime for which he spent one year in jail. Also, he has been in several accidents, suffering injuries to his head and his back. He complains frequently of back pains.

Within the last five months, Ralph has been in jail twice and also in the state mental hospital. He was jailed on charges of driving while intoxicated. While there, he committed acts that were taken to be suicidal gestures. The first time, he cut his wrists superficially, and the second time, he slashed his throat with a razor blade.

Both times, Ralph was brought straight from the jail to the mental hospital. The second incident occurred only three days before his jail term was to be completed.

A case review was undertaken after three weeks at the mental hospital. Admission notes were reviewed: Ralph was unclean, nonverbal, depressed, and lacking in judgment. He claimed to be suffering from alcohol withdrawal at the time of admission. The doctor who admitted him said that Ralph looked "psychotic" at the time.

A number of features of Ralph's situation came out during the case review. During his previous stay at the mental hospital, he had received shock treatments and was heavily sedated most of the time. He was given Thorazine, a tranquilizer used to control psychotic behaviors and calm patients down, and another drug to counter the side effects of Thorazine. The two psychiatrists he saw noted that he was uncooperative and lacked understanding of his suicidal, violent, alcoholic, abusive behavior.

Today his situation remains complex. First, Ralph admits to several suicide attempts or gestures, dating back to when he was 18, but he is not willing to talk about them other than to say that he is depressed all the time. Second, he has a fiancee, whom he plans to marry within a year. She visits him regularly, dominates communication between him and the staff when she is around, and believes that he would be better off discharged. Also, she reports that he is well behaved, even gregarious, around her family. Ralph has virtually no other social contacts. She has been encouraging him to go to AA meetings and accompanies him when he does attend. In a conversation with a social worker, Ralph said he was afraid that she would press charges for a beating he gave her eight months ago.

Third, Ralph's contacts with his siblings and adoptive family have been minimal. He says he would like to live with his adoptive family, but they absolutely refuse to have anything to do with him. He has had no contact with any of his siblings in over two years. Fourth, Ralph apparently does well at skilled manual work and is only about one term short of completing training *as a mechanic at a vocational school. When asked about his plans for the future, he says that he wishes to complete his schooling, get a job, and then get married. Fifth, he was married in his late teens and fathered two children (ages 7 and 8 now) before getting divorced at age 22. However, it is unknown where this family is and what connection, if any, he has with them.*

Finally, it seems clear that Ralph is a depressed, angry person who can be dangerous to himself and others. His antisocial tendencies seem to have been established early in his life, and they are exacerbated by his alcohol problem. It is not at all clear that he has even begun to work through what was perhaps the central trauma of his childhood, his mother's suicide.

Two weeks ago Ralph was discharged and placed in a community halfway house. Ten days later he was readmitted to the mental hospital (three days ago) after he beat his roommate and then slashed his wrists. The treatment team, composed of a case manager, a nurse, a physician, a social worker, a psychologist, and a teacher, is not sure whether Ralph should be discharged again so that he can pursue the goals he articulates. The team is not convinced that he can handle life outside the hospital. The alcohol problem remains and seems to precipitate actions dangerous to Ralph and others; yet he still has goals, and apparently his fiancee remains supportive. If he were to establish a relationship with someone at a mental health center to secure help for him at his lowest points, and if he were to attend AA meetings and stop abusing alcohol, some members of the treatment team believe that he might be able to get his life together and placed in the community again (Hamlin, 1985).

These case studies describe two treatments of mental illness. As you answer the following questions, you will come to understand better the characteristics of the medical model.

- What problems did Robert Smith face? Ralph Jones?
- What treatments did Robert receive? Ralph?
- Why are these treatments classified as part of the medical model?

 ## The Public Health Model

Definition

Public health is a concept that is sometimes difficult to define. One challenge in defining it is its multidisciplinary nature, which leads to difficulty in understanding it as a whole and defining its operations. We can approach the definition of public health in three ways. One is to define it by examining its historical development, achievements, and health successes. The next section will provide a brief review of this perspective. A second approach is to examine its goal, which is to provide the opportunities and conditions for health as a basic human right. The goal is reflected in its mission: to fulfill society's interest in assuring conditions in which people can be healthy (Committee Study of the Future of Public Health, 1988). Because the concept of health has changed during the 1800s and 1900s, a third approach to defining public health reflects its dynamism and adaptability. For example, until the past few decades, health has meant the absence of disease and disability. Today, health has a more positive meaning—the capacity to live fully, which entails maintaining the physical, mental, and social reserves for coping with life's circumstances in a way that brings satisfaction (Afifi & Breslow, 1994).

The public health model bridges the medical and human service models but is more obviously linked with the medical model. Diagnosis and treatment of individuals using medicine and surgery are the core of clinical medicine. Physicians have delineated parts of the body (anatomy), how they function (physiology), their disorders (pathology), and the agents of disease (etiology). Their goal is to combat disease by repairing the breakdown of the "machinery" (Afifi & Breslow, 1994). Those physicians who are cognizant of social, environmental, and biological factors and see disease as it affects populations have moved toward the public health model.

Public health is sometimes not separable from human welfare. Improving public health means improving education, nutrition, safe food and water supplies, immunization, and maternal and child health. It is particularly difficult to dissociate ill health from poverty.

In conclusion, a number of characteristics of the public health model distinguish it from the other two service delivery models. The public health model, like the medical model, is concerned with individuals who have problems, but it extends the concept of heath care beyond the traditional medical model (Pinkstaff, 1985). In the belief that individuals' problems may be linked to other social problems, the public health model serves larger populations rather than just individuals. Societal control is a prime concern of the public health model, as it attempts to solve many of society's social problems. This model is unique in that it approaches social conditions or problems in two ways. Data are collected from the public at large as well as from examination of the individuals who have the problem in question (Pattison, 1984).

The public health model applies a multicausal approach to studying the causes or origins of problems and emphasizes prevention. The preventive component also distinguishes this model from the medical model. The general aims of the American public health service system include not only a more equal distribution of health care services to all segments of the population (including the elderly, persons with disabilities, and the impoverished), but also identification of social, nondisease problems and methods of attacking their causes and contributing factors. The objective of the public health model is to improve the present and future quality of life and to alleviate health problems that have consequences for society in general.

History

Communicable diseases, poor sanitation, and lack of medical knowledge have been community health problems since ancient times. During the colonial period in North America, smallpox, yellow fever, and cholera were major health problems. Laws such as the Massachusetts Poor Law of 1692 gave local authorities the power to remove and isolate the afflicted. By the end of the 18th century, establishment of the first dispensaries and the first local boards of health had laid the foundations for voluntary organizations and public health agencies.

In the early 1800s, people migrated from the country to urban areas around burgeoning industrial plants. Severe disease outbreaks resulted from the poor nutrition, overcrowding, filth, and excessive work requirements of the inhabitants living in these slums. In 1842, Edwin Chadwick, an English social reformer, wrote a grim account of the conditions in England's slums. This document profoundly affected the development of public health and led to the enactment of the English Public Health Act of 1848. On this side of the Atlantic, Lemuel Shattuck, a Boston city councilman, prepared a report financed by the Massachusetts legislature that presented the first plan for an integrated health program in the United States. The 1842 Chadwick Report in England and the 1850 Shattuck Report in the United States precipitated both a sanitary awakening and social reform that constituted public health at that time (Afifi & Breslow, 1994).

The social philosophies of the early 19th century impacted public health as they reflected two beliefs about disease. The first was that disease was providential. Like poverty and natural disasters such as floods, disease occurred as a result of God's wrath toward an individual. Therefore, the obvious solution to the problem was improved behavior. The second belief linked disease to the disorderly and filthy cities with their unpaved streets, poor drainage, untethered animals, and outside privies. Intuitively, people realized the impact of environmental factors on disease. Many believed that the solution was to eliminate dirt and filth to create a healthier environment.

A report by Lemuel Shattuck in 1850 declared the need for improved sanitation and disease control in Massachusetts and recommended establishment of state and local boards of health, collection of vital statistics, institution of sanitation programs, and prevention of disease (Shirreffs, 1982). Although widely ignored at the time, Shattuck's report has come to be considered the most farsighted and influential document in the history of the public health system (Committee Study of the Future of Public Health, 1988). By 1868, Massachusetts had established the first state public health department in the country.

A second important event was the organization in 1861 of the U.S. Sanitary Commission, the first major public health group in America. It is significant to the public health movement because its efforts were primarily preventive; it alerted the public to the benefits of preventive sanitary measures. Appalled by the poor conditions in army camps and hospitals, a group led by Dr. Henry Bellows, Louisa Schuyler, and Dr. Elisha Harris organized this voluntary citizen effort. A central focus of the commission was to unite all voluntary groups to aid governmental agencies in meeting the physical and spiritual needs of men in uniform. Initially, their efforts were directed toward teaching proper personal hygiene and inspecting and supervising living arrangements in camps and field hospitals. Their later efforts included re-cruiting nurses, distributing supplies, and assisting in communication be-tween soldiers and their families.

Prevention emerged as a major component of the public health movement when Dr. Louis Pasteur and Robert Koch demonstrated that germs—not God or dirt—cause disease. (See box.) The "golden age of public health" (1890–1910) included the discovery of causes for typhoid, tuberculosis, and cholera. Personal cleanliness, inoculations, serums, and hygienic laws became the basis of reform, and preventive medicine developed beyond research and lab diagnosis. Preventive medicine included a social focus, with well-organized public health education programs (Trattner, 1999). Today, the Public Health Service is part of the Department of Health and Human Services (see Figure 4-1). It focuses on interventions aimed at disease prevention and health pro-motion that shape a community's overall profile.

Industrialization and its spread around the world during the 19th and 20th centuries stimulated the problems of communicable disease; these were followed by the difficulties that accompanied epidemics of chronic disease—coronary heart disease, cancer, diabetes, and chronic obstructive lung disease. Public health responded to the first set of problems and has made strides to-

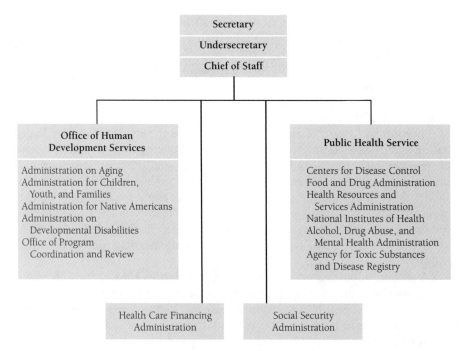

Figure 4-1 ✦ **Organization of the U.S. Department of Health and Human Services**

SOURCE: From "The Future of Public Health," by Committee Study of the Future of Public Health Insti-tute of Medicine, 1988, Washington, DC: National Academy Press.

ward controlling the second. A third group that has emerged in the past two decades consists of HIV/AIDS; domestic, school, and street violence; and substance abuse.

Many changes have occurred in public health over the years. In 1789, the Reverend Edward Wigglesworth assessed the health of Americans and produced the first American mortality tables. By 1900, influenza, pneumonia, tuberculosis, and gastrointestinal infections were the main causes of death in the United States. Average life expectancy at birth was 47 years. This statistic has seen a phenomenal rise, with life expectancy at birth extending to 68 years by 1950, a change attributable to improvements in diet and sanitation and the development of antibiotics and vaccines. By 1997, life expectancy has grown to 76.5 years. Leading causes of death are heart disease and cancer. The leading health problems are chronic diseases (*Healthy People 2000*, 1995).

The Healthy People Initiative, begun in 1979 and reformulated each decade, is the prevention agenda for the United States. It is a national effort to

The Public Health Service

The Public Health Service has a distinguished history that dates back to the late 1700s, when many merchant seamen arrived ill and unattached in American port cities that had little capacity to care for them. In 1798, adopting the British tradition of caring for sick mariners at public expense, Congress enacted a measure, which President John Adams signed into law, that provided for "the temporary relief and maintenance of sick or disabled seamen." The first hospital dedicated to the care of merchant sailors was a building purchased near Norfolk, Virginia, in 1801. The first public hospital actually built with tax revenues, however, was in Boston.

Since that time, almost 200 years ago, the Public Health Service has grown to prominence as a federal enterprise dedicated to promoting and protecting the public's health, with a mandate that often embroils its agencies in controversy. The eight agencies of the Public Health Service are the Agency for Health Care Policy and Research, the Agency for Toxic Substances and Disease Registry, the Centers for Disease Control and Prevention (CDC), the Food and Drug Administration (FDA), the Health Resources and Services Administration, the Indian Health Service, the National Institute of Health (NIH), and the Substance Abuse and Mental Health Services Administration.

SOURCE: From "Health Policy Report: Politics and Public Health," by John K. Iglehart, 1996, *Health Policy Report, 334*, p. 203.

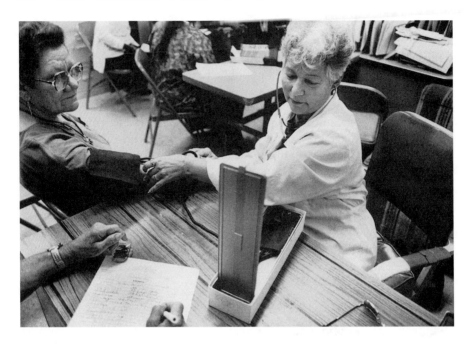

provide a vision for improving the health of all Americans and to guide decisions and actions. Led by the Public Health Service, the initial objectives for
1990 were established in 1980 and expanded for 2000 to include topics such
as HIV infection and cancer. Objectives for *Healthy People 2010* are being developed through a broad consultation process that involves many different
people, states and communities, professional organizations, and other health-
oriented groups. You can check the progress of *Healthy People 2010* on its website (http://www.health.gov/healthypeople).

The major challenge has been to shift the national emphasis to prevention,
with some of the following successes: Since the 1970s, stroke death rates have
declined by 58% and coronary heart disease death rates have declined by 49%;
a 32% decline in the death rate from car crashes is attributed to the increased
use of safety restraints. Unfortunately, cases of AIDS, tuberculosis, asthma, and
birth defects have increased.

The Internet has also greatly influenced health care. Health information
has proliferated so rapidly that no one knows for certain how many World
Wide Web health sites exist. Some estimate the number at between 10,000 and
20,000 (Medicine Online, 1999). In fact, a Harris poll published in February
1999 revealed that over 60 million people searched the Web for health information in the 12 months preceding the poll. This type of information can be a
powerful tool in coping with diseases or maintaining one's health, but often-
times fast and easy access does not equal accuracy of information. Knowing
who puts out the information, checking for frequent updates, and looking for
conformity to the Health on the New Foundation's Code of Conduct (HON
Code) are clues to the accuracy of information. (See Table 4-3.)

TABLE 4-3   ✦   SUMMARY POINTS: HISTORY OF THE PUBLIC HEALTH
MODEL

- The model fulfills society's interest in assuring healthy conditions.
- Massachusetts Poor Law of 1692 empowered governments to act to promote healthy conditions.
- Local boards of health were established by the end of the 18th century.
- English Public Health Act of 1848 was passed.
- Shattuck (1842) and Chadwick (1850) reports apprised citizens of public health problems.
- The U.S. Sanitary Commission was established in 1861.
- Massachusetts established the first state public health department in 1868.
- By the 1900s, public health adopted a social focus.
- In 1979, the Healthy People Initiative was established.
- *Healthy People 2010* is being planned.

Case Studies

The following case study illustrates historical problems that are the primary focus of the public health model. It tells of Sean O'Reilly, who lives in the 1850s in New York City. The study illustrates the living conditions that called attention to public health concerns in America. Especially in larger cities, the problems of immigrants living in poverty greatly challenged public health professionals. The second case illustrates a major public health effort today.

SEAN O'REILLY

Sean O'Reilly, age 25, was the first member of his family to emigrate from Ireland to America. He joined the great numbers of Irish who came to America in the wake of the potato blight that devastated Ireland in the middle of the 1840s. His journey, in a wooden sailing vessel from Liverpool, took 40 days. The voyage was very difficult. Like most poor immigrants, he traveled in steerage, a lower deck below the water line, reserved for third-class passengers. The space was four to six feet high and lined with two berths of wooden bunks. The floor was crowded with baggage, water, and cord wood. The only fresh air for the steerage area came from the hole in the deck for the hatchway.

After the six-week crossing, Sean emerged from steerage looking pale, weak, and 20 pounds lighter than when he started. He had not succumbed to cholera or dysentery, as had several other passengers. The starvation, filth, and crowded conditions he had encountered during the passage to America were just a continuation of the hardships he had experienced in Ireland, which had driven him to emigrate.

The ship docked in New York. Even though Sean did not feel well, he was not eligible for medical treatment from the Marine hospital on Staten Island, as he did not have a communicable disease. Nor did he have enough money to enter Bellevue, the city hospital. He ignored the "runners" who accosted him on board, trying to get him to travel to other cities for a "small" fee. He left the ship and joined hundreds of other new arrivals, mostly Irish like himself, in search of a place to live and a job.

Although Sean had been a farmer in Ireland, he felt that the land had somehow rejected him. He wanted to stay with other Irishmen, near the sea, so he decided to remain in New York City. Sean found work before he found lodging. The first night, he slept in an alley, and the next day he joined a construction gang, moving earth to build roads in the city. The men he met at work suggested that he live with them in a tenement building that housed other newly arrived Irish immigrants. His first Saturday night in America, he was invited to and attended a "kitchen racquet" (get-acquainted party) organized by the family who lived downstairs.

Housing was the most difficult problem Sean faced; laborers' jobs, the sort of work he could do, were plentiful but irregular. Slum lords who took advantage of immigrants in dire need of housing crowded families into small, filthy, dimly lit, poorly ventilated tenements situated on narrow, unpaved streets with inadequate drainage. Partly because there was no integrated health program or municipal board of health, the city was disorderly, dirty, and disease ridden.

From the time he landed, Sean became part of the considerable Irish community in New York. He shared two rooms with a family of six. His living conditions never significantly improved. He held several jobs constructing roads, buildings, and sewage ditches. The jobs involved long hours, hazardous working conditions, low wages, and frequent short periods of unemployment.

Any money he made beyond bare living expenses went to the church and to his small account in the Emigrant Industrial Savings Bank of New York. This account enabled him to bring his family to America through the system known as "one bringing another," in which each immigrant worked and saved for a prepaid ticket for the next member of his family to come to America. By the late 1850s, most of Sean's family had joined him in New York.

REMOTE AREA MEDICAL VOLUNTEER CORPS

Remote Area Medical (RAM) Volunteer Corps is a charitable organization with no paid employees, but uses an airborne force of volunteers dedicated to serving mankind and providing free health care, veterinary services, and technical and educational assistance in remote and rural areas of the United States and around the world. Its history is deeply rooted in the adventuresome nature of its dreamer, designer, and founder, Stan Brock. He lived for many years in the Amazon region of Guyana, South America, where he managed the world's largest tropical ranch. The only medical care was many days' walk away in Georgetown, the nearest city. After ranch owners acquired a small aircraft, he would transport sick or injured people and fly in basic medical necessities. He became a sort of "jungle quack," doing his best to get aid to the rain forest dwellers. When he left there to cohost the Wild Kingdom *television series, he traveled extensively, still discovering people who were medically helpless all over the world. He vowed that some day he would find a way to take medical care to people who had none.*

The vow became reality when RAM was incorporated in March 1985 and subsequently received tax-exempt charity status by the Internal Revenue Service. Since then, there have been as many as 34 yearly expeditions, serving thousands of people and animals on a conservative budget amounting to over $7.5 million. There is a medical record on every person and animal treated. RAM has used the services of over 3,500 volunteers from throughout the United States, Canada, Europe, and South America.

RAM volunteer health care delivery teams consist of physicians and surgeons of all specialties, nurses, dentists, dental assistants, optometrists, opticians, technicians, veterinarians, and administrative and logistical support personnel who travel to destinations as far away as India or who work here in the United States. Team members pay their own expenses and are asked to procure medicines and other supplies. A team might have as few as 10 members or as many as 40.

One of RAM's first expeditions was to Hancock County, Tennessee, where it launched the Rural America program. Expeditions to American destinations now comprise over half of the schedule. On Native American reservations, RAM veterinary volunteers hold spaying and neutering clinics, inoculate pets, and treat over 4,800 livestock a year. In answer to the ever-present crisis of animal overpopulation, RAM also conducts two-day weekend "Fix-a-Pet" clinics in rural counties of Appalachia. A typical Appalachian dental and vision care clinic for people is also open on Saturday and Sunday in communities suffering from a lack of providers and/or having a large unemployed or uninsured population. Hosts of such services are county health departments, housing authorities, humane societies, regional health agencies, or private primary care facilities.

RAM teams go only where they are invited. Word of mouth, an expedition nearby, a news article, and often unknown sources familiarize a group or community with its services and frequently generate invitations. The team carefully assesses the area's needs, visits the site, and when appropriate, arranges an expedition. In addition to activity in this country, RAM has programs underway in Guatemala, Haiti/Dominican Republic, India, and South America. Foreign expeditions can be ten days to three weeks in length, during which team members might treat as many as 4,000 patients.

RAM medical services run the gamut from a basic blood pressure check to full-scale surgery. Operating teams repair cleft lips and palates, remove cataracts, correct eye muscle problems, and perform trauma surgical procedures. Internal medicine, family practice, or emergency specialists provide treatment for skin disorders, intestinal parasites, tropical diseases, and routine ailments and injuries. Dental teams offer emergency extractions and restorative work. Eye care professionals check visual acuity, examine for ocular disease, and dispense free eyeglasses. Thousands of pairs of eyeglasses a year are secured from the Lions Club Eyeglass Recycling program and carried overseas. In this country, RAM's portable optical lab enables skilled technicians to make new glasses to prescription on site.

All providers strive to educate patients, their family members, and the community about the basics of oral and physical health, first aid, hygiene, food handling, clean water, animal management, and self-care.

> *Remote Area Medical is unique in the scope of services it offers, the frequency with which teams are dispatched, its local and international focus, the variety of destinations selected yearly, and the success of its multifaceted mission. It is truly a relief organization by people of the world for people of the world.*

The following questions will help you clarify the role of public health today.

- How do the public health problems in the last case study compare with those Sean O'Reilly encountered?
- How do these two case studies illustrate what you have read about the history of the public health model?
- How do the solutions in public health in the 1850s differ from those today?

 ## The Human Service Model

Definition

A primary focus of the human service model is to provide services that help individuals solve their problems. As Table 4-4 shows, this model differs considerably from the medical model and the public health model. According to the human service model, problems are an expected and even necessary part of everyday life. They occur because human existence is a complex process, involving interaction with other individuals, groups, institutions, and the environment. The human service model considers the problem of the individual within the context of the environment. If an individual must be temporarily removed from the environment to provide effective treatment, then treatment within the context of the environment will continue once the individual reenters that environment.

Individuals are one of the *clients* of the human service system. Clients can include smaller groups such as families, larger geographic populations such as neighborhoods or communities, and populations having problems in common such as the homeless and substance abusers.

The primary method of treatment or service is problem solving, a process focused on the here and now. Problem-solving models range from three to six phases. Generally, the flow of all these models begins with problem identification and advances to decision making and implementation (McClam & Woodside, 1994). It is important, however, to remember that these three phases are not truly discrete units of activity. During problem solving, the boundaries between the various phases and activities become blurred. For example, "problem definition and goal setting are directly related, and the generation of alternatives can occur early in the goal-setting process" (McClam & Woodside, 1994, p. 12). Another example is evaluation, which is not always distinct from implementation and, in fact, occurs throughout the process. (See Table 4-5.)

TABLE 4-4 ♦ AN OVERVIEW OF THREE MODELS OF SERVICE DELIVERY

	View of the problem	Who is the client?	Who is the worker?	Where does treatment occur?	Method of treatment	Goal of treatment
Medical	Individual has a physiologically based illness or disease	Individual who receives services is called *patient*	Trained professional in health sciences (doctor, nurse, dentist, psychiatrist)	Office Institution	Diagnosis Treatment Behavioral prescription Medication Psychoanalysis	Return individual to prior state
Public health	Individual, groups, and society have disease or illness. Environmental and social pressures also contribute to problem	Individuals and special populations or geographic areas (community, neighborhood, state, nation) can be clients	Public health training combines medical knowledge with community action skills	Office Community	Medical diagnosis Prescription Education Mobilization of resources Advocacy for special populations	Prevention Social action
Human services	"Problems in living" problems may be internal, environmental, and/or intrapersonal	Individuals, families, special populations, and environment can be clients	Volunteer Paraprofessional Entry-level human worker who works with abuse, rehabilitation, education, etc. Professionals (rehabilitation or mental health counselor, social worker, psychologist)	Offices/agencies/ institutions serving individuals, families, children Community	Problem-solving process	Enhance client's well-being, quality of life Teach client problem-solving skills Prevention

....

TABLE 4-5 ✦ SUMMARY POINTS: THE PROBLEM-SOLVING PROCESS

- Process focuses on here and now.
- Phases or steps range from three to six.
- Process begins with problem identification.
- Process then moves to decision-making stage.
- Process terminates in implementation.
- Evaluation is important throughout the process.

....

The first phase, problem identification, is particularly critical to the entire process because identification of the problem directs the phases that follow. This phase also includes preparing to solve the problem, a step that often occurs before the client enters the process. Decision making follows problem identification and includes setting goals, generating alternatives, and making a decision. After a decision is made, the third phase, problem resolution, begins. Activities in this stage are planning, implementing, and evaluating the solution.

The problem-solving approach is used in this model for several reasons. First, the process provides a systematic way of thinking about complex situations. Problem identification suggests ways to describe situations in clear, understandable terms, encouraging the client and the worker to prioritize the problems that need to be addressed and discouraging impulsive, reactive behaviors. Second, the effectiveness of the process can be assessed at each stage. If the worker or the client discovers new information or if the problem or the environment changes, then the process can be revised. Third, clients can learn this problem-solving process and use it themselves when they no longer require services. Clients have the opportunity to improve their own problem-solving skills by working with a human service worker to solve problems and by rehearsing the behaviors under the worker's direction. Fourth, the outcomes of the process support the philosophy of human services by fostering client self-esteem and sense of personal responsibility as clients work successfully through the process. In addition, the results of the process improve the quality of life for the client. Fifth, the approach is a tool for identifying other problems that may occur and determining strategies to prevent future problems. (See Table 4-6.)

Philosophy

In its broadest sense, the philosophy of human services was solidified during the 1940s. It included the following beliefs:

- People had the right to expect their society, through its technology and other resources, to prevent their deprivation and provide for their basic human needs.
- The society, through its government, had the irrevocable responsibility for providing people with adequate human services.

TABLE 4-6 ✦ SUMMARY POINTS: HISTORY OF THE HUMAN
SERVICE MODEL

- 1940s—Development of human service philosophy occurs.
- 1950–1990—Community mental health movement expands definition of "good care."
- 1960s—Medical profession recognizes importance of human service goals.
- 1990s—Human service educators recognize common human service themes.

- Meeting people's needs comprehensively and effectively required an understanding of the "whole person" and his [or her] relationship to [the] environment.
- Meeting the "whole person's" needs meant that the resources of many disciplines should be cooperatively mobilized for him [or her] (Eriksen, 1981, p. 53).

Other factors contributed to the development of a human service model. One factor was the community mental health center movement, which grew out of the public health model (Rapoport, 1962). This movement broadened the definitions of care, services, recipients, and goals of intervention (English, Kritzler, & Scherl, 1984). A second contributing factor was the medical field's recognition of the goals of the human service field. The medical profession began stressing patient responsibility for diet, exercise, recreation, and rest. A third contributing factor was the support of President Jimmy Carter, who publicized the fact that Americans did not have access to adequate mental health care. This was attributed to residence, gender, race, and age. Carter's understanding of the mental health dilemma reflects the human service philosophy of the 1940s, with its emphasis on both the responsibilities of society and the importance of working with the whole person.

Most authors agree that a model of human service delivery should include the following characteristics or themes (Burger & Youkeles, 2000; Eriksen, 1981; Harris & Maloney, 1999; Mandell & Schram, 1997a; Mehr, 1998):

1. The *generic focus* is critical in both human service training and delivery. This focus allows for the application of basic helping skills to serving different populations and for other models to provide services to clients most effectively.
2. Services should be accessible, comprehensive, and coordinated. Prevention, restitution, and rehabilitation are equally important parts of an *integrated* service system.
3. The *problem-solving approach* emphasizes the here and now. Included in this approach are the acts of helping the client solve the problem and teaching the client problem-solving skills.
4. Taking into consideration the impact of social institutions, social systems, and social problems, the model works with the person and

the environment. Treating the *whole person* is best accomplished when the worker recognizes client needs in relation to others and to the environment.

5. Human services is *accountable to the consumer.* Clients are active participants in the human service model, making decisions, taking action, and accepting responsibility for themselves.

Case Study

The following case study illustrates several concepts you have read about in this chapter. It presents four possible clients who are experiencing problems and who have different perspectives on their problems. This situation also illustrates both the individual and the family as clients. Let us focus first on the human service model of service delivery.

Consider yourself the human service professional who has received the following case. As you read it, think about these questions:

- How have Susan, Ted, Justin, and Matthew solved problems in the past?
- How do you think each person in the case study will define the problems?
- As you consider problem solving as a systematic way of thinking, how would you as a human service professional approach the problem Susan faces?
- How will the themes and characteristics of human services guide your work with this case?

Susan and Ted met in college, where she was studying to be a teacher and he was studying to be an engineer. Ted was from an upper-middle-class family; Susan, from a religious, working-class family. Even while they were dating, Ted was a heavy "social drinker," but Susan ignored his drinking. She wanted to marry a man with a college education and have a large family. She came from a small, close-knit family and had only one sister. She remembered her family as having few luxuries while she was growing up, but much love and nurturance. Ted's family was also small, but not close. Ted had no contact with his family, even though they lived in the same town as the university.

During Ted and Susan's sophomore year, Susan's grades began to fall. She was on a partial scholarship and was in danger of losing it. She dropped out of school and moved out of the dorm into an apartment with Ted. Then Susan became pregnant. Ted dropped out of school and got a job as a draftsperson for a small local firm. They married.

Leaving behind a happy, carefree life without responsibility, they now faced an uncertain future. Susan tried to be the "perfect wife" her mother had been. She was determined to work before the baby was born and assume the role of homemaker. Ted began drinking heavily. He lost several jobs during Susan's pregnancy and often took his anger out on her by hitting her and keeping her constantly tense and fearful. He turned to drugs, and the relationship de-

teriorated further. After losing several more jobs, Ted had to take a menial, low-paying job just to make ends meet, and his resentment increased. He spent more time away from home, leaving Susan with only the money she was earning for food or transportation. She was alone and depressed but did not confide in her family, because she did not want to upset them.

Often Ted was away for days. As Susan's pregnancy progressed, he became more violent. Once, he beat her so badly that he cracked two of her ribs and broke her nose. He also attempted to strangle her. She told no one and lied to her doctor, coworker, and friends about the injuries. Ted "came to his senses" and tried to make amends, but he began drinking heavily once again and in a fit of rage kicked her in the stomach, bringing on labor. Susan delivered a son in the sixth month of her pregnancy. Justin weighed 3 pounds, 2 ounces, and had difficulty breathing. He was placed in an intensive-care nursery for six weeks before his parents could take him home. During this time, Susan worked and Justin continued to be sickly, suffering from chronic ear infections and colic. Ted had trouble adjusting to his new son, so Susan quit her job and took care of him alone.

Justin had many health problems and was constantly under the care of physicians. He was often hospitalized with pneumonia and severe dehydration. When Justin was 14 months old, Ted deserted them. Susan had no money, no job, and no car. She turned to her parents for a small loan and got a job in a department store making minimum wage. She had to work, but it angered her to leave Justin with a baby-sitter. Being a single parent was difficult. By the time she paid the rent, the bills, and the baby-sitter, there was no money left. She was desperately unhappy but determined to make the best of things.

Several months later, Ted returned. He had a new job making good money and was ready to "work things out." He continued to drink, and he still beat her, but she now wanted him at any cost. He soon learned this fact. One year later, Susan had another son, Matthew. At this point, Ted and Susan bought a house in a small town near the university and proceeded to raise their family. For Ted, this consisted of nightly bouts with the bottle in front of a television set and of forcing himself sexually on Susan. The years passed, and Susan continued to put up with his drinking and rapes. Eventually, Ted's drinking became uncontrollable, and he started abusing the children. One night he came home late, pulled a gun, and shot at Susan. A neighbor called the police; he was handcuffed and arrested. Ted's father, who had previously been completely out of the picture, now came to Ted's aid by paying his bail. This became a regular routine. Each time Ted was out of jail, he would return home to drink and terrorize Susan and the children. After six months, Susan told Ted she wanted a divorce. He became enraged and threatened her. She persisted and engaged a lawyer. Her intention was to return to the university to finish her education and continue with her plans to be a teacher. She had less than two years to go and was confident that with child support, income from a job, and financial aid, this plan was feasible. Until the divorce, Ted refused to leave the house. The boys suffered terribly, seeing their mother beaten and their father handcuffed and taken to jail in a police car.

Currently, the youngest child, Matthew, now 14, works part time while attending high school as a sophomore. He is doing poorly in school but is managing to pass his courses. He likes his job and the money he makes. He is able to help pay for some of the things the family needs. He no longer has plans for college and, indeed, intends to continue working at the pizza restaurant if and when he graduates from high school. Although Matthew's grades have recently dropped from an A to C and D, Justin's grades have suffered the most. He is now failing all his classes and has developed severe behavioral and emotional problems. He skips school, refuses to do his homework, and "hangs out with the wrong crowd." He takes drugs at home and school and sells drugs to his classmates. Justin is extremely depressed and hostile. He carries a knife to school and threatens classmates with it. During one incident, when the victim's parents pressed charges, Justin was suspended from school and referred to the juvenile correctional department. He was placed in a program for adolescents who are dependent on alcohol or drugs. School officials realize that Justin "has problems" but have offered Susan no guidance or support, taking action only when Justin's behavior is life threatening.

Justin received correctional treatment in a private residential hospital. One condition of Justin's admission into the hospital was coverage under his father's insurance plan. As Justin started to improve slightly, Susan discovered that the boys were not, and never had been, covered by their father's insurance. She did not tell the hospital personnel for fear that Justin would be dropped from the program. She felt that the program was his only hope. She has now received bills totaling more than $8,000 that she is expected to pay. She knows she will soon have to admit to the hospital that she cannot pay.

Susan is in trouble financially. She receives free medical aid from the university student clinic but has to find the money for her children's medical care. Last Christmas, a church she joined took up a collection for her and the children and bought them $200 worth of groceries. She requested one month of subsidized utilities from the local utilities company but is eligible for this assistance only one time. She is concerned that she will not be able to afford utilities this month. Ted pays child support only sporadically, and he moves from town to town. Susan never knows where she can find him in case of an emergency and is not certain he would even help. Ted continues to have visitation rights, because he "sometimes" pays child support. She is furious about this privilege but keeps thinking he will eventually take more responsibility for his children. Constantly depressed because of this situation, Susan also fears that bill collectors will start to hound her and that, if an emergency occurs, she will not be able to handle it. She does not know what to do.

As you think about these clients' needs from the human service perspective, you quickly realize that $200 for groceries and one month of subsidized utilities solve only immediate problems. The larger problems that Susan, Ted, Justin, and Matthew face are much more complex and will require comprehensive, coordinated service delivery.

You have learned in this chapter that human service professionals use three primary models of service delivery. In taking charge of this case, you will function within the context of the human service model. To promote the well-being of the whole person and to provide the comprehensive services necessary to that end, you may rely on professionals whose service delivery is guided by the public health model or by the medical model. To minimize duplication of services and to promote coordinated service delivery, you need to maintain active links with other professionals who may work with the same clients as you do.

Now that you are familiar with the history of Susan, Ted, Matthew, and Justin, review the problem-solving process. Select one of the individuals in the case study as your client and ask yourself the following questions:

- What is the mind-set of this client now?
- What problems and subproblems does the client face?
- What alternatives are possible to solve these problems?
- How would you as the helping professional use the human services model in this case?
- How might professionals from the public health model or the medical model facilitate the delivery of services your client needs?

Using models is a helpful way of identifying the different approaches to clients' problems. The distinctions among the models are not arbitrary, for each has a separate history and has developed in response to different social needs. From the human service perspective, however, each model has a part in the problem-solving process. The worker is responsible for blending the models and the treatments or services they represent in response to client needs. Indeed, one strength of human services is the focus on clients' needs and the flexibility to use approaches from various models to meet those needs.

 Things to Remember

1. Three different models represent orientations in service delivery: the medical model, the public health model, and the human service model.
2. Underlying each of the three models is a set of philosophical assumptions that guide the delivery of services and shape beliefs about the causes of problems, their treatment, and the role of the professional in the model.
3. The medical model views the person coming for help as a *patient* whose problem is diagnosed as a disease or sickness and treated by a physician or service provider who prescribes a treatment or cure for the "disease."
4. At the turn of the 20th century, Mary Richmond, author of *Social Diagnosis,* used the medical model to describe social casework.

5. Until the end of the 19th century, insanity was socially defined, but when psychiatry emerged as a medical specialty, insanity became a medical label.

6. Psychotropic drugs are now among the most widely used treatments for mental disorders. Psychopharmacology, the study of the effects of drugs on mental health, is an area of interest to human service professionals.

7. The public health model, like the medical model, focuses on individuals and larger populations; it attempts to solve many of society's social problems.

8. Communicable diseases, poor sanitation, and lack of medical knowledge have been primary community health problems since ancient times. Laws such as the Massachusetts Poor Law of 1692 in North America and the Public Health Act of 1848 in Britain initiated efforts to improve public health conditions.

9. The U.S. Sanitary Commission was the first major public health group in the United States. Its efforts were primarily preventive, alerting the public to the benefits of preventive sanitary measures.

10. A primary focus of the human service model is to provide services that help individuals solve their problems, including a consideration of client problems within the context of their environments.

11. Individuals are among the clients of the human service system, as are small groups, larger geographic populations, populations defined by lifestyle, and populations that have problems in common.

12. The primary method of treatment is problem solving, a process focused on the here and now and encompassing three phases: problem identification, decision making, and problem resolution.

13. The human service philosophy emphasizes both the responsibilities of society and the importance of working with the whole person.

14. Themes characteristic of human service delivery are its generic focus; accessible, integrated services; problem-solving approach; treatment of the whole person; and accountability to the consumer.

15. Using models is a helpful way to identify the different approaches to clients' problems.

Additional Readings: Focus on Mental Illness

Gibbons, K. (1995). *Sights unseen.* New York: Putnam.
The subject of this novel is a manic-depressive mother and the havoc she wreaks on her family.

Neugeboren, J. (1998). *Imagining Robert: My brother, madness, and survival: A memoir.* New York: Henry Holt.
A novelist describes his younger brother's 30-year battle with mental illness, and his own struggle to navigate the nightmarish system of mistreatment and inattentive care that dooms many victims of schizophrenia and manic-depressive disorder.

Slater, Lauren. (1999). *Prozac diary.* New York: Penguin Books.

Lauren Slater, patient, therapist, and author of *Welcome to My Country,* shares what it is like to be cured by America's preeminent selective serotonin reuptake inhibitor.

Simon, C. (1998). *Mad house: Growing up in the shadow of mentally ill siblings.* New York: Penguin Books.

Boston Globe reporter Clea Simon shares her experiences of growing up with two mentally ill siblings as well as conversations with other siblings of mentally ill people about such concerns as the value of individual versus group therapy, what to look for in support groups, and their fears of bearing mentally ill children.

Winerip, M. (1994). *9 Highland Road.* New York: Pantheon Books.

This book was written after the author spent two years following the daily lives of the residents and their 24-hour-a-day counselors in this group home. Winerip spent time talking with them; eating with them; following them into and out of psychiatric hospital wards, day programs, schools, and jobs; reading their records; visiting their families; and talking with their social workers and psychiatrists.

QUESTIONS TO CONSIDER

1. What types of problems lead people to human services?

2. How do people find help?

3. What are helpers like? What are the different ways of categorizing professionals who deliver human services?

4. How do human service professionals provide services to those who want or need them?

PART TWO

Clients and Helpers in Human Services

Part Two focuses on the people who are involved in the practice of human services, either as recipients or as service providers. Chapter 5 introduces the client or consumer—who may be an individual, a group, or a population—and gives examples of these different types. The chapter examines how they get help, barriers they encounter, and their perspective on help.

Chapter 6 shifts to the human service professional, the provider of human services, with an examination of helpers' motivations, values, and characteristics. It also provides an overview of the categories of human service professionals and insights about them. The chapter concludes with a description of the roles and responsibilities of human service professionals.

The primary purpose of Part Two is to further refine the definition of human services by considering the individuals who are involved in service delivery. As you read the two chapters in this part, think about the Questions to Consider.

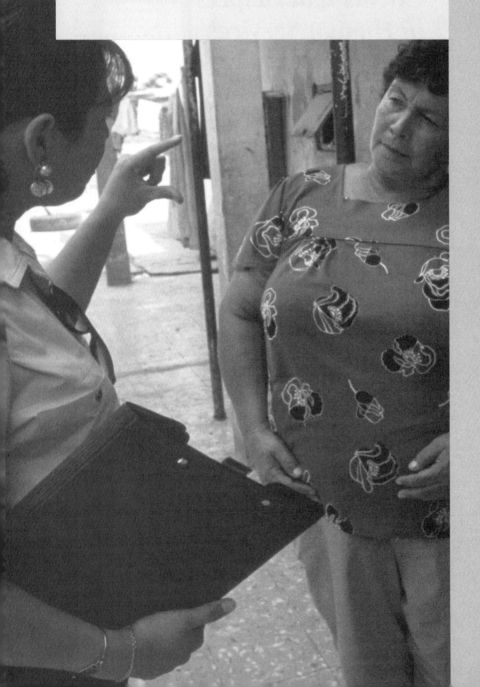

Chapter 5

The Client

The purpose of this chapter is to explore the recipient of human services. This individual may be called a client, a consumer, or a customer. We have elected to use the term "client" since it is most often used in agency settings. Understanding the client is critical to any study of human services. Indeed, the client is the reason there are helpers and a helping process. Part One has already established that some people, in some circumstances, need assistance from others to survive and to develop the ability to help themselves.

In an effort to define the term *client* comprehensively, this chapter introduces several ways of thinking about the user of human services. One way of viewing the client is to study the meaning of the phrase "working with the whole person." This guiding principle in human services focuses on the many components that define an individual and the areas of support a helper must consider when providing assistance.

Describing the problems that clients experience is also an important consideration in defining the client. Problems can be considered in various ways. Several possible theories can be used to define the problems and difficulties that confront individuals. The developmental theory approaches problems from the life span perspective and defines them in terms of life crises or tasks that occur during a lifetime. The situational perspective describes problems that occur from accidents and other traumatic points in time. Meeting human needs, both physical and psychological, is another approach taken to explain the problems that individuals encounter. Finally, one theory posits that social change has a primary effect on the problems individuals experience. Each of these perspectives is defined and its impact on the delivery of human services is described in this chapter.

The term *client* has many meanings. In some cases, clients are individuals; in others, the client may be a small group such as a family, or even a larger population such as the residents of a geographic area. In this chapter you will meet several individuals who are clients: Rufus, who has been in a motorcycle accident; two individuals who share first-person accounts as victims of random violence and nonphysical assault; Elizabeth, a homeless teenager; and a pregnant teenager who is involved in a gang. In the international arena, you will also read about the lives of children who are victims of war and poverty. These accounts will illustrate the concepts introduced in this chapter.

Finally, in defining the client, we explore the experience of getting help from the client's perspective. Sometimes it is difficult for human service professionals who themselves have never been clients to understand thoroughly what it is like to ask for and receive services. We discuss the many ways of getting help, the barriers to be surmounted, clients' expectations, and their evaluation of services.

 ## The Whole Person

Clients enter the human service delivery system as individuals with multifaceted perspectives that include psychological, biological, social, financial, educational, vocational, and spiritual components. These perspectives are integrated within the individual to form the "whole person" that the human service professional encounters. During the helping process, the professional is continually aware that the client does not simply represent "a housing issue," "a food stamp dilemma," or "a child care consideration." Problems for clients are rarely single issues, and the human service professional should approach each client with the expectation of more than one problem. In fact, one problem can cause, influence, or at the very least be related to other difficulties.

The case of Rufus is a good example of how problems in one area influence problems in other areas. The following is from the official record.

> The client, a 38-year-old white male, was involved in a motor vehicle accident while riding his motorcycle. He sustained severe head injury, multiple orthopedic fractures, and cardiac arrest at the scene of the accident . . . evaluated the client in an acute rehabilitation facility 18 months after injury. The client had completed the acute rehabilitation phase of recovery, but because of funding issues, discharge had been delayed. The client was nonverbal . . . although he had some automatic activity of daily living, ambulation and communication functioning. The client needed 24-hour supervision for activity and safety. He was newly married, and his wife worked full time. (McBride, 1992, p. 72)

Rufus was involved in a motorcycle accident and the initial concerns for him were physical. He sustained multiple injuries and experienced cardiac arrest on-site, so attention to his physical well-being was of primary importance. Once his physical condition stabilized, human service professionals involved with planning and providing his care—using the "whole person" perspective—established the following treatment plan that addressed other issues.

> *Current treatment plan.* Client receives 0.5 hour of occupational therapy 1 day a week. Client receives physical therapy for 2 hours per day, 5 days per week or as tolerated. Client has not been able to be tested by speech therapist nor does he respond to attempted intervention.
> *Immobility.* Client is at risk for complications due to immobility. . . .
> *Nutrition.* Client's usual weight is approximately 190 lbs. Client has a very poor appetite . . . current weight is approximately 170 lbs.
> *Verbal communication.* According to therapists and physician, client appears to withdraw from social stimulation . . . been observed to read a newspaper . . . consistently not engaged in eye contact or verbalized with therapists. . . .
> *Bladder and bowel impairment.* Client is incontinent of urine . . . and of bowels.
> *Self-care deficit.* Client is able to assist in bathing and dressing activities . . . he has not demonstrated any consistency in follow-through in step-by-step procedures . . .

Psychological assessment. Client has been consistently followed by a psychiatrist while in the acute rehabilitation facility. Multiple medical regimens have been utilized. . . .

Potential injury. Client is at risk for potential injury . . . appears to need 24-hour supervision and care. . . .

Family/parenting. Client was newly married prior to injury . . . on home visits . . . major problems included mobility . . . and client's behavior. (McBride, 1992, p. 73)

This treatment plan illustrates a multiproblem client who is receiving help in the human service delivery system. Note that, in this case, severe physical problems affect other areas, such as psychological functioning, relationships with family, vocational limitations, and financial difficulties. Although the financial and vocational are not addressed specifically in the treatment plan, advocates for the client are currently trying to find financial resources for him as he does not have long-term care benefits or home care benefits. Vocational needs are addressed by recognizing that the client will not be able to work and will need 24-hour supervision or care.

As a human service professional working with clients, the critical point to remember is that the client is an individual made up of psychological, social, economic, educational, vocational, and spiritual dimensions and possibly will have needs in many of those areas. Even if a client appears only to be looking for housing, the helper realizes that the client may possibly have other difficulties such as unemployment, illiteracy, or a lack of child care. If single problems are solved with little attention to the other difficulties the client is experiencing, then that person may not be able to become self-sufficient.

A majority of clients enter the human service delivery system because they are experiencing problems. Those problems can be defined in many ways.

Perceptions of Client Problems

Problems are a normal part of life. This concept is central to understanding who a client is and what problems the client encounters. As you recall from Chapter 1, the "problems in living" approach, which is basic to our definition of human services, has been a major factor in shaping the human service model (as described in Chapter 4).

Defining Problems

Several definitions of *problem* are useful in discussing problems in living. For example, Epstein (1981) defined a problem as "a situation that is causing trouble, discomfort, difficulty" (p. 170). *Webster's Third New International Dictionary* (1986) expands that definition to include "an unsettled matter demanding solution or decision and requiring considerable thought or skill for its proper solution or decision" (p. 1807). These definitions suggest that problems in living can have two components: a description of the problem and a course of action leading to its resolution. First, the problem is described as a situation, event, or condition that is troublesome for the client. It can be as simple as a pregnant 20-year-old married woman's request for information about prenatal care programs or as complex as an unmarried, pregnant 15-year-old's need for counseling. The second component occurs in several stages: The problem is identified and discussed, solutions are formulated and implemented, and the results are evaluated.

One complicating factor in identifying and resolving problems is the difficulty of predicting what an individual will experience as a problem. Factors such as the cultural values of the society and the developmental needs of the individual influence how problems are defined. For example, an increasingly common problem in this society is care of the elderly. The extended family that once cared for elderly relatives has been replaced by the smaller nuclear family, a unit whose living space and lifestyle are sometimes not suitable for the care of others. American society also tends to view the elderly as people who have already made their contributions and have retired from productive activity. In some cultures, the elderly continue to work; in others, the elderly have a high status though they have stopped working. Pinpointing a problem is also hard in this example because of the difficulty of predicting when elderly individuals will need care and what care they will require. Some people live in nursing homes at age 65, unable to manage independent lives; others are living alone with minimal support at the age of 90.

How clients view their own situations and what they perceive to be problems are important factors in problem identification. Epstein (1981) suggested that client problems have two components. First, the person lacks the resources to solve the problem, and second, the person lacks skills to do so. Given Epstein's definition, the client and the helper may disagree about the client's situation. For example, the helper may believe the client lacks resources or skills, while the client may perceive no problem at all. In the client's environment, unemployment, poor school attendance, and illiteracy may be normal conditions among neighbors and family members. The client experiences these conditions as a way of life, not as situations that must be corrected or problems that need to be solved. The helper, on the other hand, may view these conditions as problems that should be faced and resolved.

Even if clients recognize the existence of problems, there is no guarantee that they will seek assistance. If they do ask themselves whether help will alleviate the problems they have, they may conclude that it will not. They may see the condition as something to be endured, or they may feel that having the difficulty is preferable to seeking assistance. (See Table 5-1.)

TABLE 5-1 ✦ SUMMARY POINTS: CLIENT PROBLEMS

- It is difficult to predict what an individual will experience as a problem.
- The individual perspective is part of the problem definition.
- A person often lacks resource or skills, or both, to solve problems.
- No guarantee exists that an individual will seek help.

Understanding Client Problems

Despite the difficulties of identification, problems are still a useful way to address the identity and needs of the client. It is because individuals have unmet needs that they come in contact with the human service delivery system. The system uses a variety of conceptual frameworks to aid in identifying problems. This section introduces models to address three types of problems: developmental and situational problems, hierarchical needs, and needs created by social change.

A DEVELOPMENTAL PERSPECTIVE

According to developmental theorists, individuals engage in certain tasks or activities at different points in their lives. Describing the developmental process, Sheehy (1995) said, "We continue to develop by stages and to confront predictable crises, or passages, between each stage" (p. xi). Of the same process Levinson (1978) wrote: "An incomplete, highly dependent child grows in complex biological, psychological, and social ways to become, in greater or lesser degree, an independent responsible adult" (p. 1). The change of dependent children into independent adults was studied by Erik H. Erikson, a psychoanalyst and expert in adult development, whose major contribution to the understanding of human development was his description of the "eight stages of man" (Erikson, 1963). Erikson's stages model is one of many perspectives on development. His stages, summarized in the list that follows, reflect the tasks through which individuals work during the different stages.

> *Basic trust versus basic mistrust.* Infants learn to trust in an environment that consistently provides for their needs—that is, one in which the caretaker is sensitive to the needs of the infant. A person who does not experience this warmth and caring in infancy will have difficulty trusting others in later years.
>
> *Autonomy versus shame and doubt.* In this stage, the toddler wishes to "let go" and try new things but does not know the alternatives and consequences of such actions. The child at this stage needs both urging to try new things and gentle protection from the consequences of his or her lack of experience. A toddler who does not experience such support may later be reluctant to try new things and may doubt his or her abilities.
>
> *Initiative versus guilt.* The child who moves beyond the stage of autonomy is able to define a task and work to complete it. *Initiative* means cooperative effort, enthusiasm for new things, and acceptance of responsibility. When a person experiences success at this stage, he or she will generally become an adult who is willing to accept moral responsibility and takes pleasure in developing his or her abilities. A child who does not develop the ability to take initiative becomes an adult who is unable to take risks and meet new challenges.

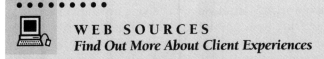

WEB SOURCES
Find Out More About Client Experiences

http://www.isl.net/~hoffcomp/shirley.html

This site explains the progression of Pick's disease as experienced by Shirley Hoffman. The narrative is written by her husband and describes both of their points of view. Symptoms of Pick's disease are similar to Alzheimer's disease and are often misdiagnosed.

http://www.isl.net/~hoffcomp/morris.html

Morris Friedell is a professor of sociology and has been diagnosed with Pick's disease. He describes the early symptoms of the disease, the path to diagnosis, and the prognosis for his life.

http://members.aol.com/depress/mystory/html

Deborah Deren tells a compelling story of her experience and continuing battle with depression. She provides the reader with details about her early experiences, diagnosis, and current struggles. She represents individuals who have successfully battled this disease.

http://www.mentalhealth.com/story/p52.html

This site provides stories of individuals who are struggling with mental health issues. The stories briefly describes experiences of mental illness.

http:www.jersey.net/~joebur/personal.html

This site explains Lyme disease and the disastrous effects it has on the lives of the individuals it strikes. Personal stories are from children, young men and women, and older adults. They also include a parents' description of the loss of their child.

http://canceranswers.org/stories

Presented at this website are stories of four women who are breast cancer survivors. They explain the effects the diagnosis and treatment have had on their lives and the lives of their families. The stories are very different, representing varying reactions and decisions made once the cancer was diagnosed.

http://www.fvpf.org/stories/story_karen.html

Stories best describe the experience of domestic violence. This site includes stories of parent against parent, while others describe the abused wife's point of view. These poignant stories illustrate the tragedies and suffering associated with domestic violence.

http://www.caregiver.on.ca/cgps.html

This site discusses the prices that caregivers pay for helping members of the family.

Industry versus inferiority. In this period of growth, the child begins to experience life as a worker and provider. Receiving instruction and evaluation (in the culture, in school), the child learns to enjoy work and develops good work skills, such as the ability to concentrate and to manipulate the tools of the society. If the child does not develop a sense of being capable, he or she may later have a fear of inadequacy, resulting in poor performance, low expectations, or both.

Identity versus role confusion. In this stage, the adolescent begins to combine the identity formed in the previous stages with the work he or she must accomplish in the future. The stage is complicated by physical growth and sexual maturation. The adolescent rebels against those who previously provided support and relies on peers and heroes and heroines for guidance and care. During this stage, the individual struggles to make sense of an adult world in terms of childhood experiences.

Intimacy versus isolation. The young adult, having formed an identity during the previous stage, desires to establish intimate relationships that may include the components of mutual love, sexual intimacy, and parenting. An inability to establish intimacy with others may result in isolation.

Generativity versus stagnation. The adult assumes the responsibility for "parenting" the next generation, guided by the children's needs, as described for the previous stages. This parenting responsibility is required of all adults, not just those who are biological parents. During this stage, acceptance of this role helps the adult avoid stagnation and loss of purpose.

Ego integrity versus despair. The ego integrity that is possible at this stage represents the culmination of the successful development of identity through the previous seven stages. The older adult understands and accepts life as it has been experienced, assumes responsibility for that life, and accepts death as the final part of the life cycle.

Developmental theorists view life as a *process* from birth until death, from the beginning to the end. Although everyone goes through the same developmental stages, individuals experience these stages in different ways. Development may be affected by the social context in which the individual lives—the home, family, community, culture, country, and sociopolitical climate. A person's characteristics, including traits, wishes, values, and childhood experiences, may also influence the way that person experiences each stage. Determining the stage on which the individual is working is sometimes difficult. Moving from task to task and from developmental stage to developmental stage are not activities as discrete as having a birthday or completing a list of jobs or chores. Sometimes an individual is deeply focused on the tasks of a certain developmental stage, but there are also times of transition between stages, when the tasks are being completed and the individual is only beginning to formulate the questions that will signal the next stage (Levinson, 1978).

An individual is deeply focused on a specific developmental stage at a time of intense questioning and exploring. A developmental stage begins when the tasks of that stage are of primary importance, and the stage ends when the individual's focus has changed (Levinson, 1978). For example, a toddler who has learned to walk may want to explore every nook and cranny at one instant but be paralyzed by a new environment a moment later. When the child's focus changes from the independence of walking to the independence of exploring new environments, his or her developmental tasks have changed.

There is a dimension of quality to the completion of developmental tasks. Even if a task is finished, it is not necessarily finished well. As mentioned earlier, developmental tasks are addressed within the individual's social context, and that context may not support individual development. In addition, how the individual has completed previous developmental tasks affects his or her work on the next stage. An individual may not reach the next stage with the necessary skills or confidence to continue developing.

Sheehy (1995) suggested that, in Western culture, the "normal activities and tasks for each stage are changing." Citing examples of 9-year-old girls developing breasts, 9-year-old boys carrying guns to school, 40-year-old women having their first children, and 50-year-old men being forced into retirement, Sheehy sees a life cycle that has changed. Puberty is earlier, adolescence is extended into the 20s, middle age extends well into the 50s, and the activities of the elderly are broadening. According to a recent population study, there has been a ten-year shift in the life stages. When developmental theories are used to identify problems that individuals experience, an important point to remember is that these traditional stages are changing. Even the concept of "elderly" or "being old" is shifting as we see increasing longevity.

One way to understand the concept of defining problems by theories of psychosocial development is to study specific examples, such as the relationship of middle-aged mothers and adolescent daughters, which follows. It illustrates the developmental tasks of individuals in the *identity* (adolescent daughter) and the *generativity* (middle-aged mother) stages. Bassoff (1987) explained the problems that may arise when individuals work on particular tasks in their developmental stage and described how additional problems can develop when individuals in a family are focused on the tasks of different stages.

Adolescent development is a difficult period for young people, who are involved in a struggle for identity. Family harmony and individual well-being are threatened during this adolescent rebellion. Mother–daughter relationships are particularly vulnerable, because the daughter rejects not only adults in general but in particular the one adult with whom she has greatest similarity—her mother. The daughter's developmental tasks in the identity stage focus on separation from parents, which involves a growing independence. The adolescent daughter rejects her previous world of family and forms her own world with personally chosen friends of both sexes.

During this time, the middle-age mother is involved in developmental tasks of her own, as she reassesses her purpose in life. She is facing the end of her power as the "giver"—relinquishing her role as a primary caregiver in the family. (This assessment applies both to women who remained home to raise their children and to those who held outside jobs and pursued careers while raising their children.) The mother must change roles and develop new ways of relating to her family and friends. Time that had been devoted to caregiving tasks is now freed up, and she may begin to use that time for her own personal growth and development. Also in this stage, the mother begins to understand that life is not perfect and tries to view relationships and situations more realistically.

An ideal situation exists when the daughter and the mother can grow together. During this time, each may be involved in developmental tasks that can complement the other's. When the tasks are in step, the mother allows the daughter to separate, for two reasons. The mother understands that the daughter's separation is a necessary (albeit difficult) growth process for the daughter. Also, the mother does not feel personally hurt when the daughter rejects her, because the mother is attempting to reduce her role as caregiver and to relinquish the power as "giver" that she has held over others. The mother uses her daughter's questioning as an occasion to reevaluate her own life plans and purposes. The daughter is allowed to rebel and to reject the family and the tradition it represents without losing the basic support of the family. At the same time, the daughter is given more control and autonomy; as she separates, she also assumes more responsibility for her actions (Bassoff, 1987).

Unfortunately, most individuals do not operate in the world of the ideal. Problems arise when, as in this example, individuals are engaged in difficult developmental tasks. If the mother is feeling insecure about losing her primary role as a caregiver, she may continue to smother the daughter and resist any independent actions the daughter takes. When the daughter rebels, the mother, who views herself primarily as a caregiver, feels personally rejected by the daughter. The daughter may intensify her rebellion by running away, acting out in school, and verbally and physically abusing the mother. The daughter may also refuse to assume any responsibility for her behavior. Pressure from the mother–daughter conflict not only can ruin that relationship but also can threaten the stability of relationships with other family members.

The problem just described is one example of the problems in living that arise as individuals work on developmental tasks. Using a developmental model to view problems may be helpful to the human service worker, because it provides the worker with a basic understanding of the process of growth and change that individuals normally experience. Workers can use Erikson's stages to help describe problems in terms of current tasks that require the client's focus, as well as to determine whether the previous developmental tasks have been adequately completed.

Human service professionals can also use developmental models to provide a framework for identifying problems not regarded as normal. For example, certain problems associated with mental illness (such as hallucinations and delusions) and with criminal behavior (such as aggressive, violent behavior) are labeled deviant. In any attempt to account for this deviance, Erikson's developmental model is a starting point for identifying whether a problem can be

TABLE 5-2 ✦ SUMMARY POINTS: ERIKSON'S DEVELOPMENTAL
PERSPECTIVE

- Individuals engage in certain tasks or activities at different times during their life.
- Stages are experienced differently by each person.
- The social context affects movement through developmental stages.
- Traditional stages are changing as society changes.

categorized as a problem in living or as a departure from the expected. With clients who have very serious problems not classified as problems in living, it may be necessary to use several problem identification models. (See Table 5-2.)

A SITUATIONAL PERSPECTIVE

Another way of viewing problems in living is from the situational perspective. Problems resulting from accidents, violent crimes, natural disasters, and major changes in life—such as a move, job change, or divorce—are all defined as situational problems. The characteristics of these problems are very different from those of the developmental problems discussed in the preceding section. First, these problems usually occur because the individual is in a particular place at a particular time. It is difficult for individuals to "be in the world" without experiencing some situational problems. Such problems can occur even if the individual has not done anything to contribute to or cause them. In such cases, individual responsibility begins once the situation has occurred and is identified as a problem situation. Linking situational problems with a specific event may be difficult because the event might be only a marker of a more complex situation. For example, with divorce or a geographic move, there are obviously contributing factors that precede the event. However, the problem may still be characterized as situational because of the existence of the marker—a clear problem on which the client and the human service professional can focus.

Another characteristic of situational problems is that they can lead to short-term or long-term difficulties, or both. Most such problems require, at a minimum, immediate action. The complexity and quantity of assistance required depend on the severity of the problem and the state of the client when the situation occurs. Situational problems may require additional help after the short-term assistance has been provided. Yet another characteristic is that individuals experiencing situational problems are often viewed as victims— persons who suffer injury from their own fault or that of others. One of the first responsibilities of the helper is to move the client from the role of victim to the status of taking responsibility for personal actions and thoughts.

I first became involved with human services in January. As a victim of aggravated assault, attempted murder, and mayhem in a case of random violence, my situation was severe. As the result of the assault, I was blinded in my right eye and impaired in my left eye. The first person I saw was my physician, who gave me the prognosis and told me what medical treatment I would need, including surgery. The second person was a hospital administrator, who told me I had no major insurance that would cover my needs and the costs of surgery. The third person I talked to gave me hope. He was a case manager who worked with victims of violent crime. He talked with me for two hours about what legal processes were involved, how to apply for assistance, and whom to see in the different agencies. He told me to have faith in the system. And he told me that his job was to help link me to services that I need and then monitor progress.

Violent crime, such as the assault just described, is a situational problem experienced by Americans every day. Problems also include the unreported violence that occurs behind the doors of homes, workplaces, and institutions and the nonphysical assaults that go unreported. The emotional sufferings of these victims can be the most serious result. One explanation for this finding is the damage that occurs after the crime to previously psychologically healthy individuals. After the crime, even healthy individuals are likely to experience depression, anger, shame, and anxiety. They begin to question their previous sense of social order and to redefine their ideas of fairness and justice. Women in particular experience a sharp increase in physical and psychological stress after such victimization, feeling both powerless and helpless. The following account describes the fear and terror that accompanied a nonphysical assault.

It was an ordinary day like any other, exceptionally cold and dreary. The walk to class was an ordinary walk, exceptionally quick in order to keep warm from the cold. Few walkers were walking so the pace and the tempo were the only interests keeping me alert. A hand, his hand, dipped to below his belt whereupon he unzipped his pants. Odd, I thought. In order to keep warm, I kept walking. Not only was he unzipping his pants but he was showing me the most private part of his body. The only tempo I felt now was that of pounding beating inside my chest in sheer and utter panic. I was moved to another place, another time, another element. I panicked. I was terrified. What would he do from here? The ordinary day became a tangled net of confused thoughts, options. Where do I go? Where was he? Where did he go? Was he behind me? Watching me? Would he try to get me, touch me, hurt me? The numbers were all mixed up in my head. They were simple numbers. I know them. The police dispatch woman talked me through the incident quicker than it happened. Sirens, lights flashed, and uniformed men pounced. Safety. Was it safe? Am I safe? Can I move? Breathe? Walk? Think? Was it a dream? Did this just happen to me? The litany of questions confirmed my story as truth. The story was told again. And again. And yet again. The story will be told a fourth time on Tuesday to a judge and then again to an administrative hearing board for the university. My story. Will he be convicted? Will he go to jail? Will he be ex-

*pelled from this university? He never touched me, yet he scarred me irrepara-
bly. The terror and the fear will never escape me.* (Willis, 1999)

Another situation that creates problems is unemployment. Corporate downsizing, closing of mills and factories, and the high rate of small-business failures are factors that have made unemployment a situational crisis for many individuals. One example is Don Harris of Joliet, Illinois.

As the morning sun glints off the windshield of his rusty brown van, Don Harris crosses the hump of the steel drawbridge on the Des Plaines River into Joliet, Illinois, with a load of magazines he delivers for $72 each week. The job helps Mr. Harris soothe a stung pride. After 26 years with one company, he recently lost a $29,000 position as a grocery-store manager and had to resort to food stamps. (Tyson, 1995, p. 10)

These new unemployed are finding it difficult to secure jobs comparable to the ones they lost. Many are now working in retail outlets and shopping malls. Their jobs are part time or temporary, pay less than their previous jobs, have fewer benefits, and often provide less job satisfaction. Overall, the affected individuals feel ashamed and unappreciated. The situation also creates economic difficulty that the whole family faces as the chief breadwinner's ability to provide the basics such as food, clothing, and shelter is threatened. (See Table 5-3.)

MEETING HUMAN NEEDS

Another way of defining human problems is to identify basic human needs and ask, "Which of these are being met and which are not being met?" Abraham Maslow developed a hierarchy of needs that is helpful in the problem identification process. Maslow's hierarchy begins with the most basic of physical human needs and ends with the need of individuals to become self-actualized, to strive to develop their understanding of themselves and their environment (see Figure 5-1).

According to Maslow, these needs exist in a hierarchy, which means that individuals cannot address higher-order needs until their most basic needs have been met. If an individual is hungry, cold, scared, or in a life-threatening situation, this person will have difficulty concentrating on love and belonging

TABLE 5-3   ✦   SUMMARY POINTS: SITUATIONAL PROBLEMS

- Such situations occur because an individual is in a particular place at a particular time.
- Problems can lead to short- or long-term difficulties or both.
- Experience results in a variety of feelings for the person.
- A person experiencing situational problems is often viewed as a victim.

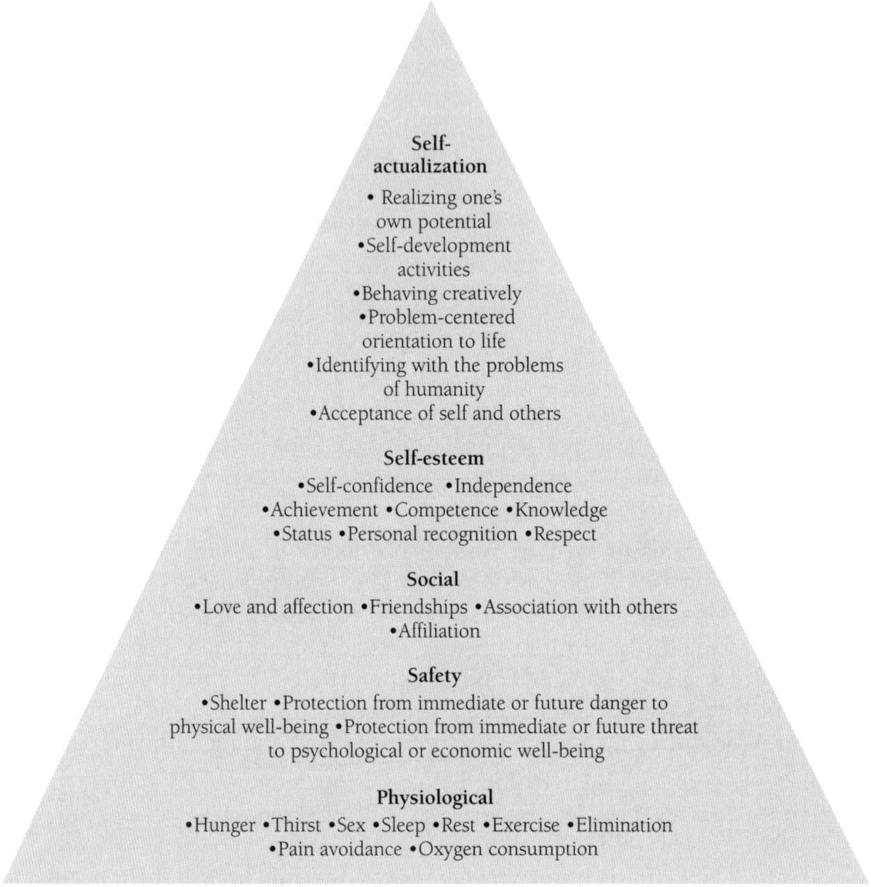

Self-actualization

• Realizing one's
own potential
•Self-development
activities
•Behaving creatively
•Problem-centered
orientation to life
•Identifying with the problems
of humanity
•Acceptance of self and others

Self-esteem
•Self-confidence •Independence
•Achievement •Competence •Knowledge
•Status •Personal recognition •Respect

Social
•Love and affection •Friendships •Association with others
•Affiliation

Safety
•Shelter •Protection from immediate or future danger to
physical well-being •Protection from immediate or future threat
to psychological or economic well-being

Physiological
•Hunger •Thirst •Sex •Sleep •Rest •Exercise •Elimination
•Pain avoidance •Oxygen consumption

Figure 5-1   ✦   Maslow's hierarchy of needs

SOURCE: Adapted from *Fundamentals of Psychology*, by A. Haber and R. P. Runyon, p. 304. Copyright ©
1983 by McGraw-Hill Publishing. Adapted by permission.

needs. Likewise, people who get little acceptance or respect from others will have difficulty involving themselves in activities that will lead to self-actualization. Brammer (1999) suggested that the needs can be divided into two categories: "D" needs (*deficiency* needs) and "B" needs (*being* needs). "D" needs comprise the first four levels, wherein an individual seeks to achieve calm and satisfaction. After these "D" needs are met, the individual seeks to achieve the "B" needs and concentrates on developing the self.

The importance of meeting basic needs is a primary consideration in the case of child abuse and neglect. According to Child Abuse and Neglect National Statistics, in 1997, child protective services agencies investigated 2 million reports alleging maltreatment of almost 3 million children (National Clearinghouse on Child Abuse and Neglect Information, 2000). When children are abused and neglected, many of their basic needs are threatened, including their physical, safety, social, and self-esteem needs. Even though experts agree on the needs that are not being met, they have not always agreed on the way to restore children to a supportive environment.

During the l960s and 1970s, the emphasis was on removing the child from the home and placing the child in foster care. During the 1980s, the approach was to leave children in the home and provide services to parents that helped them better meet their children's needs. Today, the debate continues about whether foster care or family reunification is the best approach to meet the children's basic needs.

On a larger scale, natural disasters such as hurricanes, tornadoes, floods, and earthquakes may result in human needs by many people at the same time. Immediate needs may be physiological, safety, or both (e.g., food, clothing, shelter, and water). When these needs are met, concern shifts to higher-order needs. Moving from a shelter to more permanent housing, returning to school and jobs, and dealing with the longer-term emotional effects of a large-scale disaster will be the focus of many victims.

SOCIAL CHANGE AND ITS EFFECTS

Axelson (1999) suggested another view of the problems of human existence. Human beings experience problems not just because of their needs as individuals but also as a result of rapid social changes, the breakdown of many traditional forms of society, and conflicts between old and new values. In this century, many changes have occurred rapidly in society—sometimes explosively. Rapid social change leaves individuals in unfamiliar situations. Often, people do not have the skills, self-confidence, and support from others to adjust to changing demands. You can imagine the alienation and isolation experienced by people who retain the "old" way or who are no longer part of the mainstream of society as a result of changing urban areas and population shifts to suburbia. The homeless constitute one such group. Today that definition has expanded to include children, individuals with a dual diagnosis of mental illness and substance abuse, and those who live in the rural areas.

Homeless people have a variety of needs. This group can serve to illustrate the developmental and situational perspectives, as well as the approaches of Maslow and Axelson. Most people know there are homeless individuals, either from seeing coverage of their situation in the media or actually seeing homeless people in their community. In the discussion that follows, you will see that the homeless have multiple needs. Very basic survival needs come first; without a home, existence becomes a struggle to secure food, shelter, rest, and safety. However, homeless people also need recognition and acceptance by the community.

Few people choose to be homeless, yet many individuals find themselves in this situation as the result of rapid social change, unemployment, fire and flood disasters, or eviction. The homeless are single men and women and poor elderly who have lost their marginal housing, ex-offenders, single-parent

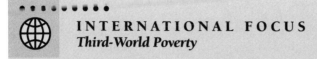

INTERNATIONAL FOCUS
Third-World Poverty

The following case study illustrates the effects of poverty on the physical and mental development of some citizens of the world. As you read about Fatima, Jaime, and Francisco, consider the following questions:

1. Which of Maslow's needs have been met? Which have not been met?
2. What are the consequences of these unmet needs?
3. How do the unmet needs influence Francisco's ability to develop according to Erickson's model?

HOW PEOPLE UNDERDEVELOP

Francisco's mother, Fatima, is small for her age. She is visibly weak, distant, yet easily irritated by the children. Years of pregnancy and menstruation, along with an iron-poor diet of maize, have made her chronically anaemic. Her husband, Jaime, is a landless laborer, with a low, erratic income barely enough to keep them all alive and clothed. No one eats enough, and when there's not enough to go round Fatima goes without, even when she's pregnant. And that is frequently, as the couple uses no form of contraception. They have had ten children, six of whom survived to adulthood.

Fatima went through several periods of undernourishment while Francisco was in her womb. There were times when Jaime could not get regular work and everyone went hungry. Fatima also had several attacks of stress and anxiety when Jaime beat her. Francisco probably suffered his first bout of growth retardation, both mental and physical, before he even saw the light of day.

He was born underweight, and his brain was already smaller than normal size. For the first few months he was breast-fed and suffered few infections, as he was partly protected by the antibodies in his mother's milk. Then he was weaned onto thin gruels and soups, taken off the breast and put onto tinned evaporated milk, thinned down with polluted water from the well. His diet, in itself, was inadequate. Then he started to get more and more infections, fever, bronchitis, measles and regular bouts of gastroenteritis. With well-fed children these pass within a few days; but in his case they went on for weeks and sometimes a month or more. In these periods he could tolerate no milk and few solids, and so was given weak broths, tea or sugar water. By now he was 25 percent un-

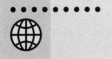

derweight. Because of poor nutrition, he was even more susceptible to infection, and each time he was ill, he lost appetite, and ate even less. Then he got bronchitis which developed into pneumonia. But Fatima borrowed money off a relative, went to town and got antibiotics for him.

So he survived. But malnutrition made him withdrawn and apathetic. His mother got no reward from playing with him, so he received little of the stimulation his brain needed to develop properly. As he grew older, infections grew less frequent, but by the time he went to school, aged eight, he was already a year behind normal physical development and two years behind mentally. The school, in any case, was a poor one, with only three classes, no equipment, and a poorly qualified teacher. As Francisco was continually worried about whether and what he was going to eat that day, he was distracted, unable to concentrate, and seemed to show little interest in schoolwork. The teacher confirmed that he was a slow learner, and could not seem to get the hang of math or reading and writing. As the family was poor, they did not want to keep him on at school. He was doing so badly anyway that there seemed no point. He did a year, then was away for three years helping an uncle who had a farm, then did another year, then left for good, barely able to read or write more than a few letters. He soon forgot what little he had learned. So, like his father, he began tramping round the local ranches asking for work. Without any educational qualifications or skills, that was all he could ever hope for. And because so many were in the same boat, pay was low. When he was twenty-two he married a local girl, Graciela, aged only fifteen. She too had been undernourished and was illiterate. She soon became pregnant and had to feed another organism inside her before she herself had fully developed. Graciela had heard about family planning from a friend, but Francisco would not let her use it and anyway she was not sure she wanted to. So, by the age of only twenty-five, Graciela already had five children and had lost two. The children had every prospect of growing up much as Franciso and Graciela did, overpopulating, underfed, in poor health and illiterate.

households, runaway youths, "throwaway" youths (abandoned by their families or victims of family abuse), young people who have moved out of foster care, women escaping from domestic violence, undocumented and legal immigrants, Native Americans leaving the reservation after federal cutbacks and unemployment, alcoholics and drug abusers, ex-psychiatric patients, and the so-called "new poor" who are victims of unemployment and changes in the job market (Rivlin, 1986, p. 4).

Accurate statistics describing the homeless have been difficult to obtain; the very nature of the problem makes counting difficult. In many cases, homelessness is a temporary circumstance rather than a permanent condition. The National Coalition for the Homeless (1997) suggests a better measure of the magnitude of homelessness is the number of people who experience homelessness over time, not the number of homeless people. It is estimated that 760,00 people are homeless on any given night, and 1.2 to 2 million people experience homelessness during one year. (National Law Center on Homelessness and Poverty, 1999).

People are homeless for any number of reasons. One is that the technological society in which we live has eliminated many unskilled and semiskilled jobs; downsizing and closing of factories has been the direct cause of job loss. In fact, employment-related problems such as unemployment and low wages represent the primary reason why individuals are homeless. A second reason is urban renewal or gentrification, which many municipal governments promote as a way to revitalize the downtown areas of cities. This movement has brought a decrease in low-cost housing, displacing individuals without providing any alternative affordable homes. Even in Atlanta, Georgia, in preparation for the 1996 Olympics, a new ordinance was passed prohibiting living on the streets, and there was stricter enforcement of the antiloitering and panhandling ordinances (Smothers, 1996). The changing structure of the American family has also contributed to the growth of this population. Because the nuclear family is more isolated than in previous generations, such events as divorce and the death of a spouse have forced individuals (and in some cases, whole families) to adapt to a lower level of survival. Finally, deinstitutionalization, which many blame for most of the homeless population, in fact accounts for only 20% or 30% of this group (Kondrates, 1991; Nooe, 2001; Torrey, 1997).

The plight of people who are homeless for one or more of these reasons continues to be a problem as the number of public support programs decreases. As this group becomes more visible and society better understands their situation, perhaps more assistance will become available to help them reenter the mainstream of life. Today, almost one-half of all psychiatric patients are substance abusers and are categorized as dually diagnosed individuals who are difficult to serve. They have greater risk than any other single group for rehospitalization, violence, suicide, poor self-care, and homelessness (Blankertz & Cnaan, 1995). The homeless individuals who are dually diagnosed also have high rates of interaction with the criminal justice system and have few family relationships they can use for support. Because of their history of medical noncompliance, they are never stable enough to receive services for any substantial length of time and they usually enter the human services delivery system only in a crisis (Blankertz & Cnaan, 1995).

Families with young children are among the fastest growing segments of homeless. Although some are without family and friends, many have relatives or other social ties, but they believe those in their support network would not "take them in" for more than a day or two. Urban schools are struggling to provide educational opportunities for homeless children. The schools are faced with a challenge to educate during a time when children do not have a stable home and do not know where they will be living from day to day. There is also a growing number of teens who are homeless and not living with a parent or older adult.

Many refer to children in homeless situations as victims for they have "high rates of developmental lag, academic failure, shyness, dependent behavior, aggression, short attention span, withdrawal, depression, and anxiety" (Nord & Luloff, 1995, p. 462). The following story illustrates one teen's experience. Elizabeth became homeless when her parents threw her out of the house with only the clothes on her back.

From April to October, Elizabeth lived in eight different places. She has lived in houses and trailers, with friends and alone. She lived in a friend's trailer by herself during the summer. He used the trailer every weekend, so she would have to move out during the weekends. Elizabeth lived with some friends for a couple of weeks, then would have to find a new place. She lived with one boyfriend and his parents for over a month. Currently, she lives with a boyfriend and his two siblings; she has lived there for 2 weeks. "I'm very embarrassed about my situation and I always try to hide it from the other kids. It's really not my fault, but I feel guilty," she says. "I don't have hardly any clothes so I don't feel I look as good as the other girls at school. If some of the people I lived with hadn't given me a few clothes I wouldn't have anything to wear." (Nord & Luloff, 1995, p. 469)

Homelessness, once thought of as an urban problem, has now become a serious problem for those in the rural areas. Research indicates that families, single mothers, and children comprise the largest group of people who are homeless in rural areas (Vissing, 1996). Not as much is known about the rural homeless as the urban homeless. More information is needed to determine whether the rural homeless experience is different from the urban one in order to address the needs of this group. (See Table 5-4.)

TABLE 5-4 ✦ SUMMARY POINTS: HOMELESSNESS

- Basic survival, security and safety, and recognition and acceptance are needs.
- Homelessness results for a variety of reasons.
- An accurate measure of the magnitude of homelessness is the number of people who are homeless over time rather than one night.
- Families with young children, dually diagnosed individuals, teenagers, and rural individuals comprise large groups of homeless.

To improve your understanding of how human service workers understand this complex client group—the homeless—think of some homeless people in your community. As this group becomes more numerous and more visible, you may see them sleeping beside buildings or rummaging through
garbage cans. Think of an individual you have seen, and describe his or her
physical appearance. How old do you think this person is? How do you imagine this person spends an average day? Where in your community does this
person stay at night? How might this individual fit into the categories of the
homeless as described? Identify five problems that your homeless individual
has. Which problems are represented in Maslow's hierarchy? Which problems
are associated with rapid social change?

• • • • • • • • • •

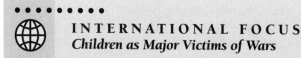

INTERNATIONAL FOCUS
Children as Major Victims of Wars

A report issued by UNICEF in 1996 says that children are now the major victims of war. According to the report, during the last ten years, over
2 million children have been killed in wars that have devastated civilian
populations. The report also stated that from 4 to 5 million children have
been disabled, 12 million are homeless, and over 1 million have lost or
become separated from their parents. In addition, over 10 million of
these children are suffering psychological effects resulting in trauma
caused by their war experiences. The report proposes that an antiwar
agenda be adopted that targets improving and protecting the lives of
young children (Crossette, 1995).
   Some recommendations are as follows:

  • Raise the age of military involvement from 15 to 18 years of age.
  • Draft a child impact statement each time economic sanctions are consid-
    ered internationally.
  • Outlaw land mines, which maim or kill children.
  • Prosecute those who commit war crimes against children.
  • Allow children to reside in "zones of peace" where they can receive food
    and medicine during wartime.
  • Impose limited cease fires to protect and serve children's needs.
  • When war is over, provide rehabilitative services to children.

A poignant story of one young Vietnam girl's experience illustrates
the pain that children experience (Sciolino, 1996). Documented on film
by American journalist Nick Ut, 9-year-old Phan Thi Kim Phuc was running into the camera; she was naked and her arms were waving, she was
caught by the lens screaming in agony with napalm burns over her body.
In June 1972, there was fighting between the North and South Viet-

Clients as Individuals, Groups, and Populations

This chapter has presented approaches to identifying problems through understanding human needs. This section examines three ways to think about the term *client,* using a brief client history to illustrate different perspectives about client identity.

In many cases, the client will be an individual. In fact, most of us will think about each of our clients as one person. In the following case history, you will read one person's account of her life. Think about her as your client. As you read, make note of the facts you learn about her and her situation. What are

namese troops in the Central Highlands of the South. The order was made to drop napalm bombs and they fell near a pagoda where Phan Thi Kim Phuc and her family were hiding. Two of her brothers were killed and she and another brother survived but were badly burned. The photographer took her to the hospital where she spent the next 14 months in rehabilitation. She had numerous grafts in an attempt to rebuild her body. During that time she was in intense pain and the medical staff said that she fainted and lost consciousness whenever her wounds were touched or washed. The world lost sight of her until a Dutch film crew found her in 1984. Later she moved to Cuba and tried to study, but she had to quit after she developed severe asthma attacks and diabetes that impaired her sight. In Cuba, she married a fellow Vietnamese man and traveled to Moscow for the honeymoon. When the plane landed in Newfoundland for refueling, they did not reboard. She sought her freedom in Canada, where she and her husband for a time were on welfare. Today he holds two jobs. She recently returned to the United States in an effort to forgive those who injured her and others in her country (Sciolino, 1996).

Today, Phan is still not free of reminders of the war. She has constant problems with asthma, diabetes, and migraine headaches. She also does not have sweat or oil glands and is in constant pain. "When the weather changes, the pain comes—like I am cut, cut . . . I try to keep down my pain, thinking, thinking to control my pain. I ask my husband, 'Tell me stories, funny stories, or ask me something,' so I have to answer him. And that is the way I can live day by day. And I never think something sad" (Sciolino, 1996, p. A8). But she says that she is blessed, for she is a wife and a mother of a son, 3-year-old Thomas. She says that in her house she is always smiling.

her problems? Using the models discussed in the previous section, apply what you have learned to help you understand her situation.

When I was 12 years old, my mother and her boyfriend left me with my grand-mother and never returned. Momma told me they would be gone for the week-end and would pick me up on Monday. That was four years ago. My grand-mother tried to do right by me, but she is old and can't get around very well. After Momma left, I was angry, hurt, and sad. How can a mother leave her child and never want to see her again? I managed to finish the school year, but my grades were down and I was absent a lot. The guidance counselor at my school talked to me about the importance of staying in school and working hard. That might be important to kids who have a family, but I was alone. School was just a place for other kids to make fun of me and call my mother names. When kids laughed at me, I wanted to die. I couldn't take it. I started fighting back. I was suspended from school for "consistent and persistent, dis-ruptive behavior." It wasn't my fault that I had to fight. I only went off when kids picked on me or laughed at me. Why am I the one getting suspended?

Over the summer vacation, I met Victor. He was really nice to me. He was in a gang. He told me the gang would protect me from anyone who tried to mess with me. The school couldn't make that promise. Me and Victor started off as friends, but we got closer. I had sex with Victor on my 13th birthday. He said it would be really special. It wasn't. It hurt like hell. Not only that, but I got pregnant. Victor said not to worry, the gang family would be the baby's family. I really didn't want to get involved with the gang, but I felt like I didn't have any choice now with the baby coming. Victor was right about being protected. Once I joined the gang, nobody bothered me or laughed at me anymore. I moved out of my grandmother's house and lived with Victor. I guess Granny didn't care because she never came after me.

Things were good for a while. Soon after I got pregnant, Victor changed. He was distant and not around at night anymore. Even though I was Victor's girlfriend, I had to have sex with all the guys in the gang. Having sex with all the gang bangers in one night is called "pulling a train." They "pulled trains" on me until I got big with the baby. Victor stopped having sex with me, but he said he still loved me and wanted to be with me and the baby. I didn't believe him. I knew he was sleeping with a lot of other girls. I wanted to go home to Granny's but Victor went crazy when I talked about leaving. We had a huge fight. Victor covered my mouth with his hand while he held a knife to my stom-ach. He cut a "V" on my arm with a knife and said if I left he would do more than "scratch me on the arm" next time.

I didn't have to go to school because I was pregnant. The school sent a teacher to our apartment once a week to help me keep up. I told her she was wasting her time. I didn't want to go back to school, but she came every week. She also made arrangements for me to see a doctor for prenatal care check-ups at the health department. They gave me free food vouchers there to buy cereal, cheese, and milk. Victor liked it when I came home with the food vouchers. He used them to get weed. That was OK with me cause I liked to smoke pot. I was getting high as often as I could. When I was stoned, I could forget about all the shit in my life.

One night I was with Victor at a party. His fellas were getting too wild. They wanted Victor to be the shooter at a drive-by. He didn't have to do it, but I could tell he was not going to back down from a challenge. Victor didn't even say good-by to me. I somehow knew I would never see him again. None of those guys came back. They shot up the wrong 'hood. The boys they wanted to pop found out they were planning a drive-by and were waiting for them. Victor shot up the crack house but when they tried to drive away, their car crashed into the curb. Before they could turn around, the other guys started shooting up the car. They shot Victor. I don't know how many times. Then they pulled Victor and his crew out of the car and crushed their faces with baseball bats. The police came too late. Victor was dead. I guess I should have been more upset. It really seemed more like a dream.

That was four years ago. I had my baby, but he was very small and sick when he was born. I named him Victor and call him Little Vic. We live in a group home for single teen mothers. I get a lot of help from the houseparents. They take good care of me and my little boy. I go to school here and want to get my GED. Little Vic has something called "developmental delays" and goes to a special school for special needs children. My life is not great but it's getting better.

If we think about clients as individuals, then there are several clients in this situation. The young woman who is sharing her story is a client and is in fact, currently receiving services to help her with her education, housing, and parenting. Her son, little Victor, is also a client with special needs that may be both physical and mental. He is attending a special school. At some point, Victor, the father, may have been a client, but he is now dead. In any case, these individuals have needs and problems that they are unable to address alone. If they became our clients, we would use the concept of the whole person introduced earlier in this chapter to assess their needs and problems, think about the four models that would help us understand their situations, and consider ways to access the services that are needed.

Another way to think about this case is to consider a broader definition of client—groups as clients. Examples of such groups may be a couple, a family, or several individuals who share a similar situation or problem. In this case history, we might think of Granny, little Victor, and his mother as a family unit that might be a client. It is also possible to think about Victor's gang as a client group who needs human services. If we focus on the gang as a potential client group, then we would need to understand the gang culture which might include the structure of gangs, the ways of identifying gang members, and why and how kids join gangs.

We can also think of larger groups as clients—neighborhoods, cities or counties, problem populations, or geographic regions. In this case history, we

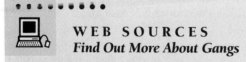

WEB SOURCES
Find Out More About Gangs

http://www.gangsorus.com/gangs.htm

The focus of this site is to provide general knowledge about the backgrounds and other aspects of some familiar street and prison gangs. Links include gang court, gang laws, girls and gangs, street gangs, and prison gangs.

http://www.novagate.com/novasurf/gang.html

The Gang Awareness page at this site lists a number of resources across the United States that will increase the viewer's awareness of gangs.

http://www.iir.com/nygc/maininfo.htm

The National Youth Gang Center is one of five major components of a comprehensive, coordinated response to the gang problem by the Office of Juvenile Justice and Delinquency Prevention. Topics include gang information, the Rural Gang Initiative, legislation, literature, and strategies.

http://www.lunaweb.com/memgang.htm

This site is an example of a community's response to the gang problem. The Memphis Police Department promotes gang awareness by providing answers to often-asked questions, suggestions for public participation, and a list of resources.

might consider gangs as a client group that is a community or a national or societal problem. For example, the United States has seen rapid proliferation of youth gangs since 1980. Their presence is felt in communities in several ways, including their dress, language, colors, and music. Perhaps of greatest concern though is the increase in violence and crime. Assaults and batteries, drug-related crimes, auto thefts, home invasions, drive-by shootings, graffiti, and an increase in truancy and school dropouts are associated with gangs. One response to community needs is the National Youth Gang Center, which is funded by the U.S. Department of Justice's Office of Juvenile Justice and Delinquency Prevention. The center assists state and local jurisdictions in the collection, analysis, and exchange of information on gang-related demographics, legislation, literature, research, and promising program strategies. Their website (www.iir.com/nygc) provides current information. See web sources for more information.

 ## Getting Help

Having discussed *what* problems clients face and *who* the clients are, we now address the question of *how* clients get help. The answer is not simply that clients experience problems and then find the appropriate human service agency, because people do not always use the services they need. Gross and

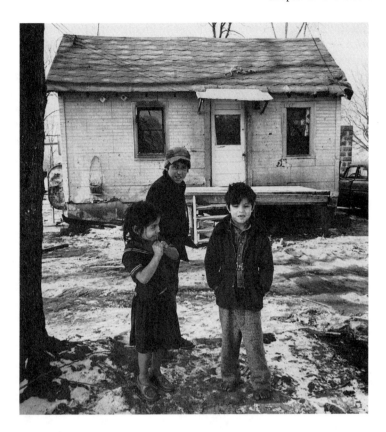

McMullen (1982), in describing the help-seeking process, raised the following questions: "Why don't people use available services? Why don't they ask for what they need if it is not available?" These are questions we continue to ask today. A discussion of the conditions under which clients enter the human service system, the barriers clients experience as they enter the system, and clients' perspectives on human services immediately before and after receiving assistance will provide answers to these questions.

Ways of Getting Help

As stated, people do not experience problems and automatically go directly to the appropriate human services agency. Individuals can become involved with the human service delivery system in several ways, including self-referral and referral by other professionals. Clients can also be forced to receive services or can receive services inadvertently as members of a larger population.

REFERRAL

Referral, a common method of getting help, includes self-referral and referral by others. According to Boy and Pine (1968), "a counseling relationship that has been initiated by the client is built on a firmer footing than one into which he has been forced" (p. 144). Individuals may voluntarily seek assistance from human services agencies because they are desperate and confused. They have experienced a traumatic event or are in a situation so intolerable that they can no longer ignore it. Self-referral typically occurs when clients have tried every way they know to cope, to no avail, and have no other ideas about how to address their problems. Some potential clients have heard about services from their friends and neighbors or through television, radio, or billboard advertising and know exactly what their problem is and where to go. Others in desperate condition stop at the first agency available, regardless of its function, hoping that someone will be able to refer them to the right service.

Another type of referral is from another professional to a human service agency. Ministers, physicians, mental health workers, and other helping professionals often see an individual who needs assistance for problems beyond their expertise. The referring professional first assesses the client's complex situation and then refers this person to one or more additional human service agencies. For such a referral to be successful, the referring professional must help the potential client clarify problems and begin to provide some alternative solutions. (Referral may be one of those solutions.) This action may preempt the next professional's work, but it assures the client that the referring professional is not just "passing the buck." The referring professional should also provide the potential client with as much information as possible about the agency to which the referral has been made. If the client is somewhat reluctant to go to another professional for help, more assistance from the referring professional will increase the probability that the referral will be successful.

INVOLUNTARY PLACEMENT IN THE SYSTEM

Another way of getting into the human service system is to be placed in the system by others. *Involuntary* clients—referred by schools, prisons, courts, marriage counselors, protective services, and the juvenile justice system—are potentially difficult to work with because they have not chosen to receive services. The service to which they are referred usually offers only part of the treatment they are to receive. Their cooperation and participation in that service is often monitored, and decisions about subsequent treatment (including release from treatment) are partially based on their observed attitudes and progress. This creates some pressure on the clients to treat the referral seriously.

One example of the use of involuntary referral of clients is the case of child abuse. The decision to allow a child to remain in or return to a home may be contingent on agreement by one or both parents to receive counseling services. For another example, the juvenile court may order involuntary services for first offenders. Depending on the crime and the circumstances, judges often sentence juveniles to receive counseling, to perform tasks in the social services, or to assume other responsibilities related to their crimes. A third example involves individuals incarcerated for crimes. Much of their time in prison is programmed by others, and they have little say over their treatment.

Involuntary clients and voluntary clients may feel very differently about human services. Someone else has decided that the involuntary clients need assistance; they have not admitted that they need help and probably would not have chosen the human services they are receiving if they had decided to seek help on their own. They are often embarrassed or angry that someone else has decided what they need and has sent them to receive the services in question. Because they have not chosen the assistance, they may also feel trapped. Their alternatives are much more limited than those of voluntary clients. If they do not like the treatment or the worker, they may have little ability to change the helping situation.

INADVERTENT SERVICES

Another way of entering the human service system is to be part of a larger population that is targeted for services. In this situation, receipt of services does not depend on the individual's need or ability to qualify for the services, and the client does not have to ask for them. Although inadvertent services can often help the client, they also have their limitations. Ideally, before services are provided to a large population, the consumers using the services are consulted. However, some of the clients receiving the services may not have had any input about the type of service provided or the manner in which it is delivered. In such cases, the services provided may seem useless to the client. Services that clients receive inadvertently include the redevelopment of low-cost housing; neighborhood crime watch programs; shelters for the homeless, AIDS victims, or the elderly; and emergency help for disaster areas.

Many clients who need help do not receive the services they need, nor do they seek them for a variety of reasons. Barriers that clients experience are discussed next, including how they view the problem, the cost of the resources, and the reluctance to use friends as helpers. Reading a description of these barriers may be frustrating, because the problems are presented from the client's point of view, without any discussion of how helpers can overcome such client barriers. We have chosen to separate client barriers from helper responses to retain the focus on the client. Subsequent chapters will provide a human service response to such barriers.

Barriers to Seeking Help

In discussing barriers, one of the first factors to consider is how the client views the problem. If the client considers the problem too difficult to solve, too overwhelming to consider, or too embarrassing to admit, then this person is less likely to seek help. Clients who perceive the problem this way may consider the process of seeking help a burden or a waste of time. From the client's perspective, the problem cannot be solved even by experts.

If the client is embarrassed at having the problem, seeking help means admitting to others that there is a problem. The very nature of many problems in living involves a reluctance to admit to having problems. Spouses in troubled marriages may be reluctant to talk about their difficulties because parents and

Mental Health Facts

WHAT TO WATCH FOR

Even when you try your best, you will still experience periods of frustration and unhappiness. Usually, with time, you will overcome your distress. But you should learn to recognize when your problems—or those of your loved ones—are too much to handle alone. You can help yourself, your family, and your friends by knowing when to ask for professional help. Some of the warning signs include these:

Undue, prolonged anxiety. This is an anxiety out of proportion to any identifiable reason or cause. Of course, all of us experience problems that make us tense and anxious. But a deep, continuing anxiety—a state of constant tension and fear that fastens itself to one cause after another—is a signal that help is needed. Unrelieved anxiety not only causes mental anguish but can also lead to physical problems.

Prolonged or severe depression. Depression strongly affects thinking, feelings, and behavior. Feelings of inadequacy, helplessness, hopelessness, undue pessimism, and loss of confidence are symptomatic of depression. Changes in behavior patterns are a key sign that depression may be getting out of hand and help should be sought.

Depressed individuals often withdraw from friends they normally enjoy, from loved ones, and from the usual occupation and hobbies that give pleasure. Their eating and sleeping habits change. Some suffer from loss of appetite and insomnia; others seek solace in overeating and sleeping.

Other symptoms of depression include low energy; chronic fatigue; decreased effectiveness at school, work, or home; and loss of sexual interest. Depressed individuals are those most likely to think of suicide as a solution, although people with other mental and emotional disturbances may also be suicidal. During periods of crisis, people should be with others, avoiding isolation.

Abrupt changes in mood and behavior. These changes do not include deliberate steps a person adopts for self-improvement. They refer to changes in mood and behavior that reflect serious alterations in an individual's normal habits or ways of thinking. For example, the exceptionally frugal man or woman who suddenly begins gambling away large sums of money may be experiencing emotional problems.

Tension-caused physical symptoms. Some bodily ailments and complaints have no physical cause, such as a daily headache, a migraine induced by tension, nausea, pains, and other complaints. These symptoms,

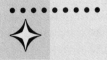

including pain, are very real. But only a physician is qualified to determine whether they are caused by distress rather than physical malfunctioning. Because medical tests may reveal an organic cause, any persistent physical ailment should be checked by a doctor.

If any warning signs are severe or long lasting, professional help may be needed. If the true cause of the problem can be identified, often the symptoms can be relieved.

HOW TO FIND HELP

There are many services available to persons experiencing mental and emotional problems:

- Mental health associations provide information about mental health resources available in your community.
- Professional associations usually have state or local chapters that can help in finding an appropriate professional in the community. These include the state psychological and psychiatric associations or medical societies.
- Family service agencies provide information, referrals, and counseling for individuals and families.
- Self-help organizations, such as the National Alliance for the Mentally Ill, Recovery, Inc., and Alcoholics Anonymous, can provide assistance.
- State and local departments of social services, city or county health departments, or county medical associations and others, including Veterans Administration hospitals, school counseling programs, and private clinics, can also provide help.

TWO IMPORTANT TIPS

How much you are helped depends on the "fit" between your personality and that of the therapist. It pays to seek help from another if you feel dissatisfied or unaided by a particular therapist.

If you have a mental or emotional problem from time to time or over a long period, try not to be unduly discouraged. Most of us experience some symptoms of stress in the course of living. When stress or its symptoms seem more severe than usual, help should be sought. *Remember, you are not alone.*

SOURCE: National Institute of Mental Health, 1985.*You are not alone: Facts about metal health and mental illness* (DHHS Publication No. ADM 85–1178). Washington, DC: U.S. Government Printing Office.

significant others have warned them about the trouble this could cause them. Abused children, spouses, and parents keep the abuse quiet because making an accusation would cause great disruption and because they, the abused, feel that the situation is ultimately their fault. Men in this society are less likely to seek help than women experiencing similar problems because men are socialized to solve problems on their own.

Another barrier is the individual's perception of the human service professional. Such workers are viewed as strangers and experts—two categories that establish immediate barriers for those in need. The helping process requires the individual in need to talk about personal issues and concerns with someone unknown. For many individuals in our society, the "stranger" evokes distrust and suspicion. The expert commands respect but also fear. The client initially sees the expert as an "accomplished" person who has little in common with individuals who have overwhelming problems. Fears of the stranger and the expert are barriers that prevent individual clients from seeking services and from trusting workers in the initial stages of the helping process.

Three barriers are directly related to available client resources: money to pay for the services, transportation to reach the place of service delivery, and the time and distance involved in traveling to receive the services. For the disabled, architectural barriers may present additional problems. Many clients may be ready and willing to seek assistance but cannot determine a way to surmount the problems of paying for services or of finding time and transportation to receive them. One solution to the inability to pay is to provide services to poorer clients on a realistic sliding scale. Transportation is a difficult problem for rural clients who live miles from the nearest population center. Equally vulnerable are clients who live in smaller cities without mass transportation or in larger cities with expensive mass transportation. Other clients cannot use services because they work long hours or are caring for children or an elderly parent. Unless service hours are extended and house care relief is provided, services may be inaccessible (from the client's perspective) even if they are affordable and nearby. What makes these barriers particularly frustrating for the clients is that they add one more set of problems to an already troubled situation.

The psychological costs of seeking help are also serious barriers. Some clients view help as effecting an immediate loss of their freedom; they fear that helpers will demand changes in their behavior, lifestyle, and work habits. They do not want to lose what little freedom they have. Clients also fear that they will ultimately have to assume responsibility for their problems, and this may frighten them. When clients admit that they need help and seek assistance, they are also afraid that they will be considered inadequate. When a person seeks help, it is a signal to others that the individual cannot solve problems alone and that his or her efforts have failed. To admit such "failure" is very difficult. Sometimes there is considerable pressure from peers not to seek help, especially if the peers see themselves as having a similar problem. Finally, clients resist seeking help because they fear being indebted to a human service worker or agency. Asking for and receiving help means giving the worker the power of a caregiver. Clients feel

TABLE 5-5 ✦ SUMMARY POINTS: BARRIERS TO HELP

- Client's perspective of the situation
- Embarrassment
- Reluctance to admit to having a problem
- Perceptions of the helper
- Cost of services
- Transportation
- Time
- Fear

pressed to live up to the worker's expectations and they fear disappointing the worker if little or no change takes place in their lives. (See Table 5-5.)

BARRIERS TO FRIENDS AS HELPERS

The barriers are very real to individuals who are experiencing problems in living and choose not to seek help. Besides being reluctant to seek the help of professional workers, such individuals often hesitate to seek out informal help from family and friends. This reluctance stems from their own fears and fear of the reactions of others. Some of the barriers to seeking help from significant others are similar to the barriers to seeking professional services. Telling friends about their problems may cause a loss of face; reputations and good appearances may suffer if others know about the problems. People want others to think well of them. It is a common worry that once others know about their problems, then they will lose friendships or respect. People also fear that the disclosure will be a burden to those who have been told—that the problems might upset the listener or place him or her in an uncomfortable situation. To impose on friends might violate the "rules" of the friendship.

Another reason individuals do not ask their friends for help is that they do not find them helpful. Many friends do not know how to respond appropriately, offering only advice, authoritarian "shoulds," and cliches. Many friends also cannot be trusted. What the individual experiencing problems considers confidential may be considered public information by the friend. Most potential clients do not want their problems to be common knowledge in their own environment.

THE RELUCTANT CLIENT

Reluctance, in its many forms, may have its positive characteristics, although many experienced helpers believe that establishing a bond with a client is easier if the client wants and seeks help. Client reluctance is to be respected. Reluctance is often self-protective, designed to maintain personal integrity. Part of the helping process requires clients to admit there is a problem, to share information about themselves and their environment, and to engage with the helper to change their behaviors and then evaluate the change. This process requires an inner strength that potential clients may lack at the beginning of the process.

The Client's Perspective

Once individuals have decided to use the human service system to seek solutions to their problems, they become voluntary clients, categorized by Perlman (1975) in three ways. *Buffeted* clients are those with multiple problems, who come often for services and use them to address their various problems. *Problem solvers* are those clients who use the services less often but for a range of different problems. *Resource seekers* are those clients who do not use the services often and come to the human service system for the resolution of just one problem. Buffeted clients and resource seekers perceive the nature of problems and the nature of services differently. Buffeted people see the human service system as a place to get help with their many problems. They perceive the system as equipped to handle a variety of the problems they experience. Resource seekers, in contrast, see the human service system as available on a more limited basis for assistance with one specific kind of problem.

Client Expectations

To understand clients, we must know what each expects from both the human service system and the service professional and how each person perceives that same system after receiving help. Today's clients are focusing more than ever on the quality of care they will receive. The following discussion of client perceptions before and after receiving services is based on the results of several studies of client perception of the juvenile justice system, family services, protective services, and services to unmarried mothers. Although the information was collected from clients requiring different services, the results are surprisingly similar.

First, many clients imagine that the helper will have an unbiased attitude toward them and will have experience in working with the problems they are experiencing. The helper will understand the problems because he or she will have the client's point of view. The potential clients who were studied also expect the helper to listen, help them decide what to do, and help them do whatever needs to be done. Clients also expect the helper to assist them in dealing directly with the environment.

Clients also have clear expectations of how the helper should behave. According to a survey, clients expect helpers to tell them what they should do. Helping professionals should be able to understand what clients say, provide them with necessary information, and offer an opinion of their own if it differs from the clients' opinions. In other words, the helper is expected to take a very active role in the helping process.

Clients also have ideas about what they expect from the helping process. These expectations fall into three categories (Franklin, 1995; Kenny, 1995; Maluccio, 1979; Toczek-McPeake & Matthews, 1995). First, clients want to find a cure or straighten out a situation. They are looking for quick solutions and quick answers. Second, if they want change, they define results as change

• • • • • • • • •

Getting Help: One Client's Perspective

I needed help, and I had mixed feelings. I felt guilty needing help. It probably had something to do with the way I was raised. If you're strong enough, you shouldn't be having emotional problems. The barriers to getting help were mostly internal. I didn't feel like it was okay to be as angry or depressed as I was. I felt I should just snap out of it. There's a family history of breakdowns. I really don't know if it's hereditary. Some people thought that was an excuse.

I really didn't have any contact with a human service worker until the second time I was hospitalized, and I think that she was the one who was instrumental in getting me the help I needed to get out. She was the first one who told me there was even any way out at all, that I might be able to get an education. I think she was helpful because she had been through a divorce and had a child, so she knew firsthand what it was like—the fear of being alone, providing for children, and the hurt that you go through in a divorce. She understood. And while she was very helpful, on the other hand, I got to where I didn't look forward to talking with her because our sessions turned into discussions of the things she had experienced. So it was good for me on one hand, and then again, I wanted to back away after a while.

I also had one doctor who put me on so many medications, I gained weight until I weighed over 200 pounds, which was just making me more depressed. I had to go for a physical, and the doctor said one of those medications shouldn't even be mixed with the others. That added to the depression, so I took myself off everything and I lay down to die. And my husband would have allowed it. It seemed like the depression was in cycles, too. I'd be depressed and I'd want to die, and then I'd get angry. When I got angry the last time, I was the one who called the doctor and said I needed help.

in self and change in others. Third, their ideas about what changes should occur are concrete rather than general or abstract.

When asked about the problems they were experiencing and what services they needed, the clients again answered in concrete terms (Kenny, 1995; Mayer & Timms, 1969; Morse, Calsyn, Allen, & Kenny, 1994; Toczek-McPeake & Matthews, 1995). For clients, the lack of resources and the need for tangible goods and services were the most important. Of secondary importance was the need to solve intrapersonal and interpersonal problems. Clients defined problems in practical terms and were reluctant to define something as a problem if they thought it could not be resolved.

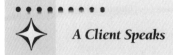

A Client Speaks

ABOUT BEING A CLIENT

When I chose to be a client, I didn't think there was any hope for me as far as my disease of alcoholism was concerned. I thought that I didn't have a choice, that I would end up one day dying as an alcoholic. And I didn't know anything about AA or about treatment centers. One day I stumbled on this information from another alcoholic who was still practicing his disease, and he told me they had a treatment program for veterans. At that point, I was in school, I was trying to get some education to better myself, and I was sick and tired of trying to fight this disease on my own. I wasn't getting anywhere with it. I might go two or three days, but then the next thing I know I'm back out there again. When exams came around, I got test anxiety, and just to relieve that pressure I would take a drink, saying to myself, "I'm just gonna take a couple of drinks." But I would drink until I'd get sick. And I decided that it was time for me to try something, 'cause what I was doing was not helping. So I called the hospital and they set up an appointment. I really didn't know what to expect when I got there. I was kind of fearful. I thought it was a place where you go to dry out and get back on your feet and then they send you back out. But it was not that way. They educated us about the disease of alcoholism and that people were beginning to accept it as a disease, and that there was hope for the alcoholic. I started to feel a little better, because until then I didn't think there was any hope for me. And I found out that I had a choice. I had a choice to drink, or to go to AA meetings to get help.

ABOUT THE FIRST DAY IN THE HOSPITAL

What stands out for me the first day I went to the hospital was that I was not alone. I thought I was the Lone Ranger, and I saw that I was not the only person suffering with this disease. I felt a sense of hope. Because everybody I talked to said, "I understand how you feel. You should have seen me three weeks ago. I was worse than you." So, my first day, my first week there, I started seeing other people coming in like I came in, and some of them were worse than I was, some were not, but when you see them that first day, you say, "Man, that was me two weeks ago." Then when they leave, you look at them, and there is no comparison. They begin to look like human beings—not just drunks that have low self-esteem and no future. The biggest thing that stood out was that I wasn't alone. For years I thought I was the only one out there.

ABOUT BARRIERS TO GETTING HELP

I think the biggest barrier is myself. I don't think it's anything out there, because wherever I go, there I am, and I still have those same problems. The world is not gonna change; you can't change other people, places, and things.

ABOUT HUMAN SERVICE WORKERS

The majority of the workers are compassionate people and are very understanding. The ones that I find are not understanding are the ones that have not experienced this disease. They don't know what alcoholism is all about. The last time that I went in treatment, I had a doctor who told me about willpower, and he did not want to admit me to the hospital on a Sunday evening. He told me to go downtown and get a motel and come in Monday to be admitted. The secretary, however, said, "We will make an appointment with you Monday, and if you think that you won't be able to make it, detox is open 24 hours a day. You can come up there, and we'll admit you in detox." But the doctor was being real tough. I think that if he had been an alcoholic, he would have admitted me, because they had beds. I even walked over to the unit and talked to the nurse on duty. She said that she had two or three beds available, but he told me that he was not gonna admit me. At first he said he was. He said, "I have to call over there and find out if they have any beds, and if they do, then we'll see what we can do for you." I don't know if he called or not, but he didn't admit me. But getting back to what I was saying, people who have been through alcoholism understand and they can see through all your cunning, manipulative ways.

ABOUT GETTING HELP

I think the biggest thing for any person seeking help, or anyone who is in an institution, is to break out of the denial stage. I think that is the biggest downfall for everybody, for any client. That was my biggest problem for years. I knew I had a problem, but I would not admit it. I always said, "No, it was just circumstances, I was at the wrong place at the wrong time," or "I just had one beer too many." I was in denial for a long time. And today sometimes I'm in denial about certain things, but the key to that is awareness; today I'm aware of what my downfalls are, and what I need to do to make life better. If you really and truly want to

(continued)

A Client Speaks (continued)

do something about your problem, you have to be totally honest with yourself, because you can't be honest with other people until you start being honest with yourself. And once you start being honest, you got to be open-minded, be able to take criticism from other people, and in my case, I needed to stop being passive and start being assertive and not letting people control my feelings.

ABOUT BEING A VIETNAM VETERAN

I was over there for a period of 90 days in Saigon, Thailand, and Korea. I was in the air force and I didn't have a rifle, I had an IBM computer. Life centered around the NCO club. That's where I started my drinking. I had a lot of fear when I went over there, a fear of dying. The first place I went was Da Nang in 1970. Every day we had rockets coming in, and I was afraid all the time that I was over there, and I first started drinking to relieve all of my fears—the nervousness and the worry that the next one was gonna hit this barracks. When I first went over there, every time that siren would go off, I would take cover. After a period of time, I got into drinking, and any time that siren would go off, we'd sit there and continue to drink. It's a part of my life sometimes I really don't like to talk about. We have a veterans' group at the hospital, and I told them that I didn't think that I was qualified to sit in with those who were out there in the field and are now suffering from posttraumatic stress syndrome. Every time they see a Vietnamese, something just goes off and all they see is just that person, and they're ready to fight, ready to kill them right here in America today. I'm fortunate that I don't have to go through that. But coming back here to the United States and saying that you're a veteran, putting on your veteran's cap, and feeling proud that you served your country, and then someone spits in your face and calls you a baby killer when we were over there taking orders, I don't know what this world's coming to. It makes me angry, it makes me angry.

Client Evaluations of Services

Clients today are much more sophisticated in the area of client satisfaction. They are acquainted with issues of access and quality of services, and many of them provide feedback to agencies and service providers by filling out satisfaction surveys and questionnaires after they have received services. Because of the current climate of accountability, clients are more vocal about what they expect and what will satisfy them.

The clients' views of services after the process were consistent with their prior expectations. The most positive outcomes, in their view, were the practical improvements in their lives, such as better living conditions, food, and clothing, as well as intangible improvements, such as increased self-confidence, assumption of new roles, acquisition of new skills, and solution of their problems in living. Helper activities that they viewed as particularly helpful were the ones that went beyond talking with them. They praised workers for helping them get something, taking them somewhere, talking with someone for them, seeing someone with them, and referring them. Most clients considered the outcomes of the helping experience to be very positive, viewed the workers as helpful and fair, and believed that things were better for them after the service than before. Most perceived at least some improvement or the potential for improvement in their situations.

Several research studies have examined the factors that are linked to client satisfaction and client dissatisfaction. The following description of those factors represents a summary of this research (Frager, Coyne, Lyle, Coulter, Graham, Sargent, & Allen, 1999; Franklin, 1995; Gariti, Alterman, Holub-Beyer, & Volpicelli, 1995; Haines, Petit, & Lefrancois, 1999; Kenny, 1995; Morse, Calsyn, Allen, & Kenny, 1994; O'Donnell, Parker, Proberts, Matthews, Fisher, Johnson, & Hadzi-Pavlovic, 1999; Offer, 1998–1999; Toczek-McPeake, & Matthews, 1995; Winefield & Barlow, 1995). The factors are related to client expectations before services, as described previously.

SATISFACTION
1. The client's satisfaction is linked to the client's perceptions of the helper. Specifically, the clients were more satisfied with the services they received if they perceived the worker as having similar values, if the helper accurately perceived their needs, and if they perceived the worker as an expert with experience in the problem area.
2. The clients also wanted to have a good relationship with their human service professional. For them that meant that the helper spent time with them, listened to their problems, and provided emotional support. This also included being called prior to appointments and receiving follow-up contacts.
3. The clients wanted to participate in the process of helping, especially if they were long-term clients. They wanted to have input into the decisions about their treatment. They also based their satisfaction on the amount and accuracy of the information that they received.
4. Satisfaction is also linked to the helper's ability to solve problems and the amount of change the clients thought occurred during the helping process. Clients also expressed a willingness to return for help if the need were to arise. They measured their satisfaction based on the number of outcomes that were met and the ways in which their treatment plan was followed.
5. These clients also stated that their environment had been supportive and that they themselves were independent and proactive in seeking solutions to their problems.

Conversely, those clients who expressed dissatisfaction can be described as follows:

DISSATISFACTION

1. Dissatisfaction arose when clients wanted material assistance from the helper, but the helper wanted to focus on personal and interpersonal problems. There was a clash between the helper's and the clients' expectations.
2. The clients who were dissatisfied received unwanted advice and help. They also thought the helper did not have the skills to assist them with their problems, was inaccessible, and never understood their problems.
3. Clients were also dissatisfied when they were not clear about their problems and their treatment plan; that is, they could not articulate precisely what the problem was or what intervention was proposed to resolve it.

 ## Things to Remember

1. The term *client* includes more than just individuals; a client may be a small group such as a family, or a larger population such as the residents of a geographic area.
2. Definitions of problem suggest that "problems in living" can have two components: a description of the problem and a course of action for resolving the problem.
3. A way of defining human problems is Abraham Maslow's hierarchy of needs, which begins with the most basic of physical human needs and ends with the need of individuals to become self-actualized.
4. Human beings experience similar problems, not just because of their individual needs but also as a result of rapid social changes, the breakdown of many traditional forms of society, and conflicts between old and new values.
5. Individuals can become involved with the human service delivery system in several ways, including self-referral, referral by other professionals, or involuntary placement.
6. Self-referral occurs when individuals have tried every way they know to cope, to no avail, and have no other ideas about how to address their problems.
7. Ministers, physicians, mental health workers, and other helping professionals often see an individual who needs assistance for problems beyond their expertise, and after assessing the client's situation, refer the client to one or more additional human services agencies.
8. Client expectations fall into three categories: to find a cure or straighten out a situation, to define results as change in themselves and change in others, and to describe what changes should occur as concrete rather than general or abstract.
9. From the clients' perspective, positive outcomes were the practical improvements in their lives, such as better living conditions, food

and clothing, and intangible improvements including increased self-confidence, assumption of new roles, acquisition of new skills, and solution of their problems in living.

10. Clients' satisfaction is linked to their perceptions of the helping professional and of the relationship, the worker's ability to solve problems, and the amount of change the clients thought occurred during the helping process.

11. Conversely, clients who expressed dissatisfaction did so because they wanted material assistance from the helper or they received unwanted advice and help.

Additional Readings: Focus on Clients

Dash, L. (1996). *Rosa Lee: A mother and her family in urban America.* New York: Basic Books.
For four years the author followed Rosa Lee Cunningham, her eight children, and five grandchildren, in an effort to capture life in the growing black underclass.

Dryfoos, J. G. (1998). *Safe passage: Making it through adolescence in a risky society.* New York: Oxford University Press.
Child advocate Joy Dryfoos examines hundreds of successful programs that are models to help children face such obstacles as failing schools, dangerous streets, drug abuse, and teen pregnancy.

Knapp, C. (1996). *Drinking: A love story.* New York: Dial Press.
The author began drinking at age 14 and drank for years until a series of personal crises forced her to confront her alcoholism.

Parent, M. (1998). *Turning stones: My days and nights with children at risk.* New York: Fawcett Books.
The author, a caseworker for Emergency Children's Services in New York, writes about eight cases that illustrate how society allows extremes of child abuse to happen.

Schwarz, J. E., & Volgy, T. J. (1993). *Forgotten Americans.* New York: W. W. Norton & Co.
The authors examine a relatively new category of the impoverished: the working poor.

Simon, P., & Burns, E. (1997). *The corner: A year in the life of an inner-city neighborhood.* New York: Broadway Books.
This book follows a small group of people who are struggling to survive the drug market that fuels their world—an inner-city neighborhood in Baltimore.

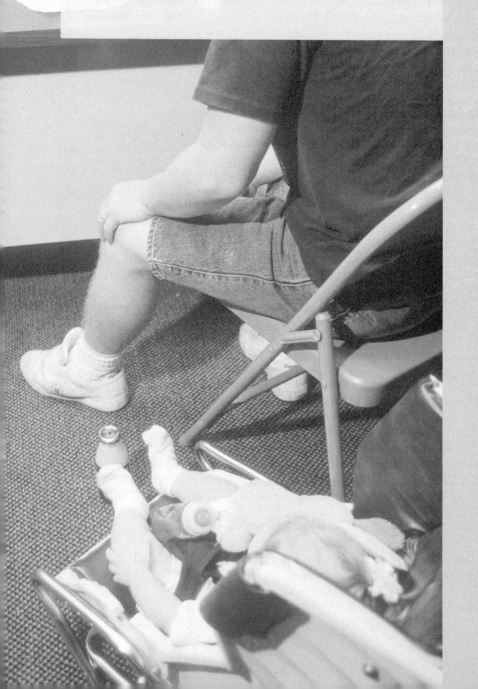

Chapter 6

The Human Service Professional

Helping means assisting other people to understand, overcome, or cope with problems. The *helper* is the person who offers this assistance. This chapter's discussion of the motivations for choosing a helping profession, the values and philosophies of helpers, and the special characteristics and traits helpers have will assist in establishing an identity for the helper. We also define workers as human service professionals, as well as introduce other professionals with whom they may interact. An important key to understanding human service professionals is an awareness of the many roles they engage in as they work with their clients and with other professionals.

In this chapter you will meet two human service professionals, Beth Bruce and Carmen Rodriguez. Beth is a case manager at a mental health center and has previous experience working with the elderly and adolescents. Carmen is a vocational evaluator for a state agency. She has varied responsibilities related to preparing clients for and finding gainful employment.

Who Is the Helper?

In human services, the helper is an individual who assists others. This very broad definition includes professional helpers with extensive training, such as psychiatrists and psychologists, as well as those who have minimal training, such as volunteers and other nonprofessional helpers. Regardless of the length or intensity of the helper's training, his or her basic focus is to assist clients "to understand, overcome, or deal with external or internal problems" (Okun, 1997, p. 7), "to reach goals that are important to them" (Brammer, 1999, p. 303), to provide a "link between the traditional professional and the client" (Epstein, 1981, p. 33), or all these functions.

The human service worker is a helper who can be described in many different ways. For example, Hutchins and Cole Vaught (1997) suggested that effective helpers are people who are "together"—that is, whose thoughts, feelings, and actions are congruent. Such a helper, believing that each client is a unique individual different from all other clients, will greet each one by name, with a handshake and a smile. Others view a helping person as an individual whose life experiences most closely match those of the person to be helped (Lyon & Duke, 1981). The recovering alcoholic working with substance abusers is an example of this perspective. Still another view of the helper, and the one with which you are most familiar from your reading of this text, is the generalist human service professional who brings together knowledge and skills from a variety of disciplines to work with the client as a whole person.

Your understanding of the human service worker as a professional helper will become clearer as this section examines the reasons why individuals choose this type of work, the traits and characteristics they share, and the different categories of their actual job functions.

Motivations for Choosing a Helping Profession

Work is an important part of life in the United States. It is a valued activity that provides many individuals with a sense of identity as well as a livelihood. It is also a means for individuals to experience satisfying relationships with others, under agreeable conditions.

Understanding vocational choice is as complex and difficult a process as actually choosing a vocation. Factors that have been found to influence career choice include individuals' needs, their aptitudes and interests, and their self-concepts. Special personal or social experiences also influence the choice of a career. There have been attempts to establish a relationship between vocational choice and certain factors such as interests, values, and attitudes, but it is generally agreed that no one factor can explain or predict a person's vocational choice.

Donald Super, a leader in vocational development theory, believes that the vocational development process is one of implementing a self-concept. This occurs through the interaction of social and individual factors, the opportunity to try various roles, and the perceived amount of approval from peers and supervisors for the roles assumed. There are many other views of this process, but most theorists agree that vocational choice is a developmental process.

How do people choose helping professions as careers? Research in this area tells us that the choice is influenced by direct work experience, college courses and instructors, and the involvement of friends, acquaintances, or relatives in helping professions (Pins, 1963). Money or salary is actually a small concern compared with the goals and functions of the work itself. In other words, for individuals who choose helping as their life's work, the kind of work they will do is more important than the pay they will receive.

There are several reasons why people choose a helping profession. It is important to be aware of these motivations because each may have positive and negative aspects. One primary reason why individuals choose helping professions (and the reason that most will admit) is the desire to help others. To feel worthwhile as a result of contributing to another's growth is exciting; however, helpers must also ask themselves the following questions: To what extent am I meeting my own needs? Even more important, do my needs to feel worthwhile and to be a caring person take precedence over the client's needs?

Related to this primary motivation is the desire for self-exploration. The wish to find out more about themselves as thinking, feeling individuals leads some people to major in psychology, sociology, or human services. This is a positive factor, because these people will most likely be concerned with gaining insights into their own behaviors and improving their knowledge and skills. After employment, it may become a negative factor if the helper's needs for self-exploration or self-development take precedence over the clients' needs. When this happens, either the helper becomes the client and the client the helper, or there are two clients, neither of whose needs are met. This situation can be avoided when the helper is aware that self-exploration is a personal motivation and can be fulfilled more appropriately outside the helping relationship.

Another strong motivation for pursuing a career in helping is the desire to exert control. For those who admit to this motivation, administrative or managerial positions in helping professions are the goal. This desire may become a problem, however, if helpers seek to control or dominate clients, with the intent of making them dependent or having them conform to some standard.

For many people, the experience of being helped provides a strong demonstration of the value of helping. Such people often wish to be like those who helped them when they were clients. This appears to be especially true for the fields of teaching and medicine. Unfortunately, this noble motivation may create unrealistic expectations of what being a helper will be like. For example, unsuccessful clients do not become helpers; rather, those who have had a positive helping experience are the ones who will choose this type of profession. Because they were cooperative and motivated clients, they may expect all clients to be like they were, and they may also expect all helpers to be as competent and caring as their helper was. Such expectations of both helpers and clients are unrealistic and may leave the helper frustrated and angry. (See Table 6-1.)

Values and Philosophy

Values are important to the practice of human services because they are the criteria by which helpers and clients make choices. Every individual has a set of values. Both human service professionals and clients have sets of values. Sometimes they are similar, but often they differ; in some situations, they conflict. Human service professionals should know something about values and how they influence the relationship between the helper and the client.

Where do our values originate? Culture helps establish some values and standards of behavior (Brill, 1998). As we grow and learn through our different experiences, general guides to behavior emerge. These guides are *values,* and they give direction to our behavior (Raths, Harmin, & Simon, 1978). Because different experiences lead to different values, individuals do not have the same value systems. Also, as individuals experience more, their values may change.

What exactly are values? Values are statements of what is desirable—of the way we would like the world to be. They are not statements of fact. Three processes determine whether something is a value; collectively, they define *valuing,* the process that results in values. The three categories are explained by Raths, Harmin, and Simon (1978, p. 28):

CHOOSING
1. Freely
2. From alternatives
3. After thoughtful consideration of the consequences of each alternative

TABLE 6-1   ◆   SUMMARY POINTS: WHY INDIVIDUALS CHOOSE
TO WORK IN HELPING PROFESSIONS

Help others	Contribute to another's growth
Self-exploration	Discover more about self
Exert control	Good in administration organization
Positive role models	Inspired by help from others

My Work as a Human Service Professional

Thom Prassa, a case manager at a community health agency, describes his work and the skills necessary to be effective.

In my job, I am a strong advocate for children, which means that I listen, communicate, sell, and monitor. Once a child is remanded to state custody, we must complete an assessment and a plan of services for the child. This requires that we work with the child, the family, the court, and other agencies and professionals in the community.

Adeptness at placements is critical. Which service providers in the community are good and which are not? Who is going to be able to work effectively with these children? Case managers must have their finger on the pulse when it comes to getting these kids in the right place at the right time. Communication is also important, especially being diplomatic in the sense of getting together people who are dysfunctional. Trying to develop a creative plan of care for the child sometimes means that it is necessary to tell parents or custodial designees what their responsibilities are. What must the parents do to get the child back? In a staffing, all the participants are present, they learn what their responsibilities are, and they agree to a plan of care. Then you must sell the plan to the child, explaining what is going to happen and how the child will benefit.

Sometimes I feel like much that I do is responding to crises. We put out fires all the time. We have disruptions, suicide attempts, children who need different levels of care, decisions about what to do, and communications with the custodial designee about a child. We also talk with parents, report to foster care review boards, and make progress reports to the community. This is all an incredible responsibility but I know we make a difference in the lives of children here.

There are a number of approaches to a job like mine. I have survived the past two and a half years because of my relationship with my team members. The camaraderie in the office is excellent and we support each other. You also have to have a life outside of work—hobbies, education, and friends. Strong supervisors and coworkers who respond to your needs are also helpful. (Thom Prassa, personal communication, July 10, 1994)

PRIZING
1. Cherishing, being happy with the choice
5. Enough to be willing to affirm the choice to others

ACTING
6. Or doing something with the choice
7. Repeatedly, in some pattern of life

Values provide a basis for choice. It is important for human service professionals to know what their own values are and how they influence relationships with coworkers and the delivery of services to clients. For example, professionals who value truth will give the client as much feedback as possible from the results of an employment check or a home visitation report.

Because human service delivery is a team effort in many agencies and communities, there have to be some common values that will assist helpers in working together effectively. The following are the most commonly held values in human services: acceptance, tolerance, individuality, self-determination, and confidentiality.

The next paragraph introduces Beth Bruce, a human service professional with a variety of experiences. In this section, her experiences are used to illustrate the values that are important to the human service profession.

Beth Bruce is a human service professional at the Estes Mental Health Center, a comprehensive center serving seven counties. She has been a case manager at Estes for the past eight months and has really enjoyed her first year's work in mental health. Her first job was as a social service provider in a local nursing home, where she worked for two years. She then worked with adolescents as a teacher/counselor at a local mental health institution before joining the Estes staff. Let's see how human service values relate to Beth's experience as a human service professional.

Acceptance is the ability of the worker to be receptive to the client regardless of the way a client is dressed or what the client may have done. Workers act on the value of acceptance when they are able to maintain an attitude of goodwill toward clients and to refrain from judging them by factors such as the way they live or whether they have likable personalities.

One of the most important values that Beth holds is accepting her clients for who they are. She has worked with the elderly, teenagers, and now persons with mental illness. These populations are different, but they retain one important quality for her: They are all human beings. Her acceptance of all clients has been put to the test. She had a male client in the nursing home who had once been tried for murder and found guilty. Because Beth believed that no circumstance justifies the killing of another, she had difficulty accepting that man as a worthwhile human being.

The second value of human service work is *tolerance:* the helper's ability to be patient and fair toward each client rather than judging, blaming, or punishing the client for prior behavior. A helper who embodies this value will work with the client to plan for the future, rather than continually focusing on the client's past mistakes.

Beth works with a friend and coworker who is not very tolerant of persons with mental illness. Several times, this coworker's intolerance of client behavior has caused problems for the client. Just yesterday, a problem arose with Ms. Mendoza, a 26-year-old woman with schizophrenia who is currently receiving day treatment and lives in a group home. She refused to see her parents when they came to see her at the day treatment center. Mr. Martin, Beth's coworker, forced Ms. Mendoza to see them because he believes that family is very important and that parents have a right to see their children. Now the parents are upset because Ms. Mendoza threw a chair at them. Ms. Mendoza is upset with Mr. Martin for making her see her parents, and Mr. Martin is angry with his client because he feels he was right to insist that she see them.

Individuality is expressed in the qualities or characteristics that make each person unique, distinctive from all other persons. Lifestyle, assets, problems, previous life experiences, and feelings are some areas that make this person different. Recognizing and treating each person individually rather than stereotypically is how workers put this value into practice.

When Beth first started working with the elderly, she had had little contact with older individuals. What she knew about them she had learned from her grandparents. She thought of the elderly as lively and quick-witted like her grandmother or quiet and shy, living in the past, like her grandfather. During her first months at the nursing home, the clients she encountered continually surprised her. They represented a broad range of human attitudes, behaviors, and experiences. She learned to distinguish between the generalizations she had made about the elderly and the information she now possessed based on her experiences at the nursing home.

Deciding for oneself on a course of action or the resolution to a problem is *self-determination*. The helper allows clients to make up their own minds regarding a decision to be made or an action to be taken. The helper facilitates this action by objectively assisting clients to investigate alternatives and by remembering that the decision is theirs. In some cases, clients are limited by their situations or their choices. For example, a prison inmate may have restricted alternatives from which to choose recreational activities; however, it is the inmate's right to choose from the available alternatives.

When Beth worked with teenagers, she was constantly aware that although these clients were not of legal age, they needed to believe they had some control over their own lives. She often helped them sort out alternatives, but she constantly resisted when they asked her to give advice or to make their choices for them. She believed that they should be responsible in most situations.

The last human service value is *confidentiality.* This is the helper's assurance to clients that the helper will not discuss their cases with other people—that what they discuss between them will not be the subject of conversation with the helper's friends, family, or other clients. The exception to this is the sharing of information with supervisors or in staff meetings where the client's best interests are being served.

A speech that Beth learned early when she was working with the elderly still applies in her work with clients in community mental health. When clients ask if she will keep information confidential, she responds, "Most information that you give me I will keep to myself. I do keep records about my discussions with you to share with other colleagues who need the information. But at any time, if you tell me of your plans to hurt yourself or others, I will need to tell the appropriate people." This speech reminds Beth of the practical application of this important value.

You should consider the following questions as you think about the meaning of these values in your own life and practice.

- What kinds of client behaviors would be the most difficult for you to accept? How would you meet the challenge of working with these clients?
- When was the last time you felt uncomfortable sharing information about another person? How did you resolve the situation?

As you think about these five values in relation to yourself as a future human service professional, consider the possibility of working with many different clients. As you think about the clients listed below, place a check beside those clients who would be difficult for *you* to work with. Which values might present problems or conflicts for you? Try to respond honestly, not what you think would be socially or professionally desirable.

_____ a man with fundamental religious beliefs who refuses treatment for a life-threatening illness

_____ a same-sex couple who wants to resolve some conflicts they are having in their relationship

_____ a man who wants to leave his wife and two children to have sexual adventures with other women

_____ a young woman who wants an abortion but is seeking your help in making the decision

_____ a person who has severe burn scars on the face, shoulders, arms, and hands

_____ a man or woman from a Middle Eastern culture where the male is dominant and the female submissive

_____ a person who does not want to work

_____ a man who strongly believes the only way to bring up his children is by punishing them severely

_____ a woman who wants to leave her husband and children in order to have a career and independence, but is afraid to do it

_____ a person who is so physically attractive that you can't concentrate on what the person is saying

Values are the groundwork for creating a philosophy of helping, which in turn provides a basis for working with people. A philosophy of helping embodies beliefs about human nature, the nature of change, and the process of helping. As individuals grow and develop and as their values change, their helping philosophy and style also develop. An example is the way Beth's values translate into her philosophy of helping, which influences her human service practice. (See Table 6-2.)

Beth believes that all human beings are good and that all behavior is directed to the good. She thinks that violence to others, cruelty, and self-abuse are all behaviors that the perpetrators consider to be positive ways to meet their personal needs. She also believes that people have the capacity to change, if only they believe they can change. Hence, the helper's responsibility is to develop clients' belief in themselves and help provide alternatives for change, practical assistance, and support. Because of these views, Beth has high hopes for her clients, and she believes that her major responsibility is to educate and motivate them. She is frustrated when she works with clients who have tried to hurt others, and she is puzzled when those clients do not want to change. In spite of her frustration, she has maintained her belief in the goodness of human beings.

TABLE 6-2   ✦   SUMMARY POINTS: VALUES THAT GUIDE PRACTICE

Acceptance	Maintain goodwill and refrain from judging
Tolerance	Be patient and fair
Respect for individuality	Respect differences, avoid stereotypes
Self-determination	Help clients make decisions
Confidentiality	Will not disclose client information

Characteristics of the Helper

To be an effective helper demands the use of the helper's whole self, not just a professional segment of it. This requirement creates difficulty when one tries to generalize about the values and characteristics that helpers ought to have. Ideas differ widely about what helpers should be like and what they bring to their work with others. In this section, you will read about some of these ideas. You will also be encouraged to think about the qualities you possess that might be important to your work as a helping professional, as well as qualities you may want to develop more fully to increase your effectiveness.

Brill (1998) believes that individuals learn attitudes and behaviors as they respond to their circumstances. Some responses may even be unconscious. Through the learning process, a person internalizes these attitudes and behaviors and they become a pattern in his or her life. A major influence on how an individual reacts to these needs is culture. Families, schools, and peers are among the agents who communicate ways of behaving and help determine what an individual considers to be acceptable and unacceptable behavior in different situations.

An increasing body of research supports the concept that the personal characteristics of helpers are largely responsible for the success or failure of their helping (Brown & Srebalus, 1996). In fact, Brammer (1999) concluded from numerous studies that these personal characteristics are as significant in helping as the methods helpers use. A number of researchers have examined these characteristics, and we studied this work to identify the traits that seem to be universal in effective helpers.

Eriksen (1981) began by stating what the helping person should be able to do: "listen with understanding and act with skill, experience, information, and self-awareness" (p. 128). To do this, the helper should be self-aware, objective, professionally competent, and actively involved in the enabling process.

Okun (1997) reviewed a number of research studies and concluded that certain qualities, behaviors, and knowledge on the part of the helper most influence the behaviors, attitudes, and feelings of clients. Self-awareness, honesty, congruence, the ability to communicate, knowledge, and ethical integrity are included in her list.

Brown and Srebalus (1996) also reviewed the literature and found a consensus that effective helpers have definite traits. One way to discuss what these are is to use a framework based on the work of Brammer (1999) and Combs (1969), which suggests two sets of attitudes: one related to self and the other to how one treats another person. The traits they consider important are personal congruence, empathy, cultural sensitivity, genuineness, respect, and communication.

All the characteristics mentioned are important ones for helpers. Many other perspectives can be studied, but this brief discussion shows that certain characteristics tend to be common to most studies. In preparing this text, we have reviewed a number of perspectives. Our guiding question was, "What characteristics are important for the beginning human service professional?" We identified the following qualities as important: self-awareness, the ability to communicate, empathy, and professional commitment. Each of these is discussed in depth to

The Task of Philosophy

Whether we recognize it or not, all facets of our behavior, the way we treat other people, our choices and decisions, our reactions, our values, our responsibilities or lack of it, are embedded in a philosophical base. Whether or not we are philosophically aware, we function one way or another depending on what we believe. Our philosophical beliefs are more often than not only vaguely sensed, more shadow than substance. Asked to delineate our philosophical tenets, most of us would deny ever having considered the subject. And yet our philosophical beliefs determine our response to our environment and to the individuals who people it.

Consider, for example, how one would react if he believed on the one hand that man is essentially good, or on the other, that man is essentially evil; if he were an idealist or a pragmatist; if he believed man to be a rational being or a nonrational being; if he believed in free will and freedom of choice or if he believed in determinism and predestination; if he operated from a scientific base or from a religious one.

Man is essentially good. Man is essentially evil.	Trust in man, individually and collectively. Distrust.
Idealist	Search for the absolute, the perfect in terms of goodness, truth, etc.
Pragmatist	Concentration on the present; "what works is good, useful."
Man is a rational being.	If man has the facts, he will solve his problems and work through to a logical conclusion.
Man is a nonrational being.	Emotions play a major role in man's decisions; information alone won't guarantee a solution and an end to problems.
Free will	Man has freedom to make choices, and can be the major architect of his future.
Determinism	Man is a victim of his environment, has no choices, and is the victim rather than the master of fate.
Scientific orientation	Concern with objectivity, logic, and empiricism.
Religious orientation	Concern with subjectivity, faith, and inspiration.

SOURCE: Excerpt from *Barriers and Hazards in Counseling,* by D. E. Johnson and M. J. Vestermark, pp. 39–42. Copyright © 1970 by Houghton Mifflin Company. Adapted with permission.

help understand what the quality is and why it is important for entry-level practice. (See Table 6-3.)

SELF-AWARENESS

Most authorities in the helping professions agree that helpers must know who they are because this self-knowledge affects what they do. Developing self-awareness is a lifelong process of learning about oneself by continually examining one's beliefs, attitudes, values, and behaviors. Recognizing stereotypes, biases, and cultural and gender differences are part of the self-awareness process. It is a particularly critical process for helpers because it assists them in understanding and changing their attitudes and feelings that may hinder helping. The importance of self-acceptance is underscored by the helper's use of self in the helping process.

Beth Bruce's awareness of self expanded greatly when she began to work in the field full time. As she began to learn about the culture and beliefs of others, she developed a keener sense of who she was. It seemed that, as she developed the patience to work with her first clients—who were mentally ill clients—she also became more patient with herself.

ABILITY TO COMMUNICATE

Helpers' effectiveness depends in part on their ability to communicate to the client an understanding of the client's feelings and behaviors (Okun, 1997). Listening, a critical helping skill, is the beginning of helping and is necessary for establishing trust, building rapport, and identifying the problem. Careful listening means being "tuned in" to all the nuances of the client's message, including verbal and nonverbal aspects of what is said as well as what is not said. Such focused listening enables the helper to respond with thoughts and feelings to the client's whole message.

Beth Bruce's ability to communicate was challenged when she began her work with adolescents at the hospital. These young people were aggressive, belligerent, and violent. She worked hard to listen, gain their trust, and provide them honest, constructive feedback. One of the most important skills Beth learned was to listen to the client's entire statement before formulating a response.

EMPATHY

Empathy is acceptance of another person. This quality allows the helper to see a situation or experience a feeling from the client's perspective. This may be

TABLE 6-3   ◆   SUMMARY POINTS: CHARACTERISTICS
OF EFFECTIVE HELPERS

Self-awareness	Helper understands self
Ability to communicate	Being "tuned in" to client's message
Empathy	Understand experience from client perspective
Responsibility/commitment	Devoted to well-being of others

easier for helpers who have had experiences similar to those of their clients. For example, this may explain the understanding that recovering alcoholics have for other alcoholics, widows for the recently bereaved, and parolees for the incarcerated. It does not mean, however, that helpers whose experiences are different cannot express the unconditional acceptance of the client that is a characteristic of empathy.

When Beth worked with her elderly clients, they used to tell her "you will not really understand until you are older." Beth used her communication skills to reflect feelings and content of her clients in order to demonstrate her understanding of their plight.

RESPONSIBILITY/COMMITMENT

Feeling a responsibility or commitment to improve the well-being of others is an important attribute of human service professionals. This includes attending to the needs of clients first and foremost. It also means a commitment to delivering high-quality services. In other words, workers act in the best interests of clients and do so to the best of their ability. One way that workers do this is by following a code of ethics or a set of ethical standards that guide professional behavior or conduct. Among other things, codes of ethics in the helping profession spell out what the client has a right to expect from the helper. Honesty may be one expectation of the client—a belief that the worker will be honest in answering questions or practicing only what he or she is trained to do.

Beth has been troubled by ethical dilemmas throughout her work experience. Fortunately her values have guided her practice and her supervisors have praised her responsible actions. Several examples of ethical codes and standards are presented in Chapter 9.

Typology of Human Service Professionals

Besides understanding who the human service professional is in terms of characteristics, values, and philosophy of helping, the student of human services should also know the professional categories that describe such workers. The human service profession includes several levels of workers, which may be classified in a variety of ways. Two considerations present in most categorizations are educational preparation or training and competence. The next subsection discusses categories of professional work developed by three professional educators.

Categories of Workers

The Southern Regional Education Board (SREB) identified four levels of competence in its publication, *Staff Roles for Mental Health Personnel: A History and a Rationale* (1979). Level 1 is an *entry-level* category that includes those workers who have a few weeks or months of instruction and some in-service training. These individuals may have little actual on-the-job experience. Level 2,

Maslow's View of Helping

Abraham Maslow, a man of vision, described life by taking into account "its highest aspirations." He was dedicated to encouraging development of human potential. This enthusiasm led Maslow to make statements on how people can help each other more effectively. The following written statement demonstrates his creativity and his sensitivity toward helping.

Helping? Well, I have a label for it (labels are good, they are useful for me), I call it the Bodhisattvic Version (Path). We have no good word in English for *helper*; it carries too many surplus connotations with it. I've used the Eastern conception of the Bodhisattva and transformed it a little bit for our purposes. Do you know what the word means?

There are two Buddhistic legends. In one the Buddha sat under a tree and had the great revelation he saw the truth. It's very Socratic. He saw the truth, the truth was revealed to him, and then he ascended to heaven, so to speak, to Nirvana. In another version, the Bodhisattvic Version, the Buddha sat under the tree, had a great illumination, saw the truth, ascended to the gates of heaven, and there, out of compassion for mankind, could not bear to selfishly enter heaven and came back to earth to help—on the assumption that nobody could go to heaven unless we all go to heaven.

So this is a beautiful legend, and what it means for us, I think, is to recognize that helping in the first place is a very, very hard job and the helper can be a clumsy fool—the helper can be a hurter. Very frequently it would be best to be Taoistic about helping; to keep your damn hands off is frequently the best way to help. To know when to be available and when not is to think of the helper as being available, being the consultant, rather than being the manipulator, controller, interferer, giving orders and telling people what to do, which is our choice and which is very Western. The helper comes. The helper is very frequently just a plain

the *technical/apprentice* level, includes those who have one to two years of formal training or experience. Sometimes these helpers have earned an associate arts degree. Level 3, the *associate professional* level, includes those helpers with formal training or experience, usually at the baccalaureate level. Helpers with master's or doctoral degrees are in Level 4, the *professional/specialist* level.

Another way of categorizing helpers is to divide them into two classes (Brammer, 1999). The first, the nonprofessional, includes helpers who offer unstructured assistance through friendships, family relations, and community and general human concern. The second category, the professional who provides structured helping, is the one in which we are interested. It is further divided into three categories of workers: *professional helpers, paraprofessionals,* and *volunteers and peers.* Professional helpers are characterized by certification

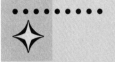

god-damn nuisance—as, for instance, anybody in the ghettos can tell you. Why should it be that the social workers, who want to help, who devote their lives to helping, should be so frequently despised and hated?

I've supposed that the Bodhisattvic kind of helping is a reliance on the self-choice of the person with you the helper being available at the wish of the other, rather than you the helper taking control of the situation and telling people what to do. This implies a kind of humility, also, because in effect what I'm asking here is that the helper become a perfect person. This is a very hard thing to do—that is, to know when to keep your hands off and when you help and when to be available and so on—especially with our young children, where frequently we do have to interfere.

What is implied, therefore, is that one of the paths to being a helper is to become a better and better person, in the psychotherapeutic sense, in the sense of maturing, evolving, becoming more fully human, and so on. If you want to help others best, improve yourself. Cure yourself. To the extent that you're neurotic when you try to help them. To the extent that you can be democratic, accepting, Taoistic, to that extent you are more likely to help better them. But this is a paradox, because one of the paths to becoming a person is by being selfish, by being within your own skin. So this paradox has to be resolved; it's kind of like the hen and the egg thing, of simultaneously, if you want to be the better helper, improving yourself and being helpful the best way you can—but doing it in the spirit of humility and of modesty rather than in the spirit of taking control.

SOURCE: Excerpt from *Abraham H. Maslow: A Memorial Volume, an International Study Project,* pp. 39–42. Copyright © 1972 by Wadsworth Publishing Company, Inc. Reprinted by permission of Brooks/Cole Publishing Co.

from professional groups, licenses by governing bodies, and degrees from educational institutions. Examples of professionals in this category are social workers, nurses, ministers, and counselors. The second group consists of paraprofessional helpers who perform some of the traditional counseling functions but also engage in broader roles, such as those of advocate and mobilizer. What distinguishes each group is the amount of formal training its members have had, their level of responsibility, and their degree of participation in policy formation. In addition, members of the professional group possess research skills, a wider theoretical background, and clinical judgment, a result of their clinical training and supervision. Tension may occur between paraprofessionals and professionals, in part because of increasing evidence that each group may be as effective as the other in delivering services.

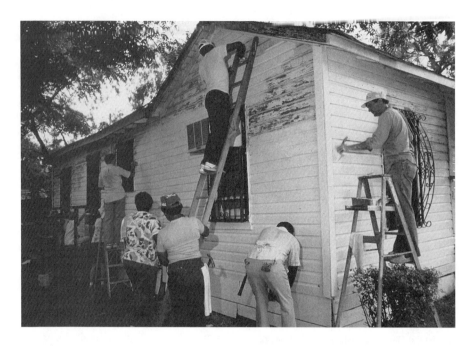

A third way to categorize helpers, similar to Brammer's (1999) system, is one proposed by Okun (1997), who categorizes workers as *professional helpers, generalist human service workers,* and *nonprofessional helpers.* Workers who are trained specialists with graduate-level training in helping theory and skills and who often have supervised clinical experience are classified as professional helpers, even though their training and credentials may vary. These professional helpers may work with generalist human service workers as part of a team, as supervisors, or as consultants. Generalist human service workers have education and training at the undergraduate level and job titles such as psychiatric technicians or aides, youth street workers, day care staff, probation officers, and church workers. Okun's third category, nonprofessional helpers, includes workers with some training in helping and little agency responsibility. They use communication skills to develop helping relationships with those people they are assisting. Included here are volunteers who work for no pay and peer helpers, who may be similar in age and experience to the clients.

The Human Service Professional

As a result of an unmet need for trained, educated workers in human services, the 1992–1993 edition of the *Occupational Outlook Handbook* included an entry on the human service worker. The latest edition continues to highlight the diversity of job titles, duties, client groups, and employment settings found in the human service profession (*Occupational Outlook Handbook,* 1998–1999). For example, the list of possible settings in which such workers may be employed includes "offices, group homes, shelters, day programs, sheltered workshops, hospitals, clinics, and in the field visiting clients" (p. 129). Examples of the variety of job titles are "social service assistant, case management aide, social work assistant, residential counselor, community support worker, alcohol or drug abuse counselor, mental health technician, child-care worker, community outreach worker, life skills counselor, and gerontology aide" (p. 129).

According to the *Occupational Outlook Handbook*, human service workers are generally under the direction of professionals who have advanced training or degrees. However, the degree of supervision they receive and the amount of responsibility they have vary a great deal, depending on their education and training, job duties, and client groups. "Some are on their own most of the time and have little direct supervision; others work under close direction" (p. 128). Those with a high school education are likely to perform clerical tasks, and those with a college degree may engage in counseling, service coordination, or management. The attainment of a bachelor's or master's degree is necessary for supervisory positions that involve greater responsibilities.

Employment opportunities include governmental, for profit, and not-for-profit settings. State and local governments employed about one in three in public welfare agencies and facilities for individuals who are mentally disabled and developmentally delayed. Another third were employed by private social or human service agencies offering a variety of services including adult day care, group meals, crisis intervention, and counseling. Many helpers supervised residents of group homes and halfway houses. They also worked in clinics, detoxification units, community mental health centers, psychiatric hospitals, day treatment programs, and sheltered workshops.

The *Occupational Outlook Handbook* (1998–1999) illustrates the diversity of settings, client groups served, and job duties. In providing direct and indirect client services, "they assess clients' needs, establish their eligibility for benefits and services, and help clients obtain them. They examine financial documents such as rent receipts and tax returns to determine whether the client is eligible for food stamps, Medicaid, welfare, and other human service programs. They also arrange for transportation and escorts, if necessary, and provide emotional support" (pp. 128–129). As service providers, they also monitor and keep case records on clients and report progress to supervisors. According to the *Handbook*:

> The variety of roles human service workers play in community settings requires a diversity of skills. They may organize and lead group activities, assist clients in need of counseling or crisis intervention, or administer a food bank or emergency fuel program. In halfway houses, group homes and government-supported housing programs, they assist adult residents who need supervision in personal hygiene and daily living skills. They review clients' records, ensure they take correct doses of medication, talk with their families, and confer with medical personnel to gain better insight into clients' backgrounds and needs. They also provide emotional support and help clients become involved in community recreation programs and other activities.

In psychiatric hospitals, rehabilitation programs, and outpatient clinics, they may help clients master everyday living skills and teach them how to communicate more effectively and get along better with others. They support the client's participation in the treatment plan, such as individual or group counseling and occupational therapy (pp. 128–129).

The job outlook for human service workers is excellent. Projections are that the number of workers will grow much faster than the average for all occupations through 2006, making it one of the most rapidly growing occupations. The rapid growth in the demand for services coupled with slower growth in resources to provide services means that employers will rely increasingly on human service workers rather than higher paid occupations.

Other Professional Helpers

As a human service professional, you will be working with a variety of other professional helpers. This section, adapted from the 1998–1999 *Occupational Outlook Handbook,* identifies the nature of the work and the training of these individuals so you will be familiar with them.

PHYSICIANS

Physicians perform medical examinations, diagnose illnesses, treat injured or diseased people, and advise patients on maintaining good health. They may be general practitioners or specialists in a particular field of medicine.

Physicians are required by all states to be licensed. It usually takes about 11 years to become a physician: 4 years of undergraduate school, 4 years of medical school, and 3 years of residency. Those who choose to specialize usually spend 3 to 5 years in training and another 2 years in preparation for practice in a specialty area.

One example of a specialist with whom you will likely be in contact is a *psychiatrist.* Concerned with the diagnosis, treatment, and prevention of mental illness, psychiatrists may be found in private offices and institutional settings, courtrooms, community-centered care facilities, and specialized medical areas such as coronary and intensive care units. They frequently act as consultants to other agencies. Psychiatrists are medical doctors who have an additional five years or more of psychiatric training and experience and are qualified to use the full range of medical techniques in treating clients. These include drugs, shock, and surgery, in addition to counseling and behavior modification techniques.

PSYCHOLOGISTS

Although their training and the kinds of treatment they use are different, psychologists are sometimes confused with psychiatrists. Psychologists study human behavior and mental processes to understand and explain people's actions.

An individual may specialize in any of several areas within psychology, including clinical, counseling, developmental, industrial-organizational, school, and social psychology. Each specialty focuses on a different aspect of human behavior. For example, the developmental psychologist is concerned with the behavioral changes people experience as they progress through life. Clinical psychologists, on the other hand, may work in hospitals, clinics, or private practice to help individuals who are mentally or emotionally disturbed adjust to life and to help medical and surgical patients deal with their illnesses and injuries. They may use interviews, diagnostic tests, and psychotherapy in their work.

Psychologists may practice with a master's degree or a doctoral degree. A master's degree prepares the person to administer and interpret tests, conduct research, and counsel patients. The doctoral degree usually requires five to seven years of graduate study and is often required for employment as a psychologist. A doctorate in psychology and two years of professional experience are generally required for licensure or certification; although requirements may vary from state to state, certification is necessary for private practice.

SOCIAL WORKERS

The focus of social workers is helping individuals, families, and groups cope with a wide variety of problems. The nature of the problem and the time and resources available determine the methods used, which may include counseling, advocacy, and referral. Social workers also function at the community level to combat social problems. For example, they may coordinate existing programs, organize fund-raising, and develop new community services.

Social workers may also specialize in various areas. Medical social workers are trained to help patients and their families cope with problems that accompany illness or rehabilitation. Those who specialize in family services counsel individuals to strengthen personal and family relationships. Corrections and child welfare are other popular areas of study and employment.

Preparation for the field of social work occurs at two levels. The baccalaureate level (BSW) is the minimum requirement, followed by the master's degree in social work (MSW), which is usually required for positions in mental health and for administrative or research positions. Training generally includes courses of study focusing on social work practice, social welfare policies, human behavior, and the social environment. Supervised field experiences are also necessary.

The National Association of Social Workers (NASW) awards certification in the form of the title ACSW, which stands for the Academy of Certified Social Workers. Licensing or registration laws have also been passed by many states to regulate social work practice.

COUNSELORS

One of the largest categories of professional helpers is counselors. Although their exact duties depend on the individuals or groups with whom they work and the agencies or settings in which they are employed, counselors help people deal with a variety of problems, including personal, social, educational, and career concerns. Examples of the different types of counselors are school and college counselors, rehabilitation counselors, employment counselors, and mental health counselors. Two with whom you may interact as a human service professional are mental health counselors and rehabilitation counselors.

The *mental health counselor* works with individuals who are dealing with problems such as drug and alcohol abuse, family conflicts, suicidal thoughts and feelings, stress management, problems with self-esteem, issues associated with aging, job and career concerns, educational decisions, and issues of mental and emotional health. Their work is not limited to individuals, however; it may involve the family of the individual. These counselors often work closely with other specialists such as psychiatrists, psychologists, clinical social workers, and psychiatric nurses.

The *rehabilitation counselor* helps people deal with the personal, social, and vocational effects of their disabilities. Disabilities may be social, mental, emotional, or physical, calling for the services of counseling, evaluation, medical care, occupational training, and job placement. Rehabilitation counselors also work with the family of the individual when necessary and frequently with other professionals such as physicians, psychologists, and occupational therapists.

Positions as a counselor usually require a master's degree in a counseling discipline or a related area. This preparation frequently includes a year or two of graduate study and a supervised counseling experience. Licensure and certification are available; requirements vary, depending on the specialty. The National Board for Certified Counselors (NBCC) and the Commission on Rehabilitation Counselor Certification (CRCC) are two national certifying bodies.

Human service workers could assume the responsibilities of social workers or counselors, or be given this title, even though they might not be specifically certified as such. The variation in the needs of agencies and the competencies of individual workers makes it difficult to establish rigid categories for function or title. However, having the title or performing the job of a mental health counselor is definitely not the same as being nationally certified. Some states and agencies will only hire workers with national certification, whereas other sites have more flexible hiring categories. (See Table 6-4.)

 ## Human Service Roles

At this point in Chapter 6, you have some idea about the identity of the human service professional and the relationship of this individual with other helping professionals. An examination of their roles further defines the human service professional.

TABLE 6-4   ♦   SUMMARY POINTS: OTHER PROFESSIONAL HELPERS

Physicians	Licensed medical professionals who provide general medical services or specialty services
Psychologists	Study human behavior to understand individual thoughts and actions
Social Workers	Help individuals, families, and groups cope with problems
Counselors	Help people deal with a variety of problems

The many human service roles to be introduced provide the framework for the helping process. In performing the various roles, the human service professional is continuously focused on the client; this client focus provides the common thread to connect the roles.

Although the roles of human service professionals are constantly evolving, the helper remains a "Jack or Jill of all trades," or, in human service terms, a generalist. The generalist knows a wide range of skills, strategies, and client groups and is able to work effectively in a number of different settings. Engaging in a variety of roles enables the human service professional to meet many client needs. What exactly do these helpers do?

Many professionals have attempted to answer this question. The Southern Regional Education Board (SREB) conducted a study in the late 1960s to define the roles and functions of human service professionals. Making use of the developmental approach, the SREB recognized that professions emerge in response to client needs. To reexamine the needs and problems that originally brought the profession into being, the SREB asked the following questions:

- Are the needs still the same?
- What are they?
- What tasks must be carried out to meet them?

As a result of this analysis, SREB identified 13 roles that human service workers could engage in to meet the needs of their clients, agencies, or communities (SREB, 1969). These 13 roles include administrator, advocate, assistant to specialist, behavior changer, broker, caregiver, community planner, consultant, data manager, evaluator, mobilizer, outreach worker, and teacher/educator.

In a more recent study, the U.S. Department of Education funded the Community Support Skills Standards Project to define the skills that human service personnel need to work in the field. The result of the work was a set of 12 broad, functional themes of work in human services. These emerged from a job analysis and are reflected in the project's report as competency areas. The areas are as follows: participant empowerment; communication; assessment; community and service networking; facilitation of services; community living skills and supports; education, training, and self-development; advocacy; vocational, educational, and career support; crisis intervention; organizational participation; and documentation (Taylor, Bradley, & Warren, 1996).

To better understand the varied roles that are assumed by the human service professional, we used the results of these two studies to categorize three areas of responsibility: providing direct service, performing administrative work, and working with the community. Next we examine these three categories and the roles that represent each area of responsibility. (See Table 6-5.)

Providing Direct Service

Providing direct service to clients is a responsibility with which many beginning professionals are familiar. This work represents the development of the helping relationship and the work that helpers do in their face-to-face encounters with

TABLE 6-5   ✦   HUMAN SERVICE ROLES

Providing direct service	Performing administrative work	Working with the community
Behavior changer	Broker	Advocate
Caregiver	Data manager	Community and service
Communicator	Evaluator	networker
Crisis intervener	Facilitator of services	Community planner
Participant empowerer	Planner	Consultant
Teacher/educator	Report writer	Mobilizer
	Resource allocator	Outreach worker

their clients. Many roles, such as behavior changer, caregiver, communicator, crisis intervener, participant empowerer, and teacher/educator, are included in the category of direct services. The following illustrate many of these roles and how human service professionals perform them.

Behavior changer—carries out a range of activities planned primarily to change clients' behavior, ranging from coaching and counseling to casework, psychotherapy, and behavior therapy.

Sun Lee Kim is a substance abuse counselor at a drug and alcohol inpatient clinic at a local hospital. Sun Lee, one of the staff group leaders, facilitates a reality therapy group each day. The purpose of this group is to encourage participants to change their communication behavior, first in the group and later in the wider context of the facility. Peer support and pressure are used to facilitate this behavior change.

Caregiver—provides services for people who need ongoing support of some kind, such as financial assistance, day care, social support, and 24-hour care.

Jim Gray works in foster care. His major responsibility is to provide support to families with foster children. One of his favorite activities is to visit foster homes to determine the success of the foster care situation and provide emotional and practical assistance to the families.

Communicator—is able to express and exchange ideas and establish relationships with a variety of individuals and groups, including clients, families, colleagues, administrators, and the public.

Dal Lam works with AIDS patients in a self-help center established by a regional hospital in a rural desert area. His responsibilities require him to communicate with different populations that include individuals who are testing HIV positive, individuals with AIDS, medical staff, insurance providers, families, and com-

munity groups. He spends much of his time in prevention work that takes him to the elementary schools, local high schools, civic meetings, and churches. His approach is always the same: clear, articulate, compassionate, and confident.

Crisis intervener—provides services for individuals, families, and communities who are experiencing a disruption in their lives with which they cannot cope. This intervention is short term, focused, and concrete.

Christy Holston works in a sexual assault crisis center and is a victim advocate. She receives four or five new clients a week, mostly women, who are dealing with issues of sexual assault, attempted rape, or rape. Some of her clients call through the hotline immediately after being assaulted, others are referred through the emergency room at the hospital, and others call to ask for help many years after the crisis.

Participant empowerer—shares with clients the responsibility for the helping relationship and the development and implementation of a plan of action. This helper ultimately encourages clients to care for themselves.

Judy Collins is a case manager for young adults who are developmentally disabled. In the program, First Steps, she works with clients to move from group home living to apartment living. She coordinates daily living training, vocational assessment and training, and first employment. Her clients participate fully in the case management process and are called "co-case managers." There is a graduation ceremony when these clients become their own "case managers."

Teacher/educator—performs a range of instructional activities, from simple coaching to teaching highly technical content, directed at individuals or groups.

Dr. Washington Lee, a physician, and Ned Wanek, a human service professional, work in a family planning clinic. They spend two mornings a week teaching classes to women and men about the reproductive system and alternative methods of family planning. In addition, they counsel individuals, provide physical exams, plan educational media, and talk to schools and community groups about family planning.

Performing Administrative Work

Performing administrative work is another important responsibility for many human service professionals. In addition to providing direct services to clients, many helpers are involved in managerial activities as they supervise or oversee processes or projects. As they work with clients, they assume administrative

responsibilities such as planning, linking clients to services, allocating resources, and evaluating. The specific administrative roles are broker, data manager, evaluator, facilitator of services, planner, report (documentation) writer,
and resource allocator.

Broker—helps people get to the existing services and helps make the services more accessible to clients.

---

*Maria Giovanni's caseload at the Office for Student Services consists primarily
of students with physical disabilities. One of her functions is to make sure these
students have their classes scheduled in accessible buildings on campus and are
able to get around campus to their classes and events. To achieve this goal, Maria
may have to help students reschedule classes or arrange for parking. She is also
"on call" to assist these students in getting other services they might need.*

Data manager—gathers, tabulates, analyzes, and synthesizes data and
evaluates programs and plans.

---

*Roosevelt Thompson is part of the staff of a local day care center. Although he
assists the child care staff when needed, his actual responsibilities are business
oriented. The day care center is privately owned but partially funded by the
city. Its clients include children referred to the center from the courts for temporary care as well as children of working parents. His concern is to see that
the center maintains an appropriate balance between referred and regular paying clients to maintain its financial stability. He continually gathers information and projects the financial needs of the day care center.*

Evaluator—assesses client or community needs and problems, whether
medical, psychiatric, social, or educational.

---

*Karen Tubbs leads a community planning organization established to assess the
community's needs in the event of a national disaster. In her coastal region, disaster means the threat of damaging winds, rain, and numerous hurricanes. Its
meetings are part of a complex process of planning for and developing resources
to begin providing human services should a hurricane strike their region.*

Facilitator of services—brokers (links the client to services) and then monitors the progress the client makes with the various helping professionals. This
helper also uses the problem-solving process when services are deficient or inappropriate.

---

*Louisa Gonzales works in a group home for young children who need a short-
term safe haven. During the time the children are in the home, Louisa spends*

many hours coordinating their care with schools, child care agencies, the health department, and the welfare department. Many times, without her services, these children would get lost in the system and would receive substandard care.

Planner—engages in making plans with both short-term and long-term clients in order to define accurately their problems and needs, develops strategies to meet the needs, and monitor the helping process.

Ruth Strauss works with families who are planning for the long-term care of aging parents. This requires careful attention to the needs and priorities of all involved. She has better luck with her families when she uses a very structured planning and decision-making model. With this model, everyone in the family has a clear understanding of the problems and the goals and can monitor the success of the plan.

Report (documentation) writer—records the activities of the agency work. This can include intake interview reports, social histories, detailed treatment plans, daily entries into case notes, requests for resources, rationale and justification for treatment for managed care, and periodic reports for managed care.

Lisa Wilhiem is a social worker in a local hospital emergency room. She is the intermediary for clients who will potentially need longer-term care. It is her responsibility to coordinate the initial requests for services to the managed care organizations or insurance companies. Although she spends several hours of her day with patients and the medical care staff, a majority of her time is spent documenting how the patient entered the health care system and what the current needs of the patient are.

Resource allocator—makes recommendations on how resources are to be spent to support the needs of the client. These recommendations are made once priorities are set and prices for services are determined.

Hoover Center, a psychiatric facility for adolescents, is developing a new program that will individualize the treatment of its clients. In the past, there was a standard treatment for all clients regardless of their problems. Because of the pressures from managed care and the limited resources available for the center, the decision has been made to ask each client's case managers to establish priorities and determine how the resources per client are to be spent. The case manager will submit a plan that will be approved by the supervisor and then submitted to the managed care organization for review and final approval.

Working with the Community

Many professionals are also very involved with their community as they develop collegial networks and work on behalf of their clients to create and improve services within the local area and beyond. The roles of advocate, community and service networker, community planner, consultant, mobilizer, and outreach worker are those which the helper assumes responsibility in the community context.

Advocate—pleads and fights for services, policies, rules, regulations, and laws on behalf of clients.

Jose Cervantes is a lawyer for a legal aid clinic in an urban area. His clients, referred by the courts, are individuals who need legal services but cannot pay for them. Most of his cases involve marital separation, divorce, custody of children, and spouse and child support. Besides handling individual cases, Jose works with politicians, judges, and other lawyers to develop a legal system that is sensitive to the needs of his clients.

Community and service networker—works actively to connect with other helpers and agencies to plan for providing better services to the community and to clients, share information, support education and training efforts, and facilitate linking clients to the services they need.

Ian DeBusk has been working for the public schools for the past 20 years. Early in his career he worked with in-school suspension programs and today he supervises school counselors in 15 high schools, 12 middle schools, and 32 elementary schools. One of his responsibilities is to help his counselors find the services their students need. Ian has colleagues within the criminal justice system, child welfare services, health department, and vocational rehabilitation agency, to name just a few. Each day he spends time on the phone and on the road helping those in his network and also asking them to help his counselors and their students.

Community planner—works with community boards and committees to ensure that community services promote mental health and self-actualization, or at least minimize emotional stress on people.

Hector Gomez is director of the local department of human services. As director, part of his responsibility is to provide leadership in human services to the city and county. He spends many evenings attending board meetings with other members of the community, discussing funding and future planning for human services.

Consultant—works with other professions and agencies regarding their handling of problems, needs, and programs.

Three members of a pediatric language lab serving young children with communication disorders have formed a consulting service as part of their job responsibilities with the lab. The focus of the service is to educate teachers and day care staff about communication disorders and help them work with children in their own facilities. The consulting activity will enable the lab to expand the impact of its services.

Mobilizer—helps to get new resources for clients and communities.

Just last week James Shabbaz, a psychiatric social worker at the research hospital, discovered that the funding for the newly formed hospice service was not being renewed. The support services provided to family members of dying patients will be difficult to replace. James has decided to schedule a meeting with hospital staff and members of local churches to assist him in thinking about alternative support for these family members.

Outreach worker—reaches out to identify people with problems, refer them to appropriate services, and follow up to make sure they continue to their maximum rehabilitation.

Greg Jones from the local mental health center travels into rural sections of a three-county area to follow up on patients who have been released from the regional mental health facility. His primary responsibilities are to provide supportive counseling, assess current progress, and make appropriate referrals.

Each job in the human service field represents a unique combination of roles and responsibilities. The following list shows the way in which roles and responsibilities can be configured.

HOME HEALTH CARE COORDINATOR
- Broker
- Data manager
- Evaluator
- Facilitator of services
- Report writer (documentation)

PAROLE OFFICER
- Broker
- Data manager
- Planner
- Report (documentation) writer

MENTAL HEALTH CASE MANAGER
- Behavior changer
- Caregiver
- Crisis intervener
- Data manager
- Evaluator
- Facilitator of services
- Report (documentation) writer
- Resource allocator

CHILD CARE PROFESSIONAL
- Advocate
- Behavior changer
- Communicator
- Report (documentation) writer
- Teacher/educator

FOOD BANK ORGANIZER
- Communicator
- Community and service networker
- Community planner
- Mobilizer
- Outreach worker

As you learn more about human services and meet human service professionals, try to determine the roles they are performing and the responsibilities they assume as they work with clients, their colleagues, and the community.

Frontline Worker or Administrator

Workers may generally be categorized as having either frontline or administrative responsibilities. Using only these two categories may oversimplify the actual responsibilities of a given helper, but the categorization is useful when you are visualizing what human service professionals actually do. The schedules that follow outline the typical day of a frontline worker and an administrator.

FRONTLINE WORKER: WOMEN'S CASE COORDINATOR (SHELTER FOR BATTERED WOMEN AND THEIR CHILDREN)

8:00 A.M. Use this time to finish what needs to be completed from the previous day if planned activities were interrupted by an emergency with a client. Read the progress notes in the case files. See clients at about 8:30—set up the appointments a day in advance. See each client two or three times each week, depending on their schedules. Be prepared for a crisis and a new client.

10:00 A.M. Go to court for orders of protection. This can last all day, depending on how many cases are on the docket. Go to court with a client for her hearing or to file for an order of protection.

11:00 A.M. If back from court, see clients or do paperwork.

12:00 noon Go to the dining room to eat with clients.

1:00 P.M. Run errands with clients; go to their homes for clothing or important documents. Get a police escort for entering the home.

3:00 P.M. Attend staff meetings once a week (usually lasting a couple of hours). During these meetings, discuss each case and service issues.

5:00 P.M. Update case notes. Set up appointments for the next day.

ADMINISTRATOR: DIRECTOR, SOCIAL SERVICES

8:00 A.M. Attend morning meetings to coordinate staff activities. Prioritize week's projects.

9:00 A.M. Check client vacancies; plan for number of admissions. Make phone calls. Gather information, review referrals, and schedule meetings and follow-up activities.

10:00 A.M. Meet with families, phone hospitals for possible admissions, meet with clients.

11:00 A.M. Meet with head administrator. Make plans, revise schedule for afternoon.

12:00 noon Eat at desk or with clients. Catch up on mail, read reports, write letters.

1:00 P.M. Discharge planning for clients. Meet with part-time staff. Reprioritize based on morning's activities.

2:00 P.M. Meet with other professionals, such as bookkeepers and nurses; contact services outside agency for information, planning, and referrals.

3:00 P.M. Complete referral book and complaint log. Make sure all tasks and written correspondence are completed. Be available to see clients and families.

4:00 P.M. Answer phone calls. Finish reports due that day. Visit with clients and families.

5:00 P.M. Complete paperwork. Plan for the next day. Answer phone calls, call people at home.

7:00 P.M. Evening visit with family or client in hospital, read mail, work on big projects to improve services, attend professional meetings.

As you can see by reading these examples, both professionals perform more than one role. Although frontline workers and administrators sometimes have similar responsiblities, each has a different focus. The frontline worker focuses on caring for the client; the administrator's primary focus is on planning and organizing services. Both have valuable responsibilities in human service delivery and share the ultimate goal of helping clients.

 ## Case Study: Meet Carmen Rodriguez

The following case study provides an example of a human service professional who is involved with many of the issues helpers encounter. As you read the case study, consider the helper's roles, values, and characteristics. Are there any potential sources of frustration for the worker? What are her expectations?

• • • • • • • • •

WEB SOURCES:
Find Out More About Helper Roles

http://www.optonline.com/comptons/ceo/00482_A.html

At this site you will find the *Compton's Encyclopedia's* entry for behavior modification. This is one of the counseling techniques that a helper in the role of behavior changer will use.

http://www.caregiver911.com/

This site provides help to those providing 24-hour services to individuals who cannot care for themselves. It provides online discussions and resources for those providing this care. Sometimes the human service professional is the caregiver; other times the professional is supporting the "at-home" 24-caregiver.

http://www.apa.org

This website of the American Psychological Association provides information for students who are interested in pursuing careers in psychology. It also offers an opportunity for users to search more specific topics such as roles.

http://www.acsu.buffalo.edu/~drstall/hndbk0.html

This site is a handbook for the caregiver of the elderly. It contains in-depth discussion of issues that caregivers (both professional and lay) face and provides suggestions for help and support. It is comprehensive and covers topics such as legal and ethical issues.

http://www.crisishotline.org/

This website is the crisis hotline in Houston, Texas. Many helping professionals are involved in crisis intervention. This site describes the services provided, including a hotline and crisis counseling.

Carmen Rodriguez has worked as a vocational evaluator for a state agency in the southwestern United States for the past four years. She considers herself a human service professional; with most of her clients, the focus of her work is much broader than just vocational counseling. She describes her job as follows.

I have been a work evaluator for the past four years. In my position, I work with clients to assist them in preparing for and finding gainful employment. One of the requirements for eligibility for services at my agency is that the individual must have a mental, physical, or emotional disability that is a handicap to employment. There must also be a reasonable expectation that the person can be gainfully employed after receiving services.

One of the aspects of my work that I like a lot is the variety of clients I encounter. They are of different ages and from varied backgrounds. I work with many Mexican Americans and Native Americans. My clients are both males and females and, as I said, they have various disabilities. Usually I work with

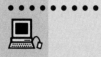

http://www.socialworkers.org

This web address accesses the National Association of Social Workers and provides information about publications, services and resources, and news and information. Career information about the profession, licensure, education, income, and jobs is also available at this site.

http://www.ssa.gov/pubs/10050.html

The Social Security Administration supports vocational rehabilitation for individuals who are disabled. The goal is to help people with disabilities get the vocational rehabilitation services they need to return to work or to go to work for the first time. The agencies to which they refer are involved in the lives of these clients and are providing the teacher/educator function. These teacher/educators provide services such as job counseling, training, and job placement.

http://www.cgr.org/human services/mental health/

One challenge of the new welfare-to-work legislation is how to link the welfare recipients with the services they need. This website outlines these brokering challenges as recognized by New York State. They advocate better brokering to enhance the success of their program.

http://aspe.hhs.gov/daltcp/reports/implees.htm

This site is prepared by the Federal Department of Health and Human Services. It outlines two approaches to long-term care. Both approaches, case management and financial control, use brokering as a major way in which clients are provided the care they need.

a client every day for a period of six to eight weeks. Because of this close contact, I feel that I get to know my clients well.

 Clients come first with me. I constantly think about what I can do for them, and I want to help them in any way I can. Sometimes their circumstances seem so poor, but I know that if I work hard enough I can make their lives better.

 Another rewarding part of my job is working with other professionals. We are all committed to meeting client needs, although at times we are limited by the purposes of our various agencies. We've found that we are much more successful working together. In fact, ten of us from different agencies meet monthly for lunch to talk about our work and find out about other services that may be available. It's also a good time to find out about new legislation and regulations and the ways agencies are dealing with funding problems or new grants.

 Another part of my work that I find particularly challenging is consulting with a variety of specialists, including psychologists, psychiatrists, and other medical specialists. It's important that I be able to speak their language to a certain extent so that I can tell them what we want them to evaluate and the kinds of information they can provide to assist us in our evaluation of the client. It's also helpful to know some of the terminology so that I can under-stand their reports. It does make me nervous to talk to these professionals, be-cause their training is different from mine. It is easier now than when I first began working here.

I guess it's pretty obvious how I feel about my work. It's rewarding and challenging, and I feel as if I learn something new each day. It may seem as if it's the perfect job, but it really isn't. There are some negative aspects to it, and probably the most frustrating is that in a bureaucracy things never seem to move as quickly as I want them to. For example, there is quite a bit of paper-work. To receive an authorization for services, I have to go through several channels. This sometimes takes days, and since I work with the client on a daily basis, I get as impatient as the client.

The other aspect of my job that I sometimes find frustrating is that clients often do not do what I would like them to do. When you work with people, it's important to realize that you don't tell them what to do. Actually, we try to teach them to take responsibility for their actions, and this involves making decisions for themselves. When they make a decision that is not in their best interest or may lead to problems or failure, it's very difficult for me not to in-tervene. I want so much for my clients to succeed, but I've learned that they are independent individuals who must live their own lives. In spite of the frustra-tions, I hope to keep this job for several years. It offers many opportunities for professional growth and gives me a chance to make a difference.

Apply what you have read in this chapter by answering the following ques-tions about Carmen Rodriguez.

- What motivates Carmen in her work?
- What do you think Carmen's philosophy is? What are her values?
- Identify the professionals with whom Carmen works.
- What human services roles does Carmen play?

Things to Remember

1. Helping means assisting people to understand, overcome, or cope with problems. A helper is one who offers such assistance.
2. The primary reason why individuals choose helping professions (and the reason most will admit) is the desire to help others. Related to this is the desire for self-exploration.
3. Values are important to the practice of human services, because they are the criteria by which human service professionals and clients make choices. Acceptance, tolerance, individuality, self-determination, and confidentiality are important values for human service professionals.

4. Characteristics that are important for the entry-level human service professional are self-awareness, the ability to communicate, empathy, and professional commitment.
5. One way of categorizing helping professionals is a three-level system: professional helpers, entry-level professionals, and nonprofessionals.
6. Human service professionals work with other professionals, including physicians, psychologists, social workers, and counselors.
7. The broad range of job titles, duties, client groups, and employment settings in human services supports the generic focus of the profession.
8. Roles and responsibilities of human service professionals can be grouped into three categories: providing direct service, performing administrative work, and working with the community.
9. Frontline workers and administrators are two more categories of human service professionals that describe the complexities of their roles.

Additional Readings: Focus on Helpers

Garrett, S. (1998). *Miles to go: Aging in rural Virginia.* Charlottesville, VA: University Press of Virginia.
From 1991 through 1995, the author followed closely the professionals involved in the Rural Elder Outreach Project in Virginia, an effort to show that communities in five central Virginia rural counties, in partnership with the University of Virginia Schools of Nursing and Medicine and two local agencies, could keep their older people at home and improve the quality of their lives.

Hilfiker, D. (1994). *Not all of us are saints: A doctor's journey with the poor.* New York: Hill and Wang.
This story tells of a physician's move from a practice in rural Minnesota to an inner-city neighborhood in Washington, D.C., and the world of poverty medicine.

Humes, E. (1996). *No matter how loud I shout: A year in the life of juvenile court.* New York: Simon & Schuster.
The author takes readers to the street with probation officers fighting to keep kids alive, into the courthouses where hope and hopelessness collide daily in epic struggles, and past the triple-steel doors of Los Angeles's Central Juvenile Hall.

Ladson-Billings, G. (1994). *The dreamkeepers: Successful teachers of African American children.* San Francisco: Jossey-Bass.
This reflective and empirical work is the story of the pedagogical practice of eight exemplary teachers that has particular significance given the changing demographics of our nation's public schools.

Manning, M. (1996). *Undercurrents: A life beneath the surface.* San Francisco: Harper.
The author, a psychologist, chronicles her own descent into blinding despair and her eventual recovery.

Parent, M. (1998). *Turning stones: My days and nights with children at risk.* New York: Harcourt Brace & Co.
The author, a caseworker for Emergency Children's Services in New York, has written this memoir about some of the abused children he has helped—or failed.

QUESTIONS TO CONSIDER

1. What is the nature of the helping process? What communication skills facilitate the process?

2. How can knowledge of systems be useful in understanding human service delivery?

3. What important ethical and professional issues must human service workers be prepared to face?

PART THREE

The Practice of Human Services

Part Three focuses on the practice of human services and the context in which helping occurs. Chapter 7 explores the helping process, introducing the skills helpers need to do their jobs well. The chapter concludes with a section on crisis intervention. Chapter 8 addresses the environment of the human service system. It begins with an examination of systems theory and its application to the helping process. The chapter then covers the referral process and ways of using the system to assist clients and the community at large. Part Three concludes with Chapter 9, "Professional Concerns." This chapter presents ethical considerations for the human service professional and describes practical applications of ethical principles. Other professional issues are also discussed: the time issue, paperwork, the dangers of encapsulation and burnout, and professional development in the field of human services. The purpose of Part Three is to refine the definition of human services (developed in Parts One and Two) by examining the helping process in actual practice. As you read the three chapters in this section, think about the questions to consider.

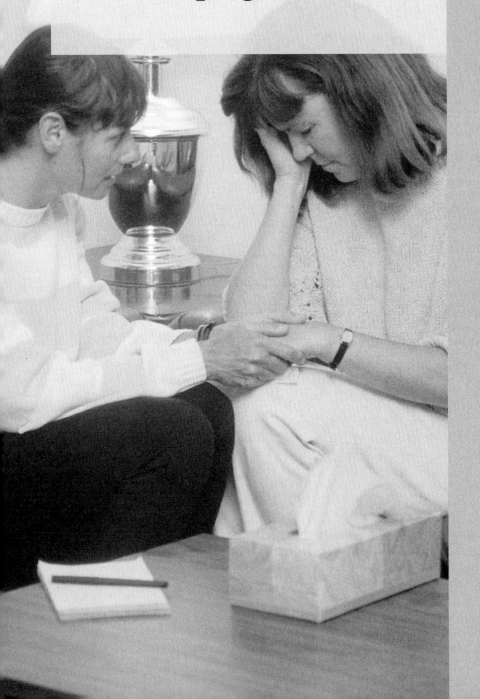

Chapter 7

The Helping Process

Helping can take many forms: "requesting information, soliciting support, making a decision, and sharing feelings" (Brammer, 1978, p. 476). Yet it is always guided by two questions: (1) What is helpful? (2) How can the needs of the client be met? In human services, assistance to the client occurs through *the helping process*. As they engage in this process, human service professionals must remember that clients are responsible for themselves and make their own decisions. Giving advice or telling someone what to do does not encourage responsibility or promote self-help, which are goals of the helping process.

The effectiveness of the helping process depends greatly on the skills of the helper, which is the focus of this chapter. The helper's ability to communicate an understanding of the client's feelings, clarify what the problem is, and provide appropriate assistance to resolve the problem contributes to the effectiveness of the process. The nature of the helping relationship, the skills of helping, groupwork, and the challenges of difficult clients will be investigated in this chapter. A look at a special human service, crisis intervention, will provide an overview of the helping process.

To illustrate some of the important concepts in this chapter, you will read about three individuals. We first renew our acquaintance with Carmen Rodriguez, the rehabilitation professional you met in Chapter 6. Then, Michiko, an international student from Japan, struggles with living in a new environment. Finally, Joan, a wife abandoned by her husband, needs support and assistance during this crisis.

 ## The Nature of the Helping Process

The helping process occurs in both formal and informal settings. In this chapter we will explore the helping that occurs in formal settings, for example, offices, institutions, agencies, street corners, and any other setting where human service workers deliver services to clients. As noted in Chapter 5, the term *client* can refer to an individual, a small group such as a family or a street gang, or a larger group such as a neighborhood or a geographic area.

The Helping Relationship

The cornerstone of helping, the medium through which help is offered, is the helping relationship. The helping process takes place within the context of a relationship that differs from others in that one person sets aside personal needs to focus on the needs of the other (or others), refraining from expressing opinions or giving advice.

Each participant brings to the relationship different perspectives and experiences. (See Figure 7-1.) Both the client and the helper bring attitudes, values, feelings, and experiences, which may be similar or may be very different. In addition, the client brings needs, problems, and expectations about what will happen, whereas the helper comes with knowledge, training, and skills to assist with the problems of the client. Matching clients with helpers is often

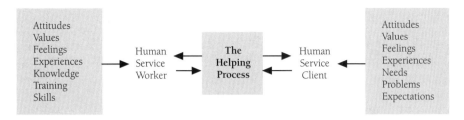

Figure 7-1 ✦ **The helping process**

random, but there is considerable evidence that compatibility between the two is important for an effective helping relationship.

Because the helper has the knowledge and expertise that the client is seeking, much of the initial responsibility for establishing the relationship rests with the helper. The importance of the characteristics, values, and philosophy of the helper are discussed in Chapter 6. As mentioned there, a growing body of research shows their importance in establishing and maintaining the helping relationship. The following questions (adapted from Rogers, 1958) may help you increase your self-awareness in relation to your own helping skills:

> Can I be perceived as trustworthy, dependable, and consistent?
> Can I express myself well enough that the client understands what I am saying?
> Can I experience attitudes of warmth, caring, liking, interest, and respect for the client?
> Can I separate my needs from those of the client?
> Am I secure enough myself to allow the client to be separate and independent from me?
> Am I able to see the world as the client does?
> Can I accept the client as he or she is?

As you begin to grasp the concept of the helping relationship and its importance to human service delivery, you may be asking yourself how it differs from other relationships. Several characteristics help make it unique (Perlman, 1979). First, helping relationships are formed for a recognized and agreed-on purpose; they are goal oriented. Second, a helping relationship is time bound, which means it usually occurs over several sessions (depending, of course, on the nature of the problem); the relationship ends when the purpose has been accomplished. Third, the helping relationship carries authority. In this sense, the word *authority* has a very different meaning from the one with which you are probably familiar. The helper's authority consists of the knowledge and skills that enable him or her to work with the client toward resolving the problem. Finally, this relationship is for the client. The focus is always on the client's problems and concerns.

• • • • • • • • •

INTERNATIONAL FOCUS
Mother Teresa and the Missionaries of Charity

Mother Teresa received God's call to serve the poorest of the poor in 1946. Her work began in Calcutta in a small way by caring for one sick and dying person she found on the streets there. Until March 1997, she was head of the Missionaries of Charity, a religious order she formed with the Vatican's blessing in 1950. The numbers of sisters and brothers in this order now total more than 4,000 worldwide. They live what they teach, not owning more than the poor they serve. Mother Teresa has won many awards, including the Nobel Peace Prize. She has founded hundreds of homes throughout the world, including four in Calcutta: Shishu Bhavan (the children's home); Prem Nivas (the center for leprosy patients in Titagarh); Nirmal Hriday (the home for the dying and destitute); and Prem Dam (the home for TB sufferers and patients with mental disabilities).

During the summer of 1995, Larry Coleman, a professor at the University of Tennessee, was with a Fulbright Hays group who visited the Mother House and three institutions in Calcutta run by the Missionaries of Charity. His account of the visit to Nirmal Hriday follows.

Noah, a Dartmouth student who volunteers with Mother Teresa, was our guide. We went to the Mother House of the Missionaries of Charity, then to Shishu Bhavan, then on to Prem Dam, and finally to the house of the dying, Nirmal Hriday. At the last place I began to shudder as one does before sobbing. I managed to accept the feeling, thereby reducing the emotional overload. Seeing children and adults in such trying circumstances and the love and caring of the sisters and volunteers to ease their suffering is a life-affirming and a life-questioning experience.

Nirmal Hriday was the original mission. It adjoins a Kali temple. Apparently, Mother Teresa took care of a monk whom no one else would care for, so she was given the house. It holds about 50 beds. As one approaches the mission, it is indistinguishable to me from other buildings in a busy shopping area. We enter through a door between two shops. Inside, a row of cots with sick and dying men is to the left on two levels. To the right is the medical and food dispensary. Volunteers were talking to the men. A blackboard provided a tally of the men, the women, the dismissed, and the dead. A short staircase descended opposite the dispensary and a long staircase went up to the roof.

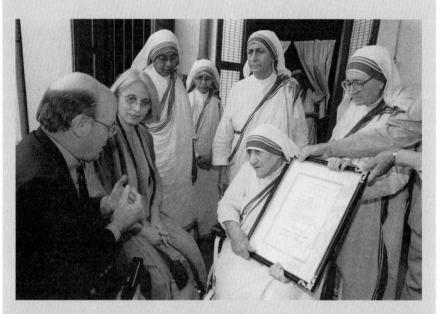

Mother Teresa accepting honorary U.S. citizenship in 1996.

Down the steps we see stone sinks in the floor, a cooking area with bright coals heating water and oil for cooking. Mounds of vegetables are evident. Separating the washing area from the food area is a narrow shelf (step) leading through a partially opened louvered door into a room with two parallel shelves. I am looking at the empty morgue. Noah commented that it is a powerfully moving experience to carry someone you know into the morgue.

Up the long staircase on the roof, sheets and clothes are drying. Volunteers are resting, either sitting on the roof in the shade or lying on the top of the outer walls of the building. Through the clothes lines and up three steps to a flat section, one could walk over to the spires of the Kali temple. At that moment I felt overwhelmed by what I had witnessed that morning. Outside the sun was shining, people were yelling, selling, sitting, etc.; inside it was quiet, softly lighted and the talking was subdued. Always contrasts in India.

Among the most poignant illustrations of helping and the helping rela-tionship is the work of Mother Teresa and the Missionaries of Charity. As you read about one American's experience, think about how the characteristics of the helping relationship apply.

Stages of the Helping Process

Usually the agency or organization with which a helper works shapes the fo-cus, the services, and the duration of the helping process. For example, voca-tional rehabilitation agencies are concerned with the work histories of clients, any disabilities that may prevent them from being employed, and their voca-tional capabilities and aspirations. Finding low-income housing, arranging adoptions, and processing applications for food stamps are not part of their services. Regardless of the focus of an agency and its services, you will find that the stages of the helping process are similar. They will include components of the problem-solving process such as identifying the problem, setting goals to resolve the problem, and determining and applying strategies designed to help the client reach those goals.

PREPARATION

Before the client arrives, the helper will want to attend to several matters. One is the *physical setting*. Are there any barriers that will prevent or make it diffi-cult to establish a relationship with the client? For example, many clients will perceive a desk as a symbol of authority, which may seem a barrier to them when the helper sits behind it. It may also be unwise to seat the client facing a window. Activities outside may distract clients and prevent them from fo-cusing on what is happening in the office. Does the physical setting ensure confidentiality? To promise the client that all matters discussed will remain be-tween the two of you means nothing if the setting is such that any discussion may be overheard by others.

Most agencies require extensive paperwork on clients. How will you han-dle note taking, filling out forms, and recording information? These decisions are best made before the client arrives. They can be handled in several ways; each helper must choose their own best method. For example, some helpers prefer taking notes while interviewing the client because it enables them to get all the facts while the client is present. Others say that taking notes while the client is talking is too difficult for them. They find that they miss important gestures and facial expressions.

The same is true of filling out forms. Some agencies require forms to be com-pleted before the client sees a human service professional. In such cases, the helper may have little choice. If there is no such policy, the worker may choose to have the client complete necessary forms before their meeting, or the helper may wish to assist the client in completing the forms, using this opportunity to establish rapport with the client and begin developing a helping relationship.

Finally, before the client arrives, the worker reviews the information about the client that is already accessible. What records are available? Is additional information needed? Based on the information available, what is the best way to approach the client? Has the helper made arrangements to have uninterrupted time with the client?

What follows is one client's description of an initial visit to a Social Security office. As you read it, pay attention to the physical setting, the workers, and the climate. What messages do those seeking services receive?

The first thing I noticed when I entered the double glass doors of the Social Security office was the back of everyone's head. I mean that there were rows of people sitting in metal folding chairs facing a blank white wall that had a door in the middle of it. All kinds of people were there—young, old, white, black, a couple of mothers with babies, some disabled. On the left side of the room was a counter with a glass partition. Three women were behind the counter. I watched the person who entered in front of me. He approached the counter and one woman told him, in a rather loud voice I thought, to take a number and sit down to wait his turn. I took number 38 before she could yell at me. As I sat there facing the blank white wall, I had a chance to observe how the agency operated. As each worker was ready for a client, she simply yelled out the number. The person then approached the counter, and there was an exchange of information, which I could plainly hear. In some cases, the individual then approached the door in the middle of the blank white wall. A buzzer sounded, unlocking the door, and the person entered. I suppose there were other workers behind the door, but I only made it to the counter. When number 38 was called, I found out I needed to write a letter to the regional office. The local office could not help me with my problem.

THE CLIENT ARRIVES

When the client enters the office, a climate of respect and acceptance is established if the client is greeted with a smile, a handshake, and an introduction. Remember that clients come with problems, feeling vulnerable, and sometimes in pain or discomfort. A helper who takes charge of the initial meeting will help the client feel at ease by giving the client time to adjust to the new situation. The use of "ice breakers" or "door openers" allows the client to become accustomed to the setting and the helper: "Did you have any trouble finding the office?" or "Parking is sometimes a problem here. I hope it wasn't for you."

Since the helping relationship is time bound and goal oriented, the helper will at some point need to inquire about the client's problem. Many clients will be eager to share their problems. Others will be reticent about discussing problems that are personal and painful; they may test the helper by sharing less important problems first. The helper can initiate problem identification in a number of ways: "Let's talk about why you're here," "Tell me what's going on," "I'm wondering what's on your mind." These are relatively nonthreatening ways of focusing on the client and the problem. Another way to do this is to have focused dialogue. After greeting the client, the helper and client can fill out the intake form together. This is a humanizing way to complete the form, and it does not require asking so many questions

During this initial stage, the helper can provide the client with information about the agency. For example, the client may want to know exactly what services the agency can provide. Other questions might concern the cost of the services, the criteria for eligibility to receive services, and the responsibilities of clients. In turn, the helper will probably have additional questions for the client. Does the client have any insurance? How did the client hear about the agency? Did someone refer the client here? What expectations does the client have for the agency and the helper?

EXPLORING THE PROBLEM

Chapter 5 discussed different perspectives on client problems. As the helper and the client begin to explore the problem, the helper should keep those perspectives in mind. The human service concepts of the whole person and the multidimensionality of problems will also guide this phase of the helping process (see box). Once the problems are identified, it is time to move to the next stage.

INTERVENTION STRATEGIES

During this stage, the helper and the client set goals and determine how those goals will be reached to resolve the problem. Should the helper find that the client's problem calls for expertise or experience that the helper does not have, the helper should refer the client to another professional who has the necessary knowledge and skills. Another reason for referral at this point arises if, once the problem has been identified, the helper has such strong feelings or biases about the situation that he or she is unable to work objectively with the client. Referral will be discussed in detail in Chapter 8.

Depending on the problem, strategies may be as simple as providing a one-time service such as pregnancy testing or as complex as working with a client who has been injured in a car wreck and is permanently disabled. In the latter case, problems may include the client's loss of ability to work a previous job, difficulties of the client and the family in adjusting to the client's disability, and barriers in the home to the client's mobility. These issues must be addressed if the client is to adjust to his or her new reality.

TERMINATION

The final stage of the helping process is termination. The relationship between the helper and the client may end in several ways. The most positive conclusion is when the services needed are provided and both participants are satisfied that the objectives have been reached. Unfortunately, not all terminations are so positive; services may be interrupted by either the helper or the client before the objectives have been reached. For example, the client moves from the area; the helper is transferred, promoted, or leaves the agency; or the client refuses to return for services (see Table 7-1).

Carl Rogers and Client-Centered Therapy

Carl Rogers, American psychologist and educator, was born on January 8, 1902, in Oak Park, Illinois. He attended the University of Wisconsin and graduated in 1924 with a degree in history. He then attended Union Theological Seminary in New York City and began to study for the ministry. He soon became influenced by a number of psychologists affiliated with Columbia University and transferred there to receive both his master's and doctoral degrees.

Rogers was initially concerned with environmental and institutional solutions to the problems of children, which he described in *The Clinical Treatment of the Problem Child* (1939). Later, he became interested in the psychotherapeutic process and gradually formulated the approach associated with his name—client-centered therapy. Client-centered therapy, or nondirective counseling, had a controversial beginning but proved to be a successful psychotherapeutic model. In *Counseling and Psychotherapy* (1942), Rogers maintained that the client knows better than anyone else what the problem is; with the help of a permissive, caring counselor, the client can find a solution to the problem. In client-centered therapy, the helper does not direct, give advice, or offer solutions and interpretations. The primary technique is "reflection of feelings." When the client speaks or acts, the helper responds by communicating perceptions of what the client means and feels. Through this "mirroring," the client can think more clearly about problems and feelings.

Rogers recognized the importance of the helper's self-awareness. He believed that the counselor's attitudes are more important than technique. Rogers considered three conditions necessary to facilitate a healthy personality change in a client. The counselor must have congruence (or genuineness); empathy (or understanding of the world as the client sees it); and unconditional positive regard or respect for the client, no matter how antisocial the client may be.

In 1942, Rogers became the first person to record, transcribe and publish verbatim a complete psychotherapy case. Recording of counseling sessions is now a common practice and an accepted part of the profession. It was largely due to the success of his book *On Becoming a Person* (1961) that the work of Carl Rogers began to attract the attention of a wider audience. Rogers has proved to be one of the most important trend setters in the field of psychotherapy. He died February 4, 1987.

SOURCE: From Taylor (1985).

TABLE 7-1   ✦   SUMMARY POINTS: HELPING STAGES

- Physical setting, paperwork, and review of information occur before the client arrives.
- When the client arrives, the helper greets the client, inquires about the problem, and provides information about the agency.
- Concepts of the whole person and the multidimensionality guide problem exploration.
- Intervention may involve referral, service provision, or both.
- Termination that is positive occurs when the needed services are provided and the objectives obtained.

In the case study that follows we visit Carmen Rodriguez, whom we met in Chapter 6. Here she discusses how she deals with many of the concepts discussed in this section.

One aspect of my work that makes it challenging is that I perform a variety of functions. For example, I always begin my work with a client with an interview. During this initial contact with the client, I try to establish rapport. I explain what we will be doing together for the next six weeks and what the schedule is like at our facility. It also helps clients to know what is expected of them. One of the best ways I've found to get this relationship off on the right foot is to talk to the client as someone I really want to get to know. I do have some background information on the client (usually an intake form, a medical evaluation, and a financial statement), and I briefly skim it before I see the client. When I meet with the client the first time, I always stand up and invite him or her in with a handshake and a smile. I leave the folder in a drawer, because I can concentrate on the client totally if I'm not distracted by reports.

After the initial meeting, I read the client's folder carefully. At that point, I usually ask myself the following questions: What do I know about this client? Does this client have a documented disability that is a handicap to employment? What evaluative information do I need to determine whether there is a reasonable expectation that this client can eventually be gainfully employed? Has this client been evaluated previously? Finally, what additional information would be helpful to best serve this client?

During the period of time that I work with the client on a daily basis, the goal is to determine what types of work the client would like to perform and what types the client is capable of performing. Sometimes these are similar, but often they are not. Staff members administer vocational tests, do some vocational counseling, and arrange for the client to try working as an employee in two or three different job settings. In most cases, I find myself going beyond these tasks. For example, many of the clients do not know about personal hygiene, so it is up to staff members to teach them about taking showers and using deodorant. Also, they may not know about proper work behavior. To succeed at a job, they must learn appropriate work habits such as being at work on time, taking limited breaks, dealing with conflicts, and getting along with other workers.

I've also discovered over the past four years that our clients often have multiple problems. Although the primary concern of our agency is vocational, clients come with other problems that affect their vocational evaluation. For example, a client may be having difficulty with a parent or guardian who is too protective. Or perhaps the client is not receiving a disability check that is due. Sometimes, clients have needs or problems that call for services from other agencies. My agency is limited to providing vocational evaluation, so if a client needs clothes or dental care, we must contact other agencies.

For the protection of the client, the agency, and the human service professional, it is necessary to maintain written case notes and documentation of services. This can be very time-consuming. I've noticed that each worker handles this task differently. What works for me is reserving the last 30 minutes of the day for updating files. I realize that these notes are important—the client may be transferred, I may change jobs, or I may be out sick—but some days it's a real chore to pull all the files and condense what's necessary into two or three sentences.

I hope to continue in my job for several more years, but eventually I would like to go back to school for further training. I want to develop my counseling skills to work with clients as individuals or groups in a more specialized way. My position as a case manager gives me practical experience and allows me to explore my career options by filling a variety of roles and working with other professionals.

An Introduction to Helping Skills

Communication is the foundation for all interpersonal relationships. Exchanging messages to understand another's perceptions, ideas, and experiences is especially important in helping relationships. Helping others will be difficult if we do not understand their problems or concerns.

In this section we introduce basic helping skills. We begin by focusing on the client's message, which means perceiving both the verbal and the nonverbal messages of the client. Next, we focus on the helper's communication by identifying the skills necessary for effective listening and responding. Finally, we discuss what the helper needs to know about cultural differences.

One person's sending a message to another person with the conscious intent of affecting the receiver's behavior is *communication* (Johnson, 1993). This process is illustrated in Figure 7-2. When the receiver interprets the message the way the sender intended, *effective communication* has taken place. When

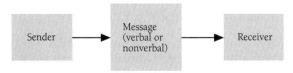

Figure 7-2 ✦ **Communication**

one person interprets the message differently from the way it was intended, the result is communication failure, the most common source of misunderstandings in interpersonal relationships.

The message that a person sends can be verbal or nonverbal. The most common example of a verbal message is the spoken word: "Hello, how are you today?" The smile and handshake or the hug accompanying that verbal greeting are nonverbal messages. The skillful helper is able to "hear" the client's behavior (the nonverbal message), as well as what is actually said (the verbal message), and to respond verbally and nonverbally to these messages (Okun, 1997). It sounds complicated, and it takes practice to communicate effectively. A good beginning is through an introduction to each component of the communication process.

Nonverbal Messages

Nonverbal behaviors (body language) include a person's posture, tone of voice, gestures, eye contact, and touch. Everyone communicates nonverbally. Each of us engages in some nonverbal behavior that we are aware of and perform intentionally. For example, when meeting someone for the first time, most of us want to make a positive first impression, so we deliberately greet that person with a smile or some other pleasant facial expression. However, we also communicate unconsciously in a nonverbal fashion. You may recall a time when you visited the doctor's office for shots and afterward wondered at the soreness in your muscles. The tension, fear, or hurt you experienced during the visit caused you to tense your muscles.

In a normal two-person conversation, more than 65% of the meaning is carried nonverbally. This fact emphasizes the importance of nonverbal communication in a helping situation. Frequently, you may find that a client's nonverbal message will provide you with valuable clues about what the client is thinking or feeling—important ideas that the client is unable to verbalize. Table 7-2 lists some common nonverbal cues and their meanings.

Another area in which nonverbal cues are important is the expression of feelings. Feelings are most often communicated nonverbally, particularly by facial expressions and tone of voice. One difficulty with "hearing" the nonverbal expression of feelings is the ambiguity of the nonverbal message. A nonverbal behavior such as crying could be interpreted in various ways; one cannot determine just from the tears on a person's face whether the person is sad, hurt, or disappointed. In fact, the person may be scared or even very happy.

Thus, we may think that nonverbal communication is a fairly straightforward process of sending and receiving messages, but it is actually a complicated mode of communication. Although they provide us with important cues about the person with whom we are conversing, nonverbal messages should be interpreted with caution.

Try this exercise: At some point today, select two people who are communicating with each other. (You may be in the library, a food-service area, or anywhere you choose.) For 10 minutes, observe the nonverbal communication of one of the participants. What behaviors do you observe? What possible interpretations can you make about the meanings of the behaviors?

TABLE 7-2 ✦ NONVERBAL CUES AND THEIR POSSIBLE MEANINGS

Cue	Meaning
Lifting an eyebrow	Disbelief
Lowering eyebrows	Uneasiness, suspicion
Lifting both eyebrows	Surprise
Eye contact	Interest, confidence
Winking an eye	Intimacy
Slapping forehead	Forgetfulness
Rubbing the nose	Puzzlement
Turning up corners of mouth	Happiness
Cocking head to one side	Friendly, human
Little or no head and/or hand movements	Cool, no emotion
Raised shoulders	Fear
Retracted shoulders	Suppressed anger
Square shoulders	Responsibility
Bowed shoulders	Carrying a burden
Shrugging shoulders	Indifference
Sitting with arms and legs crossed	Withdrawal, resistance
Clasping arms	Protection
Tapping fingers	Impatience
Fondling and touching inanimate objects	Loneliness
Leaning forward in a chair	Interest
Leaning back, arms uncrossed	Open to suggestion
Leaning back, arms crossed	Not open to suggestion
Postural change—facing away	Finished with interaction

Verbal Messages

Verbal messages consist of words spoken by a person. Such messages can be divided into a cognitive component and an affective component. The cognitive component consists of the facts of a message and reflects the person's thinking processes. This is the realm in which we are most comfortable. A cognitive message addresses such matters as who, what, where, when, and why. Consider the following statements by a coworker and try to pick out the cognitive messages.

I left work at 5:00 P.M. today. The last client I saw was Raphael Santini, and I just can't seem to get him off my mind. He is making such an effort to find a job, but he's had no luck. I couldn't believe it when he showed up today. I hardly recognized him, and I guess he could tell I was surprised, because I couldn't think of anything to say for a moment. He looked great. His hair was clean and neatly combed, and his clothes were new. He was so proud of himself, and I was proud of him too. I told him I was so pleased with the changes. I also felt good about myself, because some of my hard work with this client has paid off. I'm going to make some phone calls first thing in the morning to see what assistance I can find to help him locate a job. There's just got to be help for a motivated client like Raphael.

Some of the cognitive messages you probably identified were the speaker's leaving work at 5:00 PM ; the appointment with Raphael Santini, who is trying to find a job; and the description of his neat, clean appearance. In the cognitive realm, facts are the focus.

The affective component, the feeling part of the message, may be expressed directly or indirectly. Many clients who are unsure about what they are feeling, or who are simply uncomfortable talking about feelings, may choose to express their feelings indirectly. This means that the individual may not name the feeling at all ("Stop driving so fast!"), or they may describe it by telling what they feel like doing ("I feel like punching him in the nose"). One of the helper's main tasks may be to encourage the client to become aware of feelings and to learn to express feelings appropriately and directly: "I'm scared when you drive so fast," or "I'm angry at you for spoiling the surprise."

Review the statements about Raphael Santini. What feelings are expressed directly? In fact, there are very few, but they do include feeling "proud," "surprised," and "good." These feelings are named, and the reader clearly understands how the helper feels. Read the excerpt again, and consider the feelings that are being expressed indirectly. (It might be helpful to read it aloud.) You might identify such feelings as discouragement at Raphael's lack of success, exasperation at the job situation, disbelief at his appearance, and determination to find some type of assistance for Raphael. Determining exactly what the client (or, in this case, the helper) is feeling may be more difficult when feelings are expressed indirectly.

Listening and Responding

The way we listen and respond to the client is crucial in building a helping relationship. The first thing a helper must do before making any response to the client is to listen carefully to what the client is expressing, both verbally and nonverbally. Even though listening takes up more of a person's waking hours than any other activity, and many people consider themselves good listeners, few of us actually are. This section will introduce listening behaviors and some helper responses that promote effective helping (see Table 7-3).

THE HELPER LISTENS

The kind of listening that helpers engage in is called *responsive listening* or *active listening*. These terms describe the behaviors of helpers as they attend to both the verbal and the nonverbal communication of the client. What makes this type of listening special or different from other listening behaviors is that helpers also attend to what is not said, that is, to the underlying thoughts and feelings of the client, which are not expressed in words. Two ways of considering responsive or active listening as helping behaviors are presented here.

Egan (1998, pp. 63–64) suggested several things helpers can do to communicate to clients that they are listening. These five behaviors are presented

TABLE 7-3 ♦ HELPFUL BEHAVIORS IN COMMUNICATING

Verbal	*Nonverbal*
Mirroring feelings	Making eye contact
Clarifying	Listening
Showing a sense of humor	Smiling
Providing support	Nodding one's head
Providing information that client needs	Leaning forward
Explaining helper's role	Maintaining a relaxed posture
Sharing information about oneself	Facing the client
Being nonjudgmental	Displaying facial expression
Asking few questions	Being punctual
	Occasionally making appropriate use of gestures and touching
	Maintaining a moderate rate of speech

as a set of guidelines that helpers can follow to let their clients know they are physically present and actively involved in the helping relationship. You can easily remember the behaviors by thinking of the acronym SOLER.

S—Face the client *squarely.* This is a posture of involvement. To face away from the client or even at an angle lessens the degree of involvement.

O—Adopt an *open posture.* This is usually perceived as nondefensive. Crossing arms or legs may not communicate openness or availability.

L—*Lean toward* the other person. A natural sign of involvement, this posture is a slight forward inclination. Moving forward or backward can frighten a client or communicate lessened involvement.

E—Maintain *eye contact.* This is normal behavior for two individuals who are involved in conversation. It is different from staring.

R—Try to be *relaxed.* This means avoiding nervous habits such as fidgeting or tapping a pencil. Behaviors such as these can distract the client.

Remember that these are only guidelines. A helper's physical behavior may vary in accordance with the cultural identity of the client or what is comfortable for that particular helper.

Ivey and Ivey (1999) described *attending behavior* as another way to let the client know the helper is listening. The goal of attending behavior is to encourage the client to talk about and examine issues, problems, or concerns. Attending behavior has four dimensions: three nonverbal components and one verbal component.

1. *Visual/eye contact.* If you are going to talk to people, look at them.
2. *Vocal qualities.* Your vocal tone and speech rate indicate clearly how you feel about another person. Think of how many ways you can say, "I am really interested in what you say" just by altering your vocal tone and speech rate.

3. *Verbal tracking.* The client has come to you with a topic of concern. Do not change the subject; stick with the client's subject matter.
4. *Attentive and authentic body language.* Clients know you are interested if you face them squarely and lean slightly forward, have an expressive face, and use facilitative, encouraging gestures. In short, allow yourself to be yourself; authenticity in attending is essential (pp. 28–29).

Engaging in these behaviors encourages the client to talk, reducing the amount of talk from the helper. Benefits include communicating interest and concern to the client and increasing the worker's awareness of the client's ability to pay attention. Attending behaviors also allow the helper to modify helping behaviors to work effectively with clients who may be racially, culturally, or sexually different.

THE HELPER'S RESPONSE

Once the helper has heard the verbal and nonverbal messages of the client, it is time for the helper to speak. Remember that helpers' responses must be purposeful. Think about the characteristics of the helping relationship. This is not a casual conversation between two people, but a goal-directed exchange. Therefore, the helper must know his or her intent before speaking.

The helper has several options at this point. For example, did the helper understand what the client said? Was the message clear? Does the helper need further information to grasp the message correctly? Questions such as these will assist the helper in determining the intent of his or her response. Let us examine some of these options.

First, suppose the helper does understand the client's message and decides that the most helpful response would be one that lets the client know this. To communicate that intent, the helper may choose to *paraphrase,* to make a statement that is interchangeable with the client's own words.

CLIENT: I've been able to complete five tasks today that were on my list.
HELPER: You've had a productive day today.

The helper may determine that more than a simple paraphrase is needed to help the client become aware of or clarify feelings. In this case, a helper statement that reflects both the feeling (or affective component) and the facts (or cognitive component) is helpful. For example:

HELPER: You're really pleased that you were able to accomplish what you set out to do today.

If the helper is confused about what the client said, perhaps because the client was relating a complicated incident, the helper should ask the client for clarification. To attempt a response that will make little sense to the client and will let the client know that the helper did not understand what was said is not helpful. Responses such as "I'm not sure I understand . . ." or "I'm confused about . . ." are appropriate at this point. They also let the client know that the helper is interested enough to want to get the story right in order to be able to help.

Beginning helpers sometimes encounter situations in which clients are asking questions or seeking information that the helper does not know. Many helpers believe they should know everything and may feel embarrassed about being asked something they do not know. Unfortunately, they may attempt to answer off the tops of their heads or give an answer they believe may be correct. A better response in situations like this would be, "I do not have that information, but I do know where we can find it; let me check on that for you," or "I'm not sure about the eligibility requirements for that type of assistance, but I can refer you to someone who knows." Helpers are not supposed to have all the answers. The effective helper who wants to maintain a relationship with the client will enrich that relationship by being honest with the client.

ASKING QUESTIONS

Another technique that beginning helpers should be wary of is *questioning*. Most of us consider ourselves skilled at asking questions and find it a natural form of communication in everyday life—particularly questions that begin with the words *who, what, where, why,* and *when.* For the beginning helper, the question is the most common method of eliciting information from the client, and many helpers find themselves resorting to questions frequently. Unfortunately, one question seems to lead to another, and too many questions can interfere with the helping relationship, causing the client to feel like a witness. An overreliance on questioning, and neglecting other kinds of responses, hinders the helping process. It also creates a dependent client who has no role other than answering questions. Most questions can be rephrased as statements that elicit the same information. For example, the question "What was the last grade completed in school?" can be rephrased as "Tell me about your school experiences." In addition to discovering the final grade completed, the helper may learn how the client felt about school, whether the client enjoyed learning, and what circumstances surrounded the end of the client's educational experience.

Now that you have been alerted to the pitfalls of questioning, let us explore the time when asking questions is appropriate and how one asks good questions. Long, Paradise, and Long (1981) suggested several situations in which a question is helpful. One is to begin the interview, "How would you like to begin?" or "Could you tell me a little about yourself?" for example. A second situation occurs when specific information is needed. Asking for information to clarify ("How long have you been ill?") or to elicit examples of specific behavior ("How does that make you feel?") can provide the additional information necessary for complete understanding. Finally, questions can be useful to focus the client's attention. For example, a client who is digressing or rambling on about several problems may need the helper's assistance to focus. Such assistance can be provided by statements such as the following:

> You've mentioned several concerns that you have about your daughter. You're afraid she is using drugs, and you suspect she is not doing well in school. I guess I hear you expressing the most concern, though, about your inability to talk with her. Let's focus on that. What happens when you do try to talk with her?

Thus, there are times in a helping relationship when asking questions is appropriate and beneficial (see Table 7-4). How does one ask good questions? Egan (1998) suggested that the helper might first want to consider how the question will relate to and promote the helping relationship. Having specific objectives in mind before asking the question will help in formulating a good question.

Both closed and open questions can facilitate the development of the helping relationship when the helper has specific intentions. *Closed* questions are those that elicit facts necessary to facilitate the helping process. "How old were you when your father died?" and "How many brothers and sisters do you have?" may provide important information regarding the client's family situation if the client is having difficulties at home. Closed questions that require a "yes" or "no" answer should usually be avoided, because they lead the beginning helper to ask more and more questions.

Open questions, on the other hand, are broader, allowing the client to express thoughts, feelings, or ideas. They contribute to building rapport with the client and also assist him or her in exploring a situation, a problem, or an interaction. For example, "How did you feel after talking it over with your parents?" asks for the client's view. On the other hand, "Did you feel better after talking with your parents?" can be answered with a simple "yes" or "no," which does not enhance the helping process.

In summary, questions can be useful tools in the helping process. As with other types of responses, the key to effective questioning is knowing the intent of the question before posing it to the client. Are you seeking factual information or asking the client to offer thoughts or opinions about the topic of discussion? Considering how the question will promote the helping relationship will assist the helper in determining the appropriate strategy.

This section has been a brief introduction to helping skills. As you pursue your education and training in preparation for work in the human services, you will increase your knowledge about these skills and refine your use

---

TABLE 7-4 ✦ SUMMARY POINTS: WHEN TO ASK

- To begin the interview
- To obtain specific information
- To seek clarification
- To illicit examples of specific behavior
- To focus the client's attention

of them so that you become an effective helper. One area that requires a mastery of communications skills is working with groups of individuals. By the end of the 1980s, groups were recognized as viable means of helping individuals in a variety of settings. Groupwork flourished during the 1990s and will continue to be a major strategy in the 21st century to provide direct service to clients as well as to collaborate with colleagues and community groups. An introduction to basic group concepts and the role of communication in group work follows.

Working with Groups

Groups are natural. Since the beginning of time, individuals have banded together for survival, security, tasks, and problem solving, thus making groups a critical mode for accomplishing what needs to be done. Think about your own life—your living situation, your work, and even your leisure time. Most of these activities take place in groups. In human services, individuals also band together to accomplish tasks. Membership may be voluntary. For example, individuals with similar problems or experiences such as victims of incest or suicide survivors or children of alcoholics may work together on their problems. Involuntary membership occurs when participating in a group is mandated by some authority. Joining a group for abusive parents or one for substance abusers may be a condition for probation. In this section we will define groups, explore the skills necessary to work with a group, and consider the trends that will effect groupwork in the 21st century.

A *group* is a number of individuals who interact with each other. According to Brill (1998), groups have several characteristics. An important characteristic is the interaction that occurs among group members. This means that they participate in group meetings and discussions, share resources, give and receive help, and influence each other. Sharing common goals and values is a second characteristic. The group may be formed for an agreed upon purpose or the group may establish its own goals once members meet. The group also develops its own values, identifying what is important to the group and translating it into behavior for individuals as members of the group and for the group as a whole. Groups also have a social structure. Roles define the formal structure of the group and influence how individuals act in the group. Different group members play different roles. Examples of roles include leadership which may be a designated person or a shared role among members; the maintenance role which sees to the well-being of the group by encouraging and compromising; the facilitative/building role which helps everyone feel part of the group by initiating, seeking information and opinions, coordinating and evaluating; and blocking, a role that is aggressive, dominating, and anti group. A final characteristic of a group is cohesiveness among members. Members perceive that they belong to a group, they are interdependent in some way, and they work together to keep the group going as well as focus on common goals.

Alcoholics Anonymous (AA) is an example of a well-known group that illustrates these characteristics. Although many self-help groups formed during the late 1960s, AA is one of the more enduring ones, established in the late

Life was not very good for me about 15 years ago. I just hit rock bottom. I was a builder and an engineer by training and had established an excellent environmental consulting firm. In fact, during my consulting activities, I was fortunate enough to meet several individuals who helped me become a commercial land developer. Over a period of 5 years I amassed a fortune; I had increased my personal wealth to such a degree that I owned three homes—one in New York City; one in Lisbon, Portugal; and one in Miami, Florida. My kids attended private school; my family belonged to a prestigious country club; I was able to buy a home for my parents. All of a sudden my financial situation began to deteriorate as the business began to crumble. Because of depressed economic conditions and a recession, the land value dropped and individuals and corporations were no longer interested in land investments. Because of stressful times and other complicating factors, my wife asked me for a divorce. She kept our family home and gained custody of our three children. The two dogs stayed with her as well. It seemed that I would have to file for bankruptcy and face the losses (financially, socially, and professionally) alone.

For about 14 months I struggled with all of these problems, including lawsuits and liens against my property, and the divorce settlement. It was a terrifying time. I could not sleep; often during the lonely hours of both day and night, I would consider suicide. I always stopped because I really wanted to repay my debts and was committed to caring for my kids as well as I could. I actually lost many of my friends. They became friends of my wife. My business partners were all scrambling to recover their losses and regain their financial and social status, and I reminded them of their failures. I was living in a small apartment, which was all that I could afford, and had lost my car, my small RV, and my boat. My lawyer, who was handling the fight to avoid bankruptcy, recommended that I join a men's therapy group sponsored by Consumer Counseling Centers of America. My sister is a psychotherapist, but I have never even considered that type of help. My focus had been practical—dealing with money, homes, kids, work, and my professional life. My lawyer was so earnest about this suggestion. He was handling my case without being paid. I felt like I owed it to him to try this at least once.

At the first meeting, I was scared to death. A million times during the day I changed my mind about going. I drove up to the meeting house at 6:45 P.M. and decided once again that I would have to skip the 7:00 P.M. meeting. My hands were sweaty, I had a headache, my stomach hurt, and I had not had much sleep in months. I watched the participants enter one by one. My knees seemed to buckle as I stepped outside the car and headed for the door. The group met every week; this was an ongoing group that had been meeting for 10 years. I arrived awkwardly, sat in one

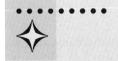

of the chairs that formed a circle. I was asked to introduce myself and then I was welcomed by the other group members and the leader, a local psychologist. Quite frankly I did not say anything during the group meeting for five months, but I did not miss a session; and from time to time I really looked forward to the meeting, since it was the one thing that I could count on each week. I also liked the camaraderie that existed within the group. By the time that I did talk in the group, I felt that I knew the other members fairly well. The first night I talked was because I was challenged by one of the group members for coming, gaining from the group, and not really being willing to give. After I finally made my first contributions, I was able to participate in the meetings, although I never had a lot to say.

One of the group rules was that we could not see each other socially. This was in part for confidentiality since we had to promise not to divulge the contents of the group discussion. We also could not acknowledge to others who participated in the group. Another rule was that each person had to be honest when he spoke. There was no "B.S." allowed or tolerated. Several times I saw members challenged when other group members thought a member was not being honest. I learned that the average amount of time in the group was approximately 16 months. There were 10 men in the group. One member had been in the group for six years. Another had joined and left after 3 months. My stay was 13 months.

It was amazing what I learned in the group. I made some incredibly good friends, people that I would have never met in any other circumstance. A few I really did not like at all; we did not share many common values. The one thing that we did share was a tragic financial encounter. Some members were like me, caught in a very difficult financial situation due to the recession. Others, it seemed, had always been troubled by financial worries. A few had declared bankruptcy at least four times; I was doing everything I could to avoid this and wanted to pay all of my debts. But our commonalities, the financial distress and the toil that it can take on an entire life perspective, held us together as a group. I felt supported, and understood.

It was difficult when I realized that it was time for me to leave the group. It was one of the group members who first raised the issue. He began very gently to remind me of how I was and how the group was when I first came. He recounted my progress and I began to feel really good about the progress that I had made. Then he said that he thought it was time for me to move on. Boy, that came as a shock and the suggestion really hurt my feelings. But once I considered the idea, I knew that he was right. My last night was sad for many of those in the group. Today I can tell you, the group is very much a part of me. Usually I don't feel free even to talk this much about the experience, since I am clear about my obligations of confidentiality. But I know that you can keep this to yourself.

1930s by founders who realized the effectiveness of individuals meeting together and interacting in such a way to support change (Gladding, 1999). Interaction among members is the foundation of AA meetings; for example, members share experiences and information. They also have a common goal which is to gain and maintain control of their lives by remaining sober. To that end, members encourage, coordinate, evaluate, support, and lead, both in regular meetings and outside meetings. These techniques are similar to those used in other self-help groups such as Parents without Partners and Weight Watchers.

Groups are formed for reasons other than self-help. Today there are specialty areas in groupwork and a set of core competencies and standards that have been established for preparation for groupwork in these areas (Association for Specialists in Group Work, 1991). Identified specialty areas include task/work groups which are focused on accomplishing identified work goals, for example, task forces, planning groups, or community organizations. The teams described in Chapter 1 are examples of this type of group. Guidance/psychoeducational groups are another type of group whose focus is education, prevention, or both. In these groups, information may be shared about AIDS, bereavement, or divorce. The goal is to prevent the development of psychological disturbances. A third type of group is counseling/interpersonal problem solving, whose focus is the resolution of problems group members face. Examples may be test anxiety, relationship difficulties, or career decision making. Psychotherapy/personality reconstruction groups are most often found in mental health facilities such as clinics or hospitals and include individuals who have serious psychological problems of long-term duration. Both abusers and victims of abuse may benefit from involvement in such a group.

What is the role of the human service professional in a group? In natural groups, such as a family or a street gang, human service professionals enter as outsiders and must make a place for themselves (Brill, 1998). They are present because a member is in trouble or there are significant problems in the group or both. In formed groups, that is, those that are organized for a specific purpose or goal, the human service professional may have responsibility for getting people involved and getting the group underway. Organizational issues such as meeting times and places, purpose, and group structure must be addressed by members before the real work of the group begins. At this point the human service professional then facilitates the work of the group toward its goal.

The foundation of all group functioning is communication skills. As stated earlier, interaction is key to the group's existence and involves the exchange of information and transmission of meaning (Johnson & Johnson, 1994). It is by means of effective communication that group members reach some understanding of one another, their goals, the division of labor, and other group tasks. Both verbal and nonverbal behaviors comprise effective communication and are every bit as complex in groups as they are in individuals. For example, silence may have many meanings: processing information, mulling over what was said, avoidance, or discomfort with the topic. Therefore, many of the points made earlier in the chapter about sending messages, listening, asking questions, and responding are critical for groupwork. In fact, the core skills identified by the Association for Specialists in Group Work (1991) include the communication skills to open and close group meetings, impart information, self-disclose, give feedback, and ask open-ended questions.

Groups are experiencing increased popularity at this time and focus on special populations. Examples are groups for individuals who are divorcing, adult offenders, overeaters, those with HIV/AIDS, adolescents, elderly living in institutions, unwed teenage fathers, and those who need support for any number of situations. This trend will continue. Other trends that will continue to effect groupwork in the 21st century are computer technology and solution-focused groups, both discussed in Chapter 3.

 ## Skills for Challenging Clients

Ideally, all clients of human services are motivated, cooperative, responsible, and like each of us; however, it is one of the challenges of this practice that not all clients fit that description. In your experience as a helper, you will likely meet clients who are different culturally, or who are resistant, silent, overly demanding, or unmotivated. They may also be different from you in other ways including background, religion, values, and life experiences.

You need to know something about these client groups because they often elicit in the helper feelings of uncertainty, hostility, and resentment. They are particularly difficult for many beginning helpers to work with, and it is important to realize that the client's behavior is not necessarily the helper's fault.

Culturally Different Clients

A recent Census Bureau report projects profound shifts in America's population that should make the country far more ethnically diverse than ever before (Friedman, 1996). By 2050, immigration patterns and differences in birth rates, combined with an overall slowdown in the growth of the country's population, will produce a United States in which 53% of the people will be non-Latino whites, down from 74% today. Latinos and Asians will grow fastest, whereas African Americans will nearly double in numbers by 2050.

As these population shifts occur, it is increasingly likely that human service professionals will encounter clients whose cultural backgrounds differ from their own. The key to working with clients who are culturally different is awareness of and sensitivity to these differences. In Tucson, Arizona, for example, Suzy Bourque at the Family Counseling Agency emphasizes the need to hire workers who appreciate different cultures. Their client population is about 30% Latino and 10% African American. Native Americans are underrepresented because they tend to take care of their own. She is constantly looking for staff who are bilingual, bicultural, and/or African American (personal communication, October 7, 1994). For the case workers at Casita Maria Settlement House in the Bronx, sometimes getting people to accept help is difficult because accepting outside help is not part of their culture (personal communication, May 4, 1994). Instead of saying to a Latino client, "You need counseling," they find that a more acceptable phrase is "Maybe you need someone to talk with." Because many of their clients are Latino, they find that they can no longer refer to them as Hispanic or Latino. Now, it is important to recognize that Latino includes people from Puerto Rico, Nicaragua, Colombia, and Honduras—and they are all different. Even human service providers from Knoxville, Tennessee, must be culturally sensitive as they work with clients from rural areas as well as Appalachia (personal communication, July 10, 1994).

Helpers must realize that culture shapes body language. Few gestures and body movements have universal meaning. For example, Arabs tend to cling or huddle together, whereas Americans like their space. Postures also vary by culture. The posture of the German male is stiffer than that of the American male, whereas the French male exhibits greater body limpness (Sielski, 1979). The direct eye contact that is so critical to standard American helping behavior may be offensive to people from Native American and Latino cultures. A helper with no knowledge of this may intend to communicate complete attention but be perceived by the culturally different client as disrespectful.

The beginning helper is cautioned against assigning too much meaning to a single gesture; instead, all means of expression—verbal, postural, facial, and cultural—should be considered. It is also wise not to generalize about cultural traits. Some Asian Americans may not like direct eye contact, yet some might.

Axelson (1999, p. 28) suggested that a multicultural approach to counseling should start with four steps to conceptualize the client who is culturally different.

1. Recognize that all human beings possess a similar capacity for thought, feeling, and behavior.
2. Be knowledgeable in several cultures; study both differences and similarities among people of different groups and their special needs and problems.
3. Gain an understanding of how the individual relates to important objects of motivation, what his or her personal constructs are, and how they are constructed to form his or her worldview.
4. Blend steps 1, 2, and 3 into an integrated picture of the distinctive person as experienced during the counseling process.

The following account, written by Michiko, a foreign student from Japan, may help you to begin thinking about culturally different clients in light of the preceding four steps.

I am a foreign student from Japan who is studying at an American university. It has been more than a month since I arrived in the States, and still I am not making American friends. I usually hang around with my Japanese buddies, so that does not help either. I hardly have any time for socializing because of all of the assignments I have to do for class. I am tense and timid around people and feel uncomfortable most of the time because I do not know how to act in pleasing, acceptable ways. I miss my friends and family and often cry when I am alone.

I have two great needs. One is to feel accepted among Americans and to adjust to the American culture. The other need is for academic excellence, since I did not come all the way from Japan just to fool around. I would like to have American friends with whom I can talk and share experiences, who will like me the way I am. I find most of my classes large and impersonal and have hardly any hope of finding a friend there. I need someone who is interested enough to get past the language barrier to get to know me. As for the academics, my professors know that I am a foreign student and they will go out of their way to help me with any difficulties I might be facing. I appreciate the attention, but that is not enough. I need help with the report assignments because I am unfamiliar with formats in English writing. I also need to be advised on study skills, because even if I prepare well in advance for a test, the grades I get are Cs and Ds.

I have many fears. I am afraid being Japanese, a racial minority, makes me less desirable as a person worth knowing in the eyes of an American. I am in constant fear of saying wrong things at the wrong moments and acting weird in front of people. My language problem still persists. Conversational English is something I find difficult, and people must speak slowly and clearly for me. I am afraid this makes me boring to talk to and hard to discuss complex subjects with. The greatest fear of all is having to go back to Japan because I could not make it academically and socially at an American university.

The young woman in this case study is one among many culturally different clients. Axelson's four steps are useful in understanding Michiko as a unique, worthwhile individual. Michiko definitely has the capacity for thought, feeling, and behavior as she attempts to function successfully in a culture foreign to her. A helper would need to learn about the Japanese culture and the ways in which it differs from and resembles American culture. Michiko has established personal goals that focus on academic and social success and is frustrated by the barriers she is experiencing. To engage effectively in the helping process with Michiko, the helper would need to explore the relevant differences between American and Japanese cultures. For example, many Asian cultures are collectivist—the individual is less important than the group. Michiko may be fearful of not succeeding academically and socially because of the disgrace it would bring to her family.

The helper would also want to adjust his or her helping behaviors to the individual of a different culture and to assess appropriate strategies of intervention. In American culture, the individual is perceived as autonomous and separate from groups. Even though a person can be a member of many groups, no one group determines identity completely. In collectivist societies, however, the individual belongs to fewer groups, but the attachment is stronger; often the individual is defined by membership in a group. Taking this information into account, the helper would choose an intervention that would focus on Michiko in relation to her group rather than an intervention designed to promote independence.

The Reluctant or Resistant Client

There are some distinctions between reluctant and resistant clients, but the principles for working with them are similar. The *reluctant* client is one who does not want to come in for help in the first place and is more or less forced to come. Such clients may be found in schools, correctional settings, court-related settings, and employment agencies (Egan, 1998). The *resistant* client may come more or less willingly but fail to carry through or participate actively in the helping process. Some of the causes of clients' reluctance and resistance are having negative attitudes about help, seeing no benefits in changing, feeling that getting help means admitting weakness or failure, and seeing no reason for going for help in the first place.

Reluctant clients may be embarrassed or angry that they are there for help. In many cases, they are there only because the court or some other authority has said they must be. These feelings are compounded by their unfamiliarity with the agency or the process. To attempt to lessen the reluctance, the helper can explain the process to the client (Ritchie, 1986). Discussing matters such as confidentiality, time limits, and expectations (for the client as well as the helper) can help demystify the process. Also, the manner in which the helper relates this can allow the client to see him or her in a role other than that of interrogator or advice giver. The following case provides an example.

Joseph came into my office with his mother and father. He sat in the chair with his arms folded. His feet did not touch the floor. He was swinging one foot and then another. He looked at his knees. I talked with his mother and father first for a few minutes and then asked them to be excused so that I could talk with Joseph alone. I am used to working with young children who do not want to see a counselor. When I work with them the first time, many say nothing during a 35–45 minute period. Some just sit and stare at me. Some stare at the floor. Others pretend to be asleep or sing quietly to themselves. On rare occasions, they try to damage the room, me, or themselves in some way. Over the 20 years that I have worked with children, five of them have never talked with me, after weekly meetings for over six months to a year. Many of them will begin to relate to me after two or three weeks, mainly through games and drawing or watching short films or videos together. Some will finally talk with me and once they get started, they cannot stop. My foremost approach is to let them know that I care about them in whatever way I can. Even for those who never spoke, I was a consistent, caring presence in their lives for an extended period of time.

Resistance is slightly different from reluctance, because resistance can occur at any time in the helping process. Clients who come to the attention of human services agencies may initially feel threatened by the referral and application procedures. Resistance may also arise later in the helping process if the client feels threatened by the subject being discussed, by the helper, or even by the helping relationship.

What is resistant behavior? Missing appointments, rejecting the helper, and inattentiveness are examples of such behavior. Clients may try to protect themselves by denying the existence of a problem, claiming it is caused by other people or situations, or distancing themselves from it.

I feel that the counselor in my school has betrayed me. We have had a good relationship ever since I came to the high school. I have worked with her one-on-one to determine my school schedule. She has conducted groups in our high school. I have participated in ones on family life, balancing a checkbook, how to apply for a job, and how to maintain healthy friendships. Today I went to see her after basketball practice. I have not been feeling well. My coach is concerned and she asked me to go to see Ms. Sharpelli. You know what she asked me? "Do you think you might be pregnant?" I walked out without saying a word to her. Even though she might be right, I promise, I will never speak to her again.

The helper can use several strategies when working with a resistant client. First, recognizing and accepting the antagonism may defuse the situation. This type of action is very different from what the client might expect; a statement such as "You probably don't want to see anyone like me" may minimize the threat to the client. Second, asking for the client's perceptions of the problem will communicate support for the client's feelings. This does not mean that the helper must accept or believe everything the client says, but it does communicate support and respect. Asking what the client wants to happen in this situation is a third strategy. It engages the client in the helping process and also emphasizes the worker's support and respect for the individual. In addition, it can provide the client with some sense of control over his or her life. Finally, for resistance that occurs later in the relationship, changing the pace or the topic may temporarily lessen feelings of threat (see Table 7-5).

The Silent Client

Particularly difficult for the beginning helper is the silent client. The uncomfortable silence may cause the helper to believe that nothing is taking place; in fact, silence can have many different meanings. It is the helper's responsibility to evaluate what a silence means so he or she can decide how to respond.

Silence can mean that the client is waiting for direction from the helper. In this case, the client may feel that it is the helper's place to determine the topic of

---

TABLE 7-5 ✦ SUMMARY POINTS: STRATEGIES FOR RESISTANCE

- Recognize and accept the antagonism.
- Ask for the client's perception of the problem.
- Ask the client for solutions.
- Change the pace or topic.

discussion or the direction in which the relationship should move. A second meaning of silence can be that the client is pondering what has been said. Resistance (discussed previously) may also manifest itself as silence; a change of pace or topic may be necessary until the client is ready to deal with what is happening.

Mr. Lopez and his wife were referred for counseling by their family physician. Mrs. Lopez is experiencing signs of dementia, and her deteriorating condition requires that Mr. Lopez be the caregiver. During the first session, Mrs. Lopez talked about her son, Enrique, and how he is learning to tie his shoes. Mr. Lopez volunteered the information that Enrique is 24 years old, lives in a neighboring state, and is a computer analyst. Other than this comment, he sat silently.

In this case Mr. Lopez may be silent for several reasons: despair over his wife's condition, confusion about her behavior, discouragement, or simply nothing to say. The helper will want to be sensitive to his behavior and to check out what he is feeling.

The Overly Demanding Client

Calling the helper at home, monopolizing time in the office, and scheduling frequent and unnecessary appointments are behaviors of an overly demanding client. Sometimes such clients become so dependent that they may want to be told what to do. When the client makes demands, the helper may become resentful of the time the client takes up and frustrated with the unsuccessful nature of the helping process. For these reasons, the helper must deal appropriately with the client's behavior.

I just called my case worker, Ms. Renfro, and she promised to come right over. I know that she usually goes to church on Sunday evenings, but I really need to see her. She is so good to me and tells me to call her whenever I need her. And she helps me all of the time. I have a regular scheduled appointment with her for 30 minutes every Tuesday morning, but I would not be able to get through a day without talking with her. Last Friday she called to tell me that she was going out of town next Tuesday and cancelled our regular Tuesday appointment. I have called her each day to urge her not to go.

Ms. Renfro will probably develop some resentment toward this client when her patience is exhausted. At some point, it will be in both their best interests for her to establish some boundaries for the relationship.

One strategy that may help with the overly demanding client is setting reasonable limits to decrease the client's dependence. Limiting client–helper contact to working hours only is one step toward decreasing dependence. A second strategy is to examine the helper's own need to be needed. Is the helper actually encouraging the demanding behavior of the client?

The Unmotivated Client

Clients who are present because someone referred them or encouraged them to seek help may be unmotivated. They may not see the need for the service and may be showing up only because some authority such as their parents, the school, or the court is forcing them to attend. Unfortunately, the unmotivated client is often unwilling to change and only goes through the motions of the helping process. The helper may find that he or she is doing most of the work in the relationship and may come to feel resentful, frustrated, and even angry. Such clients may be classed as reluctant clients, and many of the same strategies previously suggested may be helpful in establishing rapport with them. A parolee is an example of a client who must have regular meetings with a parole officer.

Many of my parolees come in to see me just because they have to. In fact, most of them come because it is one of the terms of their probation. They figure seeing me is not as bad as being returned to prison. Each day I try to see at least seven of them; and I also try to make two or three visits to see them at their work site. Most of the conversations are predictable: "How are you doing?" "Fine, I guess." "Looks like your job is going well." "Yep." "Tell me a little about your family." "They are fine." "I got some information about a new skills course . . ." "Oh." "Is there anything that I can do for you . . ." ". . . (offers no response and shrugs shoulders)." For these folks I am just a person that they must see or suffer the consequences.

 ## Crisis Intervention

Crisis intervention is a helping process that occurs at a much faster pace than other helping and incorporates many of the helping roles and skills that have been discussed in this chapter. You may find yourself engaged in crisis intervention when there is an emergency. For example, a crisis can be precipitated by suicide threats or attempts, the discovery of an unwanted pregnancy, abandonment, or natural disasters such as hurricanes or tornadoes. In this section, you will read a description of crisis intervention as a human service, including types of crises, the development of a crisis, the principles and skills of intervention, and the role of the human service professional providing this service.

Defining Crisis

Stressful events and emergencies are going to occur; individuals can probably handle some but may find themselves unable to cope with others. The inability to cope creates the potential for crisis. An individual's equilibrium is disrupted by pressures or upsets, and this imbalance results in stress so severe that the person is unable to find relief by using coping skills that have worked previously. The person is then experiencing a crisis. When identifying crises, we need to distinguish between the event or situation and the

WEB SOURCES
Find Out More About Crisis Intervention

http://www.wm.edu/TTAC/articles/articlesChallenging.htm

The Training and Technical Assistance Center (T/TAC) at the College of William and Mary is part of a statewide network funded by the Virginia Department of Education. T/TAC staff provide a variety of request-based support services and assistance to educational professionals serving school-age students with mild and moderate disabilities or transition needs in Eastern Virginia. The site describes how to develop a school-based plan for crisis intervention

http://www.indian_suicide.org/main.html

This site explores the ways that crisis intervention and suicide of Native Americans can be approached. Central to the understanding of suicide in this culture is the concept of "the center." It is critical to who they are as Native people and as individuals. "The center" refers to all those things that evolve out of our experiences and adaptation to space our very existence on this Mother Earth.

http://www.apa.org/practice/

This web page of the American Psychological Association is a link to information about a disaster response network. It includes a fact sheet, information on traumatic stress, and managing traumatic stress.

http://mel.lib.mi.us/social/SOC_crisis.html

The Michigan Electronic Library maintains a source of web links to information about crisis intervention. These links include the American Association of Suicidology, American Foundation for Suicide Prevention, convention notes about work in crisis intervention settings, Domestic Violence and Crisis Center contact information, and many other sources for assistance.

http://nrscrisisline.org/

This address is the website for the National Runaway Switchboard, a confidential hotline for runaway youth, teens in crisis, and concerned friends and family members. All services are free and available 24 hours every day.

http://www.crisishotline.org/

"Having a crisis? A crisis presents both a feeling of danger and an opportunity for growth by learning more effective coping skills. Explore strategies for working through this critical turning point." This paragraph introduces the website of the Crisis Intervention of Houston, helping people in crisis through telephone crisis counseling, referrals, intervention, postvention, and education.

http://www.edc.org/HHD/csn/

National Injury and Violence Prevention Resource Center is located in Newton, Massachusetts, providing resources and technical assistance to maternal and child health agencies and other organizations seeking to reduce unintentional injuries and violence to children and adolescents. This site provides information on the crises children face and the interventions available to them.

person's response. The crisis is the individual's emotional response to the threatening or hazardous situation rather than the situation itself.

Thus, the crisis lies in the individual's interpretation or perception of an event; the same event does not lead to crisis for all people. What one individual can handle may be a crisis for another person. For example, the houses of two neighbors were burglarized in the same afternoon by the same thief. In both burglaries, the door was kicked in, furniture overturned, and jewelry and electronics equipment stolen. Both neighbors discovered the damage when arriving home from work. Three weeks later, one neighbor has recovered from the event. She locks her doors at night, has marked her possessions, and has joined the neighborhood crime watch. The second neighbor has not recovered as well. She has yet to enjoy a good night's sleep, fears for her life each time she enters her empty house, and calls the police at least once a day. She says she is "as nervous as a cat."

Crises can be divided into two types: developmental and situational. A *developmental crisis* is an individual's response to a situation that is reasonably predictable in the life cycle. Chapter 5 explained that as individuals grow and develop, they undergo periods of major transition such as childhood to puberty, puberty to adolescence, and adolescence to adulthood. Stresses can occur at each phase. For many people, the stresses are normal developmental problems with which they are able to cope. For those who cannot cope, the stresses of these stages can have destructive effects, such as suicide attempts, rejection of others, and depression. Such reactions constitute a developmental crisis in those circumstances.

Situational or *accidental crises* do not occur with any regularity. The sudden and unpredictable nature of this type of crisis makes any preparation or individual control impossible. Examples are fire or other natural disaster, fatal illness, relocation, unplanned pregnancy, and rape. Hazardous situations such as these may cause periods of psychological and behavioral upset. A crisis may result, depending on the individual's personal and social resources at the time of the event.

The skills and strategies that helpers use to provide immediate help for a person in crisis constitute *crisis intervention.* It is short-term therapy that focuses on solving the immediate problem and helping the individual to reestablish equilibrium (Aguilera, 1998). Common practice areas of crisis intervention are childhood and adolescence, mental health problems, marital and family conflicts, emergency hospitalization, suicide prevention, and substance abuse (Aguilera, 1998).

How a Crisis Develops

Even a sudden or short-lived crisis has identifiable components that create a pattern of development. The case study that follows examines crisis in terms of its development. You may want to make note of the different roles the worker plays.

Ben and Joan Matthews and their three children (ages 9 months, 2 years, and 5 years) left their trailer in rural Illinois to drive to Florida. Ben had lost his job because the factory where he worked for minimum wage closed down. He hoped to find a job in Florida working on some of the fruit farms. The Matthews were also hoping that the climate would improve the health of the children as well as the state of their marriage.

The hope for a job did not materialize in Florida, so they headed back to their trailer in Illinois and an uncertain future. The trip home seemed plagued with problems. Two of the children became ill, the car broke down twice, and Joan and Ben argued constantly about what they should do next. A couple of times, the arguments escalated into shouting matches that ended when Ben hit Joan.

By the time the Matthews arrived in Atlanta, they had no money for food, lodging, or gas. The children were hungry and crying, the car was making a funny noise again, Joan was complaining, and Ben had a raging headache. They stopped at a fast-food place so that everyone could use the bathroom and have a drink of water. Joan gathered the children together and headed into the restaurant. When they returned, Ben and the car were gone.

According to Hoff (1995), crisis development has four identifiable phases. In the first, the person reacts to a traumatic event with increased anxiety. The individual then responds with problem-solving mechanisms to reduce or eliminate stress. Here is Joan's initial response:

Joan thinks that Ben has gone to get gas, so she returns to the restaurant. Selecting an out-of-the-way booth, she and the children sit watching and waiting for his return. After an hour, Joan begins to feel desperate. She has no money and no identification because she left her purse in the car. The children are tired and hungry, and she is becoming uncomfortable with the looks from the people at the service counter. Joan fusses with the children and tries to look natural and unworried.

In the second phase, the individual's problem-solving ability fails. The stimulus that caused the initial rise in anxiety continues. In this case, the source of Joan's anxiety does not change: Ben is still missing. Her initial attempts to deal with the situation fail, and her anxiety continues to increase because she is worried about Ben and she is worried about herself.

At this point the manager approaches and asks if he can be of any assistance. By now the children are crying. They are still hungry, are tired of sitting, and sense their mother's tension. Feeling frightened and alone, but not wanting to upset the children, Joan explains to the manager that her husband went to get some gas and that he will be back soon to pick them up. She explains about the funny noise in the car, saying that this was probably being fixed, which accounted for her husband's delay. Joan thanks the manager for his concern and tells him that her husband will surely be there shortly.

Joan leaves the restaurant and begins to check the three nearby gas stations. She does not see their car but hopes it is inside the garage. At each station, she describes Ben and the car, each attendant gives her the same response—no one has seen Ben. Joan decides to return to the restaurant.

Joan's anxiety level is increasing, and all attempts at resolution have failed. In the third phase, she uses every resource available to solve the problem and to lessen her anxiety. Joan tries several alternatives.

During the next hour, Joan becomes more and more frightened that Ben is not coming back to the restaurant. The children are very hungry and tired. Perhaps sensing her anxiety and fear, they are whining, fighting among themselves, and clinging to her. She is losing patience and raises her voice several times to tell them to be quiet and sit still. She is aware that people are staring at them, and she is afraid the manager will ask them to leave the restaurant. Realizing that it is going to be dark soon, she decides to take the children and walk to the nearest gas station, again hoping to find Ben.

There is no sign of Ben at the gas station, and the attendant still does not remember anyone fitting Ben's description. By this time, Joan is obviously very upset, and the attendant offers to let her come into the office to use the phone. She calls her mother collect in Illinois but gets a recorded message that the number is temporarily out of order. In desperation she then tries calling a neighbor of her mother's, but there is no answer. She really cannot think of anyone else to call, and she knows no one in this area.

At this point in phase three, the crisis may be prevented by redefining goals. Joan's original goal was to locate Ben or at least to wait for him to return to the restaurant. When she realizes that he is not returning, she attempts to resolve the situation by securing help from other known sources—informal helpers. The knowledge that she must get food for herself and the children as well as find shelter for the night prompts her to redefine her goal in terms of these needs.

She asks the attendant if he knows of a shelter or a church that might take them in for the night. He tells her that the shelter is on the other side of town and that he can't leave, since he is the only one at the gas station for the night. He suggests that she call the "welfare people," who might know how to get some transportation for her. She is reluctant to call them because she has heard that they take your kids away if you can't care for them. Besides, no one in her family has ever called welfare for anything. They have always been able to make it on their own.

The children are getting hungrier and more irritable, and Joan is feeling nauseous and on the verge of tears. She knows no one else to call. She doesn't want to call the welfare people, but she feels that she really has no other choice.

This is phase four. A state of crisis results when the problem remains unresolved and the tension and anxiety rise to an unbearable degree. Both social
support and internal resources to deal with the situation are lacking. All attempts on the part of the individual have failed to lessen anxiety or change the
situation (see Table 7-6).

The Helper's Role in Crisis Intervention

At this point in the case study, the human service professional becomes involved. To illustrate the steps, principles, skills, and possible outcomes of crisis intervention, the focus of the case study will shift to the perspective of the
helper. Before that happens, however, let us review some of the principles and
skills of crisis intervention so that you will understand what is happening in
the case.

TABLE 7-6   ✦   SUMMARY POINTS: CRISIS DEVELOPMENT

- Reaction to a traumatic event with increased anxiety
- Problem-solving ability fails
- Additional attempts at resolution fail and anxiety increases
- Problem remains unresolved and tension and anxiety increase to an unbearable degree

---

• • • • • • • • • •

Suicidal Behavior

- Previous suicide attempts "mini-attempts"
- Explicit statements of suicidal ideation or feelings
- Development of suicidal plan, acquiring the means, "rehearsal" behavior,
  setting a time for the attempt
- Self-inflicted injuries, such as cuts, burns, or head banging
- Reckless behavior
- Making out a will or giving away favorite possessions
- Inappropriately saying goodbye
- Verbal behavior that is ambiguous or indirect: "I'm going away on a real
  long trip." "You won't have to worry about me anymore." "I want to go to
  sleep and never wake up." "I'm so depressed, I just can't go on." "Does
  God punish suicides?" "Voices are telling me to do bad things."
- Requests for euthanasia information, inappropriate joking, stories or es-
  says on morbid themes

SOURCE: Suicidal Behavior. Retrieved September 11, 2000, from the World Wide Web:
http://www.metanoia.org/suicide/whattodo.htm.

Crisis intervention is a time-limited service. It occurs with a minimum of delay and focuses on the individual's current life situation. The helper must quickly establish trust and rapport with the client and support the client's self-esteem and self-reliance. Usually, more than one helper is involved in providing services so the client will not become dependent on a single individual. Two strategies important to crisis intervention are referral for needed services and activation of a social network for support and assistance.

The successful crisis intervention worker is one who has mastered the skills of establishing a relationship quickly with the client. Remaining calm, using common sense, and projecting self-confidence are qualities that will help the worker in a crisis situation. Effective communication skills, particularly listening and responding, are also critical for establishing trust and rapport. Nonverbally, the use of physical gestures such as holding hands or touching an arm will also facilitate the establishment of a relationship. Verbally, the worker helps the client to focus on available courses of action rather than past occurrences. These are the same skills necessary for effective communication in any helping process.

In some cases, clients may be reluctant, so the human service professional must initiate any direct action that is needed. Examples of such action are activating a support network, seeking medical help, notifying other family members or neighbors, and preventing clients from hurting themselves or others. People cannot remain in crisis forever; the duration is usually from a few days to a few weeks.

Hoff (1995) suggested several possible outcomes to a crisis. The first, a return to the precrisis state, is usually the result of effective problem solving. Both the internal strengths of the individual and the existence of social supports favor this outcome. A second possible outcome is a return to the precrisis state except that the individual acquires new skills or develops existing skills further as a result of the experience. Developing new resources and problem-solving skills are examples of ways the individual can grow. A third outcome would be behaviors such as excessive drinking, drug abuse, and blaming others. Clients may also become withdrawn, suspicious, or depressed. Extreme actions that may result are attempted or successful suicide or murder.

Returning to Joan's situation, it is now 8:00 P.M. and the office of the Department of Human Services is closed. Her call is automatically referred to the emergency child abuse line. The human service professional who is on duty frequently gets calls such as the one Joan is making, because few resources are available after 5:00 P.M. The first step in crisis intervention is to assess the nature of the precipitating event and the problem. A key question to ask in this assessment is, "What level of danger does the person pose to himself or herself or to others?"

Shirley, the helper on duty, answers the call in a pleasant but businesslike voice and introduces herself, attempting to establish a climate for positive communication. Without knowing Joan's name or location, she listens as Joan describes her situation. Then Joan asks if the helper can do anything for her family. Shirley assures Joan that she has done the right thing by calling and explains that a number of options are available to her. Before she proceeds, however, the human service professional asks Joan if she is in a safe place. Feeling some relief that someone will help her and that something can be done, Joan tells Shirley about the gas station and the attendant who has been so helpful.

After noting the phone number of the gas station, Shirley tells Joan she will make some phone calls to the women's shelter, the mission, and to a short-term foster care facility to try to arrange housing. Thirty minutes later, Shirley calls her back. There is an opening at the women's shelter, and Joan and the children can take a cab there at the shelter's expense.

When Joan arrives at the shelter, assessment continues as the caseworker and the nurse on duty take over the case from Shirley. After they eat, the nurse completes a very basic physical assessment of Joan and each of the children. Since there are no signs of physical abuse or illness, the nurse listens to Joan's story and asks a few questions. The nurse postpones a more extensive physical assessment until the next day. Joan and the children are taken to their room, where the exhausted children fall asleep immediately. Although temporarily safe, fed, and sheltered, Joan is emotionally devastated by Ben's abandonment of the family and her lack of resources to return to Illinois.

Once the initial assessment is completed, the second step, planning the intervention, begins. The purpose of this step is to restore the person to a pre-crisis state. Factors considered during this phase are the amount of disruption the crisis has caused in the person's life, the amount of time that has passed since the event, the individual's strengths and coping skills, and the presence or absence of supports in the person's life.

In the morning, the family eats breakfast, and the children are allowed to go to the playroom with the other children at the shelter. Joan meets with the nurse and the caseworker in the private office next to the playroom. They are concerned about a bruise on Joan's face, which has developed where Ben hit her the day before. Joan assures them that Ben's action was an isolated incident, caused by frustration, and that he has never hit her before. Both the caseworker and the nurse pay close attention to Joan's nonverbal and verbal communication, paraphrasing and reflecting her responses. They notice that Joan keeps wringing her hands and running her fingers through her hair. She begins to cry and tells them how Ben has deserted her and the children and that she has no idea how she will get back to Illinois. The caseworker encourages Joan to express her fears and frustrations and is supportive of the huge task Joan has before her.

She takes Joan's hand as she assures her that she can stay at the shelter for as long as she needs to and tells her that the community has many re-

sources that can help Joan get home as quickly as possible. As they begin to talk about Joan's situation, the caseworker is able to ascertain exactly what happened, when it happened, and how Joan has coped to this point. The caseworker finally decides that the primary problem is transportation home to Illinois. She also learns about Joan's mother and other family members in Illinois. Together she and Joan begin to explore some options. Joan wants to try to reach her mother's neighbor again in hopes of getting a message to her mother.

The third step in crisis intervention is implementing the intervention. In this case, it may involve only the phone call to the neighbor, who may be able to reach Joan's mother. In other cases, the intervention may be more complicated, relying on the skills, creativity, and flexibility of the worker (Aguilera, 1998). During this phase, the helper must focus on reality and identify the clients' positive coping mechanisms and support systems. Allowing clients to express feelings about situations may also be important to reduce their tensions. It may help clients deal with feelings that may have been suppressed (such as anger) or feelings that have been denied (such as grief).

The final step is the resolution of the crisis, in which the worker and the client plan for the future, reinforcing the new ways of coping. The worker also helps the client in planning for the future and preparing for any new crises that may arise. Here is how Joan's situation is resolved.

Joan is able to reach her mother, who wires money for bus fare for Joan and the children. While they are waiting for the money to arrive, Joan is able to talk with the helper expressing her feelings about what happened and verbalizing her need for continued support. In response to Joan's need for support, the caseworker gets the necessary information to refer her to a free counseling service at a mental health center near her home in Illinois. The helper also gives her a list of sources of financial aid in Illinois for her to contact when she returns home.

As you reflect on the case study, what principles of intervention are illustrated? What roles did the helper play? What skills did the helper use in this situation? How would you describe the outcome? Finally, how is the helping process followed in this example?

The Team Approach

A new trend in crisis intervention is the team approach. Members of the team are selected on the basis of their knowledge and skills. Membership on the team may also vary according to the requirements of the agency and the geographic

• • • • • • • • • •

INTERNATIONAL FOCUS
The Samaritans

The Samaritans, a British volunteer organization, was organized in 1953 to provide informal helping with crises and other problems. Present in most British communities, these volunteers befriend people with problems who are unwilling or unable to seek formal help. Having contributed to a dramatic reduction in Britain's suicide rate, The Samaritans are rapidly spreading to other countries. The seven principles and practices of the organization are as follows.

SEVEN PRINCIPLES

1. The primary aim of The Samaritans is to be available at any hour of the day or night to befriend those passing through personal crises and in imminent danger of taking their own lives.
2. The Samaritans also seek to alleviate human misery, loneliness, despair and depression by listening to and befriending those who feel that they have no one else to turn to who would understand and accept them.
3. A caller does not lose the freedom to make his own decisions, including the decision to take his own life, and is free to break contact at any time.
4. The fact that a person has asked the help of The Samaritans, together with everything he has said, is completely confidential within the organization unless permission is freely given by the caller for all or part of such information to be communicated to someone outside the Organization. A Samaritan volunteer is not permitted to accept confidences if a condition is made that not even the Director should be informed of them.
5. Samaritan volunteers in befriending callers will be guided and actively supported by experienced leaders who will have the advice, when required, of professional consultants.

limits and socioeconomic needs of the community and the clients served. The human service worker may be a member of such a team, which may also include professionals such as psychiatrists, psychologists, nurses, and social workers. According to Aguilera (1998), tasks of the human service worker include doing initial assessments, observing behavioral changes, conducting interviews, and participating in various short-term therapies. The more intensive individual, family, or group therapy would be performed by the professionals on the team. At the conclusion of the crisis intervention, the client may need to continue with professional services. If the client shows little progress after the crisis intervention, the team may recommend more traditional types of problem solving.

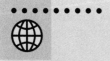

6. In appropriate cases the caller will also be invited to consider seeking professional help in such fields as medicine and social work, and material help from other agencies.
7. Samaritan volunteers are forbidden to impose their own convictions or to influence callers in regard to politics, philosophy or religion.

SEVEN PRACTICES

1. Samaritan volunteers are carefully selected and prepared by the local Branch in which they are to serve.
2. The Samaritans are available at all hours to callers, and may be contacted (anonymously if desired) by telephone or personal visit, or by letter.
3. When a caller is believed to be in danger of suicidal action, the Samaritan is particularly encouraged to ask the caller's permission for contact to be maintained during the crisis.
4. Samaritans offer longer-term befriending of callers where appropriate, while recognizing that the Branch may from time to time have to set limits.
5. Samaritans listen to those concerned about the welfare of another person, and, if satisfied that the third person is despairing, depressed or suicidal, may discreetly offer befriending.
6. Samaritans are normally known to callers only by a forename and contacts by callers made only through the Branch Centre.
7. Samaritan Branches are banded together in a legally constituted Association whose Council of Management represents all the Branches and reserves to itself the appointment of the person in charge of each Branch.

SOURCE: Excerpt from "The Principles and Practices" of *The Samaritans* (1985). Reprinted by permission of The Samaritans, Slough, England.

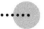 **Things to Remember**

1. Helping is always guided by two questions: (1) What is helpful? (2) How can the needs of the client be met?
2. The effectiveness of the helping process depends greatly on the helper's ability to communicate an understanding of the client's feelings, clarify what the problem is, and provide appropriate assistance to resolve the problem.
3. Formal helping takes place in human service organizations and agencies. The cornerstone of this helping, the medium through which help is offered, is the helping relationship.

4. Before the client arrives, the helper should attend to matters such as establishing the physical setting, deciding how to handle the paperwork, and determining how to gather information about the client.

5. During the helping process, the human service professional and the client set goals and determine how those goals will be reached to resolve the problem. The final stage of the helping process is termination.

6. Effective communication is especially important in helping relationships. The way a helper listens and responds to the client is crucial in building a helping relationship with that person.

7. The skillful helper is able to "hear" the client's behavior (the nonverbal message) as well as what is actually said (the verbal message) and to respond verbally and nonverbally to these messages.

8. Attending behavior is a way to let the client know that the helper is listening. There are four dimensions of attending behavior: eye contact, attentive body language, vocal qualities, and verbal tracking.

9. Once the helper has heard the verbal and nonverbal messages of the client, it is time for the helper to respond. The helper must determine his or her intent before speaking.

10. Beginning helpers should be wary of excessive questioning, which may hinder the helping process and make clients dependent.

11. Communication skills are the foundation of all group functioning as members interact to reach some understanding of each other, establish goals, determine a division of labor, and complete other tasks.

12. The key to working with culturally different clients is awareness of and sensitivity to cultural differences.

13. Among the challenging aspects of human service practice is the reality that not all clients are cooperative and willing; helpers are likely to meet the resistant client, the silent client, the overly demanding client, and the unmotivated client.

14. Crisis intervention is a helping process that occurs at a very fast pace and incorporates many of the helping roles and skills. Crises can be divided into two types: developmental and situational.

15. The skills and strategies that helpers use to provide immediate help for a person in crisis constitute crisis intervention.

Additional Readings: Focus on Helping

Gibson, G. (1999). *Gone boy: A walkabout.* New York: Kodansha International. This first-time author, an antiquarian bookseller and a father, has written a poignant and insightful chronicle of his attempts to make sense of his son's murder at the door of his college library.

Jamison, K. R. (1999). *Night falls fast: Understanding suicide.* New York: Alfred A. Knopf.
Suicide, a vast public health crisis, is the focus of this author, an internationally known authority on depressive illnesses and their treatment, who examines statistics, cases, survivors, and the media.

Meier, S. T., & Davis, S. R. (1997). *The elements of counseling.* Pacific Grove, CA: Brooks/Cole.

This book responds to the questions beginning helpers may have about the counseling process. It covers such fundamentals of counseling as explaining counseling to the client, noticing resistance, avoiding advice, listening for metaphors, and arranging the physical setting appropriately.

Verghese, A. (1994). *My own country.* New York: Vintage Books.

This author, an infectious disease specialist, recounts his life and experiences in an Appalachian town in East Tennessee as he becomes by necessity the local AIDS expert.

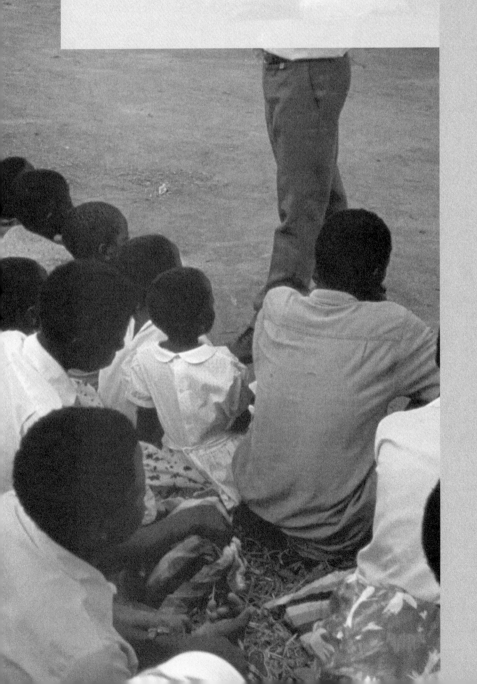

Working Within a System

Human service delivery does not occur in a vacuum. The environment in which such activities occur is critical for the human service professional. The activities occur with clients and groups in the context of their own environments, within the culture of agencies and organizations, and within the communities of rural and urban areas, the national scope, and even the global environment. It would be difficult to assist clients, to deliver effective services, and to develop needed policies and services without an understanding of the context in which we all live. This chapter will introduce the concept of the environment and its integral role in our work as human service professionals.

In this chapter, you will read about Harold, an elderly man who has been hospitalized, and Sue Ellen Draper, who is a welfare client. Their cases illustrate the concepts of general systems theory. Don Regalis and Detective Shirley Santis are human service professionals who present their perspectives on environmental influences as they work with clients.

Working within different environments can be challenging. To help you understand the issues you will confront, this chapter presents three ways to examine the context or the setting that will help define the environment more clearly. First, general systems theory is useful to explain the environment and its interactions as a whole, in other words, the broad view. Second, we will introduce a method of diagramming client life systems, useful in mapping environmental factors. Third, a model of influences can show the significant factors or components and their power upon the client and the client's environment as well as the environment within which human services are delivered.

Finally, the chapter concludes with a discussion of change at the local and community levels and with specific populations. Three international projects will illustrate successful efforts with change.

Using General Systems Theory: The Broad View

One helpful way to view the complex service delivery environment is through systems theory, the study of an organized whole. Systems theory is useful to the study of human services because it provides an organized way to describe the interactions among individuals, organizations, and the environment. The application of systems theory is not restricted to individuals and groups; it can provide a helpful perspective on any living system, including interactions among human service institutions and organizations.

Development of the theory is attributed to Ludwig Von Bertalanffy, a biologist who defined systems as elements that interact with each other (1968). The major focus of this theory is the interactions of elements in a system, including their relationships, their structures, and their interdependence. According to general systems theory, the following principles are important (Leiter & Webb, 1983):

1. Human beings are viewed as being in an environment that is an open system.

2. The human being functions as an individual and as a member of a community.
3. An individual must be viewed within the context of the immediate relationship groups (family) and within the context of the environment.
4. Human interaction is not a choice; individuals do not live in isolation.
5. General systems theory provides a representation of human social systems (groups, organizations, or communities) that are constantly interacting with one another.

Human service systems are complex and include individual clients, families or smaller groups, and the larger environment. The helping professional and the environments in which they operate are also part of these human service systems.

Understanding general systems theory can help you as a beginning human service professional in two ways. First, the theory allows you to think about individuals, groups, and organizations realistically. The definitions and models that follow present individuals, groups, and organizations, and actions in a flexible structure, which allows you to account for individuals and situations and the changes they may encounter. Second, the definitions and models presented should help you notice patterns of interaction that can improve your understanding of clients' situations (see Table 8-1).

Melson (1980) considered the following terms to be basic to an understanding of general systems theory. Following the definitions is their application to a system with which you are familiar—your school or college. Other examples focus on individuals: Harold, an 80-year-old man who has been hospitalized and will soon be released, and Detective Shirley Santis, who works in a small city gang prevention unit. These examples will help you understand the systems theory from the perspectives of an individual client and a human service professional.

The following terms are part of the systems "language":

Input—any energy (action or thought), materials (clothing, food, books), or individuals (worker, family member, neighbors, institutions, or organizations) that exist in a particular system
Transformation—the interaction or processing of inputs

TABLE 8-1 ✦ SUMMARY POINTS: WORKING WITHIN SYSTEMS

- Human service professionals do not operate in a vacuum.
- Systems theory is an organized approach to describe the interactions among individuals, organizations, and environments.
- One benefit of applying systems theory to human services is that it allows us to think realistically about individuals, groups, and organizations.
- A second benefit is that it highlights patterns of interactions that contribute to our understanding of situations.

Output—the product that results from the interaction of the inputs during the transformation

Boundary—the parameters or borders of a system that control entering and leaving the system

Now, let us consider how these terms might be used to describe what happens at your college. Think about the inputs that are part of your educational experience. These might include people (peers, instructors, administrators), materials (books, computers, films), and energy (motivation, presence, anticipation). The interaction among the inputs is the transformation that occurs in a system. In the case of your school or college, we might describe what happens during registration, at an advising appointment, or in the classroom; or we might think about extracurricular activities, intramural sports, or lectures and performances. The results or outputs of these interactions and activities are numerous. They include an educated individual, personal and social development, and preparation for a career. Finally, let us consider the concept of boundaries. There are certain requirements that must be met for you to enter and to depart this system. First, to enter the school or college you now attend, you were required to complete an application that probably included one or more of the following: an application, references, a high school transcript, and SAT or ACT scores. There are several ways people leave this system. Many leave as graduates, which means they have a certain grade point average, have completed a prescribed program of study (a major), and have no outstanding bills due the institution. Of course, there are other ways to leave and these include dropping out, expulsion, transferring, or "flunking out."

Now let us take these same systems terms and apply them to a human service situation.

Harold is an 80-year-old male who has been hospitalized for a heart bypass but is now beginning his recovery at home. He continues to live alone and take care of himself. The social service personnel from the hospital have been working with his managed care organization for the past week to plan Harold's transition from the hospital to his home. As they prepare for his discharge, they have developed a discharge plan that outlines the services he will need before he leaves the hospital and those he will need early in his home recovery. The plan calls for follow-up assessments later.

Input   The input for this case includes many actions and thoughts—both of Harold and of the hospital personnel involved in his care. Specific components of this input category are as follows:

- Harold explains his health-related goals.
- Medical and social service staff discuss Harold's needs.
- Financial arrangements are made with managed care to cover the costs of the services.

- Home health care is contracted for six weeks.
- Supplies, equipment, and medicine are purchased for Harold's home stay.
- Appropriate medical and social service contacts are scheduled with Harold.

Transformation   The transformation occurs as Harold, the hospital personnel, and other referral services actually formulate and begin implementing the plan. This interaction is shaped within the context of Harold's needs and environment, the hospital setting, and the resources and constraints of the other social service agencies involved. Complications during the transformation may include the following:

- Harold does not want strangers in his home, and he argues against the use of the home health care "old ladies," as he calls them.
- Harold is depressed one day because he is not yet feeling better. Another day, he refuses to stay in bed because he feels "great."
- Harold's great grandniece, Betsy, his only living relative, visits from a neighboring city. While she is there, she tells the hospital that Harold has no business leaving the hospital.
- Harold, the hospital social service worker, and the managed care case manager agree on home health care with reassessment every two weeks.
- Before Harold is discharged, his surgeon gets sick. The surgeon's partner works with the discharge team.

Output   In the case of Harold, the outputs resulting from the transformation or interaction of the inputs may include the following:

- Intense planning by the professional health care staff
- A written plan of Harold's discharge
- Interagency referrals to medical suppliers, druggists, and health care agencies, stating the types of services to be supplied and the dates
- Meetings with Harold and the home health care staff
- Planned assessments every two weeks and communication and review by the managed care case manager
- Medical follow-ups after six weeks and three months

Using the terms *input, transformation,* and *output* reminds the helper of the realities of the environment in which the case occurs. Using two other terms can reinforce this understanding of the context of inputs and outputs: *interdependency* and *change.*

Interdependency   One characteristic of a system is that any change in one part affects another part. When individuals become involved in the human service system, the worlds of both the workers and the clients have the potential for change. Such change occurs within the context of the environment. Because of this interdependence, completion of one task is dependent on other factors within the system (Von Bertalanffy, 1968). For example, the arrival of Harold's great grandniece, Betsy, has the potential to change the situation. She could insist that Harold is not competent to take care of himself or make decisions about his own care. The staff would then have to resolve the issue of competence. This decision could have a major impact on hospital planning, the review made by the managed care organization, and Harold's future living situation and recovery. This is only one of many inputs that could have changed the situation. For example, the availability of home health care services could have affected the planning. Although the hospital is not responsible for such services, its discharge planning is dependent on the delivery of high-quality home health care services.

Change   When input interacts within a system, two types of responses can result: homeostasis or adaptation. In the state of homeostasis, inputs are introduced, but the system withstands change and maintains itself, retaining its original state. Sometimes inputs introduce factors that contribute to major change, and adaptation results. During adaptation, the system is changed from its original state. Change can take many forms: change of organizational structure, change in patterns of interaction, or change in patterns of interdependency.

In Harold's situation, the switch of doctors had the potential to effect great change. The new surgeon could have requested a new discharge plan requiring a more lengthy hospital stay and full-time nursing care for the next six weeks. This input would have drastically altered the discharge plan and Harold's own view of his recovery. The hospital staff, as well as Harold, would have had to adapt their previous ideas about recovery. As it was, the new doctor made few changes. Homeostasis (balance) was maintained.

General systems theory provides helpers with a model for understanding and providing assistance to individual clients and families. Systematic use of the concepts of input, transformation, and output can reduce the confusing complexities of working within both the client environment and the human service system. In this next example you will see how the concepts of general systems theory are used to understand the environment of the human service professional.

Detective Shirley Santis has been on the local police force for 16 years. For the last 4 years she has worked with gangs and gang-related programs. First she was assigned the inner city as her territory, working with a unit that focused on crime reduction in the local housing projects. In reality, she patrolled the area and responded to emergencies such as domestic violence, robbery, assault, public drunkenness, loitering, and drug-related offenses. During her 3 years working this area, she had some success relating to the area inhabitants. She was able to develop a special rapport with many of the youngsters who resided in the tougher neighborhoods. Last year she was promoted to a gang prevention unit and placed on a city gang prevention task force. The work with the task force, which is the subject of this analysis from the general systems per-

spective, is challenging. The task force is expected to produce a report that includes the current status of gangs in the city and recommendations for a gang-free environment. The report is nearing the final draft stage. The committee is meeting three times this week to discuss the many differences of opinion on the nature of the problem, the recommendations, and what type of information should be made public. The report is due the week after next.

Input   For the work of Shirley Santis, input includes not only actions and thoughts of Shirley and her clients and constituents, but also other professionals with whom she works. Note that the input includes the leaders of the institutions and organizations, political pressures, financial pressures, and policy and regulations.

- As a member of the task force, Shirley contributes her understanding of gangs and gang activity in the city based on her police experience.
- In each meeting thus far, the mayor's public relations assistant insists that the document not contain details about the prevalence of gangs and their activities in the city. The mayor fears that the facts will alarm the local citizenry and stifle the economic development of the city.
- The Deputy Assistant for Probation and Parole from the Department of Corrections and the juvenile judge have recommended that gang members receive rigorous penalties for their offenses.
- The budget in the city, county, and state is stretched as it covers insurance, welfare, and education priorities. Gang prevention will have to compete for scarce dollars.
- The local citizens are frightened of the gang activity and have asked the task force to help them "take back" their homes and their neighborhoods. They will picket the next meeting if the recommendations made by the Department of Corrections are not accepted.
- The task force has heard from several consultants who have addressed gang prevention plans developed in their own cities.

Transformation   Transformation, within the context of the gang prevention task force work, occurs during this week as the task force members begin to find some agreements for the report and the recommendations that will be submitted to the mayor next week. These agreements are influenced by the status of each task force member, the recommendations that each are willing to support, those recommendations members are willing to offer for compromise, the resources available to carry out the recommendations, the personal relationships between task force members, the federal, state and local policies and regulations that must be followed, and the anticipated public reception of this plan.

- During the week, three local individuals from the gang neighborhoods contact Shirley and meet with her to talk about their ideas for the report. They press her hard to represent their ideas, since they believe that no one else will do so. Two of the individuals are parents of children who were, for a time, "wanna be" gang members. Shirley's early intervention kept them out of the local gang activity.

- Three meetings of the task force were held, but several members also met to discuss the report with each other: The deputy assistant for probation and parole and the juvenile judge met with the consultant to ask him to stress that the report must present an honest representation of the problem to the public so they can recommend strong sentencing as a deterrent to gang participation. The mayor's wife met with the deputy assistant to talk about his desire to present a positive face on the gang problem. The local school superintendent was asked by the consultant to present a five-pronged strategy from the educational perspective.
- The mayor's executive director formally presented to the task force the budgetary limits of the plan.
- At the state capital, the governor called for a "getting tough on crime" approach to criminal activity.

Output   In this case, the outputs represent the final report of the task force and the reactions from government officials, organizations and institutions within the community, the citizenry, and the gang members themselves.

- The final report represents a compromise on three issues: the presentation of the problem, the severity of sentencing for gang-related offenses, and the financial implications of the recommendations.
- The deputy assistant for probation and parole and the juvenile judge ask Shirley to help write a dissenting report, but she declines to participate.
- The mayor formally receives the report.
- The two local papers publish stories once the report is released. In one paper the headlines read, "Gangs Rule the Streets." The local weekly independent runs an in-depth look at the history of gangs in the United States, the history of gangs in the local area, gang characteristics, and current gang activity.
- The local educational association, with the help of the National Educational Association (NEA), prepares a school campaign on gang awareness, spanning elementary school through high school.
- Several task force members and other community leaders are appointed by the mayor to serve on an ad hoc committee charged with implementing the plan.
- The task force is a topic of conversation within the gangs. They scoff at the report.

Interdependency   It is clear from reading and studying the inputs, transformation, and outputs that there is a great deal of interdependency between various components of a local environment. Each of the components influences the other. In our gang prevention task force scenario, financial interdependence is illustrated clearly. The mayor worries about the honesty of the report because he does not want the city to lose the ability to attract new business and industry to the area. It is this new economic development that will support the cost of the recommendations of the task force. On the other hand, if the gang problem does not improve, the city is in danger of losing the businesses that it does have. Many agencies and programs are also worried because they know that implementing the plan will cost money. The financial resources are limited, so many of their services will be cut to fund the task force recommendations. For example, the local housing authority is asking the mayor and the new ad hoc implementation task force, "What is the gain if, by putting more police on the streets, we lose our funding and more individuals cannot find housing?" They state, "Children often turn to gangs when families cannot provide them the basics of food, shelter, and clothing."

Change   Many citizens and local leaders have a wait-and-see attitude concerning the influence of the task force upon the community. They have seen too many task force reports produced and implemented. At the local delicatessen last Saturday, several businessmen were eating breakfast when the topic of the task force was introduced. The owner of the deli expressed hope for the future of the downtown. The president of the largest bank in town announced that he intends to support the implementation task force in any way that he can. He wants to help foster positive change. Although the majority of the breakfast crowd hopes for a successful gang prevention effort, men of the group have a cynical attitude. They are not sure that change is possible. As a whole, they believe that homeostasis, where the system withstands change and maintains itself, may be the result. This means there will be no change. On the other hand, in some areas of the city, change and adaptation are already occurring. The local neighborhood citizenry where the gang activity is primarily focused, has gained a sense of community and empowerment from their attempt to influence the task force. With the help of two local churches, this group is going to continue to meet. Next week they are going to discuss a "take back the night" campaign, and the local law enforcement officials have been invited to attend.

On an individual level, another way of illustrating the influences in one's environment is the life systems diagram. Using these diagrams is another way of understanding the client's world and the influences of the human service delivery environment.

 ## Life Systems Diagram: A Practical Approach

Because many factors affect the client, human service professionals must be aware of the important parts of the client's world. Such influences can be described using a life systems diagram that illustrates the influences on the client. This is an efficient way to assess the client and the environment and helps the worker determine efficient ways to gather and think about pertinent information. Figures 8-1 and 8-2 provide a way of thinking about

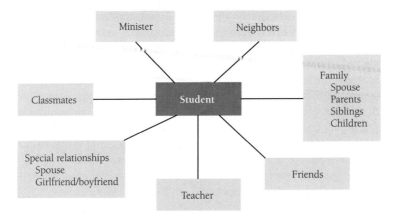

Figure 8-1   ✦   Life systems model of a student

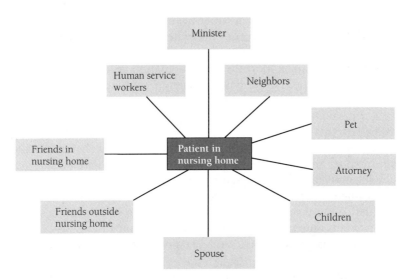

Figure 8-2   ✦   Life systems model of a nursing home patient

clients' situations. The client, whether a student, a patient in a nursing home, or a victim of a violent crime, is the central focus. Environment is considered as it relates to the client.

A model of a life system only identifies the influences in a person's life; it does not indicate relative importance. For example, Figure 8-1 represents the life system of a student. It may be similar to yours. Note that it does not suggest which influences are most important; nor does it represent the internal characteristics of the client, such as knowledge, skills, and social and religious values.

The life system of a patient in a nursing home (see Figure 8-2) is more contained than that of a student, but is equally complex. Environment is listed as

TABLE 8-2   ✦   SUMMARY POINTS: LIFE SYSTEMS OF CLIENTS

- Assesses the client and the environment
- Helps the worker determine efficient ways to gather and process information
- Focuses on the client
- Considers the environment as it relates to the client

a part of the system, because the environment of the nursing home can be specifically defined and has a major impact on the client's life. The diagram includes people from the client's previous environment and significant others from the present nursing home environment (see Table 8-2).

How do human service professionals develop life systems diagrams for their own clients—ones that will be useful to the helping process? Helpers first listen to their clients share personal experiences so they can then build the system diagram from the clients' perspectives. Using the following case, a firsthand account of a client's experience, we can practice developing a system diagram.

This case describes a student who experiences child abuse during a critical year in her life. Read the case and identify the systems, institutions, organizations, and people mentioned in the client's story. Then draw the client's life system.

When the school made allegations of child abuse against my parents, they were shocked and appalled. They considered themselves hardworking, upstanding citizens who had opened their home as foster parents to help those who are less fortunate. They saw my behavior as a case of revenge from a resentful child trying to cause problems. After the allegations were made, I was placed under the observation of a child care worker who was investigating the charges made by the school.

Except through the poor and unwanted children who lived in our home, I knew very little about human services and was apprehensive about what I should say to this woman. From our first visit, several things she did caused me even greater fear and anxiety. This woman, who was supposedly placed in my life to help make a bad situation better, seemed to always be preoccupied with irrelevant talk of what she was doing that evening. She constantly praised my parents on the commendable way they cared for the mentally retarded and other less fortunate children living in their home. It was obvious to me that I could not trust this woman who made me doubt myself and my view of what was taking place in my life. I began to wonder if I really was jealous of the foster children, if I really was an "evil little brat" who constantly got in trouble to get attention. It was as if my bruises and missing teeth were self-inflicted.

As the tension and hatred between my parents, my sister, and me became almost unbearable, I tried to reach out to this strange woman, even though I needed to hide much of the truth for the sake of my sister and me. Amazingly enough, the incidents that we discussed would later be repeated back to us by our parents. As the threats and mental torment worsened, the only emotions I felt toward this woman were betrayal and distrust.

Several months later, the school became legally involved once again, when one of my teachers found me alone and feeling quite desperate in the bathroom. After asking a lot of questions about the marks and bruises that covered my body, the teacher tucked me away in an office until she could take some action to prevent any future abuse. The child care worker was not available when the teacher called to express the urgency of the situation. When my parents arrived at the school, shouting and making violent threats, the school had to call the police to come and prevent my father from causing further trouble. A second call was placed to the worker, who was still unavailable, and my parents were escorted to the office as I was led outside to the waiting police car. I was quickly taken to a juvenile home, where I was to stay until a decision could be made by the proper authorities concerning my safety and welfare.

The previous child care worker was no longer in charge of my case because of the change in my situation. She was replaced by a man whose attitude and style were different and much more effective. After collecting a lot of information, including interviews with people who knew about my situation, he was ready to go before a judge with the question of whether I should return to my home or be placed elsewhere. In spite of everything that had happened in the past, I figured that I had nothing to lose by telling this man the whole truth, even though I expected the same attitudes and responses as the previous worker had shown me. To my surprise, this man went before the judge and took my side. He presented all the information he had gathered—a good portion of which the previous worker had disbelieved or neglected to follow up on.

The system eventually proved my innocence. Instead of being labeled a child who continuously misbehaved and could be controlled only by severe discipline, I escaped my childhood prison. I now lead a reasonably normal life, but the scars of my childhood remain an obstacle that I encounter nearly every day. At least some of this turmoil might have been avoided by more timely and appropriate action from the people in human services.

In summary, by developing a life systems diagram of a client, the human service professional can begin to understand the system or environment in which the client functions. Its advantage lies in its simplicity, for it allows the worker to describe the client's environment. Its obvious limitations are that it does not represent the chronology of events, distinguish the relative importance of system components, or describe interactions in the system.

Model of Influences: The Impact of the Environment

Another helpful way to understand the client or the human service delivery system is to study the influences of the environments in which they operate. For example, each client lives in a specific location, has friends and family, belongs to groups, and engages in certain activities. These dimensions are part of the environment that influences a client's life. With regard to the human service delivery system, the environment includes specific types of institutions and organizations, specific missions and philosophies that guide service delivery, populations served, and specific needs addressed. Other influences include how individuals within these organizations communicate formally and informally with each other.

Studying the impact of the influences on either the client or the human service delivery system environment allows the helper to better understand the reality of a situation. With an improved knowledge of the environment, the helper also can assist clients with adaptation to or alteration of their environments. By understanding the environment of the human service delivery system, helpers can use the system more effectively to meet their clients' needs. The following section defines the influences that affect individual growth and development and those factors that impact the actual delivery of human services.

Several theorists have contributed to the understanding of how the environment affects the individual. Bronfenbrenner (1979) first presented his ideas concerning influence to explain how children grow and develop. Later he and others applied the use of his theory to explain difficult environmental situations such as child abuse and violence. Many scholars and teachers have used Bronfenbrenner's ideas to develop a picture or symbolic model of an individual's environment (Huitt, 2000; LeFrancois, 1999). Figure 8-3 shows a model of influences that explains the impact the environment has upon the individual.

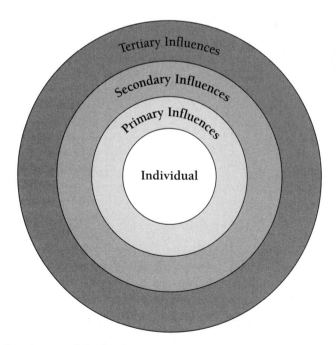

Figure 8-3 ✦ Model of influences on the individual

Model of Influences on the Individual

Using the model of influences shown in Figure 8-3, the individual is surrounded by several layers of environmental influences. The three layers include primary influences, secondary influences, and tertiary influences. The further the distance the influences are from the individual, the less influence they have. In other words, the primary environment, in most cases, has a stronger impact than either the secondary or tertiary environments.

Individual   The individual in this figure is considered from three perspectives: biological, psychological, and sociological. The biological can include the general health of the individual, any outstanding physical skills or aptitudes, or physical impairments of the individual. Psychological characteristics are factors such as self-esteem, self-concept, locus of control, resiliency, and cognitive abilities. Sociological factors include variables such as socioeconomic status, educational level of parents and grandparents, and norms of the peer group and neighborhood.

Primary influences   The most immediate and earliest influences on individuals, as children, are the family (those who interact with the child), school peers and teachers, day care or child care workers, and social and sports organizations. Family influence includes parent interactions, child care situation, presence of or absence of the mother or father or both, and age and gender of siblings. These are key variables that determine the world of the child. At times, primary influences are complicated by divorce or blended families. Physical characteristics of the environment also contribute a direct influence and can include living space and television, computer, and reading materials.

Secondary influences   Such influences are represented by the neighborhood, social organizations, and faith-based organizations. The beliefs, common roles, and norms of the community also exert an influence. For example, the neighborhood may play a significant role in the individual's life, including location (rural, suburban, urban), playmates, sense of community (involved, friendly, or isolated), traffic patterns (quiet or busy streets), and play areas.

The interactions within the secondary environment are also influences. For example, a child who lives at home and attends school is influenced by both. A child who is home-schooled has different influences.

Tertiary influences   The factors with the least influence in the life of a child are those such as international region or global changes (Huitt, 2000). For example, children in the 1950s grew up with threats of nuclear holocaust, spending time in school practicing civil defense drills, and stocking community bomb shelters with food and water. Children of the 1960s became part of a well-known rebellious generation, the baby boomers, who both protested and fought in the Vietnam War. Certain factors in this increasingly global environment will help define the children of this new millennium and shape what they believe. Such factors include increased violence in homes, schools, and the workplace, unemployment, migration to the cities, and fear of substance abuse and AIDS.

One way to better understand the model of influences is to see how a human service professional would apply it.

Don Regalis has worked with Sue Ellen Draper, a welfare client, for the past nine years. Sue Ellen has four girls: Sharon, age10; Suzie, age 8; and twins, Sarah and Sindy, age 5. Sue Ellen has always lived in this sparsely populated rural county. Welfare has been part of her family history. Her mother, Sarah McCall, raised Sue Ellen and her five brothers, Darin, Donnie, David, Drew, and Doug, on welfare. Sarah depended on both welfare and food stamps to feed and clothe the children. For years, with few services available for welfare clients in this small community, Sarah pieced together a living that combined taking in washing, using church donations, and accepting government help to provide for her children.

Don Regalis has known Sue Ellen since birth, but his first encounter with her, as a client occurred when she married and became pregnant at the age of 16. She became eligible for AFDC, since her husband, Phil, could not find work.

Don's involvement with Sarah McCall and her family, and now Sue Ellen and her family, has spanned his own career with the Department of Human Services. It has been a continuous relationship filled with successes and challenges. He is a consistent presence for this family.

Throughout the years, Don has used the model of influences to better understand Sue Ellen and her environment. The following example illustrates Don's application of the model to Sue Ellen's situation today as well as the early influences in her life.

SUE ELLEN DRAPER: THE INDIVIDUAL
- Sue Ellen is of childbearing age, slender, and attractive.
- She is a confident homemaker.
- She lacks assurance to work outside the home.
- She is able to think through difficult issues.
- She excels at accounting tasks.
- She is willing to share her skills.
- She has mechanical aptitude and ability.
- She lives in poverty.

According to Don Regalis, Sue Ellen's primary environment includes her family, neighborhood, school, and her physical environment.

SUE ELLEN DRAPER: THE PRIMARY INFLUENCES
- Sue Ellen was the youngest in the family and the only girl.
- Sue Ellen's mother focused on her to the exclusion of her brothers.
- She grew up without a father.

- She learned from her family that school was not important.
- She learned that the role of mother and homemaker was important.
- The home she lived in was small.

The larger environment in which Sue Ellen lived also affected her development. Don Regalis believes that the culture of her rural environment has had its influence.

SUE ELLEN DRAPER: THE SECONDARY INFLUENCES

- There were strong influences of neighborhood and school, which is where Sue Ellen spent a majority of her time.
- Sarah McCall's work (washing) and gregarious nature established interactions with many of the neighbors.
- Sarah McCall had multiple interactions with her neighbors since she both worked for and socialized with them.
- Sue Ellen had an active interaction within her neighborhood, helping with her mother's small business, spending coffee times in their kitchen, and providing meals and recreation space for neighborhood children, and large group summer play.
- School has the "feel" of the neighborhood.
- Teachers continually associate Sue Ellen with her five older brothers. Many are also acquainted with her mother.
- One math teacher, in particular, has been especially encouraging to Sue Ellen and two of her brothers.

Don Regalis believes that the international or global environment are more strongly influencing their community; Sue Ellen or any of her peers in this small rural county feel the impact. This knowledge helps him organize his thoughts about Sue Ellen and understand her and the pressures she experiences, and gives him ideas about her strengths. With this understanding he can better support her in the helping process.

SUE ELLEN DRAPER: THE TERTIARY INFLUENCES

- The television has always been an important part of Sue Ellen's life. She currently has a satellite dish and receives 245 channels.
- Sue Ellen has begun to lock the doors of her home and car. The increasing incidences of violence portrayed on television and at the movies has frightened her.
- One Hispanic family has moved in across the street from Sue Ellen. They do not speak English. They were brought to the community by a local church.
- Two of Sue Ellen's brothers have moved to New York City. When they return home, they describe their lives in terms that she does not understand.
- Her husband, Phil, has recently lost his job. The local mill closed because the cost of labor was too expensive.

By using the model of influences, Don Regalis is able to articulate environmental influences and to use them to work with Sue Ellen and her family.

Model of Influences: The Human Service Environment

Just as it is important for human service professionals to understand the major environmental influences for their clients, it is equally important that they know the environment of human service delivery. The model of influences, used to describe the environment of the human service professional, is shown in Figure 8-4. Similar to the model used to describe influences that impact the individual, this model represents the primary, secondary, and tertiary influences within the human service delivery system upon the human service professional.

Human service professional   The human service professional is defined by his or her attitudes, knowledge, and skills. Attitudes are represented by philosophy of helping, respect for others, self-concept and confidence as a helper, and personal and professional values such as respect for self-determination, tolerance, acceptance, and confidentiality. Knowledge includes an understanding of human behavior, the environment, familiarity with client populations, relevant methodologies of helping, and an understanding of the human service delivery system. Skills include the ability to communicate orally and in writing, the capacity to develop trust between client and helper, the competence to actively listen to clients and others, the capability to critically think and problem solve, and the ability to respond effectively in a crisis situation.

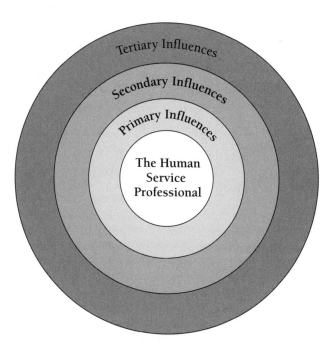

Figure 8-4   ✦   Model of environmental influences

Primary influences   The primary influences include the other professionals within the agency or organization within which the helper works, the philosophy, mission and goals of that agency, its rules and regulations, its financial goals and support, and its day-to-day activities. It also includes the physical environment of the agency, as well as the physical world that encompasses the work of the agency including modes of travel, amount of travel, and destinations.

Secondary influences   Expanding beyond the home agency, the secondary influences include organizations with which the helper has continuous or important contact. The philosophy, mission, and goals of these organizations are important. Secondary influences also include the services that the agencies provide, eligibility for these services, location, and willingness to cooperate. Included in the secondary environment are other important institutions that help shape the culture within which the professional works. These include the state, county, and local government, the financial institutions, and influential business and social organizations.

The interactions among the agencies is also a part of this secondary environment. These interactions can include communication that occurs between the members of different boards of directors at a formal town meeting, the communication between agency managers, or the day-to-day communication between frontline workers. The culture of helping within the community is also influential; for example, is there a stigma associated with poverty, welfare, substance abuse, or other human needs?

Tertiary influences   The global- and international-level influences include worldwide agendas such as "The Year of the Child" and "Healthy People 2000," which provide guidance and justification for support of special populations or areas of service. Budgeting is also influenced at the global level as the economies of our global partners have a direct bearing upon the U.S. economy. Many agencies have an international focus and their own goals and objectives are impacted by the needs as they are viewed globally. Many crisis intervention efforts focus on responding to needs created by national disasters both at home and abroad (see Table 8-3).

To view this model in action, we return to Don Regalis, the human service professional who has worked and lived in a small, rural town his entire life. When asked to use this model to describe his work environment, he wrote the following:

DON REGALIS: THE PROFESSIONAL
- I have worked in social services for the last 25 years.
- I believe that my job is to assess clients and help them "do what they want to do."
- I was educated at a college four hours away from home. This was the only time that I lived away from my community.
- The strongest value that I hold is the right of clients to determine their own goals. I believe that, at times, I do not push my clients as hard as perhaps I should.

TABLE 8-3   ✦   SUMMARY POINTS: A MODEL OF INFLUENCES

- Location, friends and family, group interaction, and activities all influence the client.
- Types of agencies, mission and goals of service delivery, populations served, and needs addressed all influence the human service professional.
- A common diagram to describe influences on both client and professional is the circle or oval.
- Individual influences include biological, psychological, and sociological aspects.
- Primary influences include the immediate and earliest influences such as family, school peers, teachers, child care workers, social environments.
- Secondary influences include the neighborhood, social organizations, and faith-based organizations.
- Tertiary influences include international or global changes.
- The human service professional is defined by attitudes, knowledge, and skills.
- Primary influences include other professionals, philosophy, mission and goals of the agency, and day-to-day activities.
- Secondary influences expand beyond the home agency.
- Tertiary influences include global and international influences including worldwide agendas.

- I know well the environment in which my clients live since I have been a member of this rural community my entire life.
- I do not have an opportunity to listen as much as I would like since my client load is so large.

The working world of Don Regalis has changed through the years, even though it seems to him his clients and their needs have remained fairly stable. He describes his primary work environment.

DON REGALIS: THE PRIMARY INFLUENCES
- I work for the Department of Human Services.
- This department is multifocused, primarily working with children and families.
- Eight people work for this office which serves one county and regions of the four surrounding counties.
- I spend two days away from the primary office visiting clients who live in the rural outlying counties.
- Each professional serves clients in at least three of the six programs that they offer.
- The goals of the agency are established by the state. The mission is to serve families and children of their service area.
- Eligibility for services becomes a problem for many of those in need in the service area, because the standards are not set locally.
- The staff operate with a cooperative spirit. Seven of the eight workers were raised in the local area.

Secondary influences are important to consider in Don's work. Since the services are so limited and the town and county so sparsely population, cooperation and communication is critical. Don provides the following information.

DON REGALIS: THE SECONDARY INFLUENCES
- Both government and nonprofit agencies serve the county.
- Several years ago I was on a steering committee that formed to coordinate services within the local area.
- The steering committee now has representatives from each organization within the town and the surrounding rural areas. Moreover, the meeting is open and professionals and local citizens are encouraged to attend. Many times most of the town comes out.
- The steering committee agenda alternates from month to month. In the first month, cooperative programming and goal setting is established. In the second month, agencies and organizations share information about agency goals and challenges. In the third month, the agenda returns to planning; and in the fourth month, the agenda is sharing information. This continues throughout the year.
- The state governance of the Children and Family Services organization requires adherence to policies and procedures that do not work well for the rural communities. I am frustrated by this situation.
- The churches in the area play a major role in providing services.
- Referrals are difficult to make because the services are so limited in this area.

The tertiary influences are more strongly felt in this rural community than ever before. Don Regalis is frustrated because this often means a loss of local control and an erosion of local values.

DON REGALIS: THE TERTIARY INFLUENCES
- Two local mills have closed in the past two years resulting in unemployment of 85 men and 65 women in the community. This means that there are fewer welfare-to-work opportunities for my clients.
- The school board conveyed a special session to discuss this violence in the school issue. Child and Family Services is trying to determine how to meet the needs of the community with regard to violence.
- Many of the students are preparing to apply to the local community college. Some parents are leery of this new focus on education.
- The newly arrived Hispanic family has visited the agency. I have not been able to offer them the services that they need.

Now that we have seen three ways in which to understand the environments of the client and the human service delivery system, it is important to focus on how the system works so it can be used effectively. Issues such as utilizing available services, understanding formal and informal networks, performing the gatekeeper role, developing services in response to community needs, and managing change are explored.

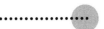 ## Using Available Services

An important part of the human service professional's responsibility is to work within the larger context of the human service delivery system and the client's environment. To facilitate this work, the professional will benefit from an understanding of the referral process and related issues. Again, applying general systems theory and the model of influences is helpful here. Referral relates directly to the interaction between the human service professional and the environment by making use of the human service network during the referral process. Thus, the helper, in seeking services for a client, facilitates the input into the human service delivery system by calling colleagues and other agencies to find the needed services, negotiating introductions and meeting times, and establishing the groundwork for the client to visit another agency. A successful referral results in the delivery of the services needed (transformation) and ends with an exit from the system. The referral process is described in this section. The primary, secondary, and tertiary influences also impact the referral process. The nature of and relationships between the agencies and the professionals within agencies contribute to the success of the referral.

Referral

One of the most important roles of a human service professional is brokering, or referring a client to another agency or service. The actual referral involves a two-step process: (1) assessing the client's problems and needs, and (2) providing the link between the client and the needed service. To understand the process of referral, the worker must know when to refer, how to refer, where to refer, and how to develop the referral. Successful brokering requires considerable time and skill. According to Crimando and Riggar (1996), effective referral is dependent on two factors: expectations and cooperation. The human service professional and the client need to understand the services that are provided by the agency or the worker who is receiving the referral. Cooperation is another key ingredient to an effective referral. All the helpers involved must keep the client's needs as the primary focus. If difficulties arise, they need to remember that the goal is to serve the client well.

To make a successful referral, the helper must have information about a service or agency. This includes its history, possible legislation that affects it, its purpose or intent, and the specific client services it provides (Crimando & Riggar, 1996). In addition, to be considered a community resource, the agency must meet the following criteria (Crimando & Riggar, 1996):

- Be able to provide the needed service
- Be willing to provide these services on referral
- Be accessible geographically
- Have reasonable eligibility standards

In other words, if the services exist but are not readily available to your clients, the agency is not a good referral source.

WHEN TO REFER

A human service professional may send a client to another professional for several reasons. The referral may be client initiated—that is, the client may request a referral. The client may realize that other services would be helpful and thus suggests a specific referral. The client may request that the referral come from the worker in order to give the client more credibility with the new service, speed up the response, or both. In another case, the client may have come to the helper in the first place specifically to ask for help in working with other agencies.

Referral may also be appropriate because the helper is not able to provide the assistance necessary to solve the client's problems. The client may present requests or have problems that the worker cannot solve, or the worker may discover that the client has a major problem that must be addressed before the others can be solved and that requires more specialized assistance than the worker can provide. Another reason for referral is that the client may be in serious psychological distress—suicidal or violent—and require intensive therapy or crisis intervention that the worker cannot provide in the human services setting. The helper may also decide to refer the client because of lack of success with that particular client; a new professional would perhaps be more effective.

HOW TO REFER

Once the helper has decided that the client needs to be referred, the complex process of referral begins. A key word in the referral process is *communication.* The following four-step process provides guidelines for linking the client with another service.

1. *Explain.* The client needs to understand why the referral is taking place. Even if the client initiates the referral, the client must understand that he or she is not just being passed on to the next human service professional. Referral is a thoughtful activity, initiated for the good of the client.
2. *Describe the services.* The client needs to be informed about the referral agency and its services. The more information the worker can give about the intake process, the services available, the fee structure, and the professionals in the agency, the more comfortable the client will be in making the initial contact.
3. *Know the contact.* Talk to the agency and get the name of the contact person, the telephone number, the address, and directions to the agency. Help the client make the appointment for the initial visit to the agency.
4. *Transmit information.* Send appropriate information about the client to the new service, always considering what that agency needs to know about the client. This will allow the agency to plan. Sometimes information can be sent electronically which speeds up the flow of information.

WHERE TO REFER

To determine where to refer the client, the human service professional must first identify the client's problems. Then the worker must find services to

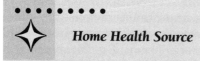

Home Health Source

Home health services are rapidly changing in the managed care environment and there are increasing demands for these services. They are one example of the emerging community-based care that is now preferred over institutional care as a method of service delivery. Home health care can be provided in homes now because of the advanced technology that allows high-quality care outside the hospital setting.

HISTORY/LEGISLATION

The roots of home health care services are in the late 1800s in New York City. The New York City Mission hired nurses to provide medical care and religious services and to teach health and sanitation to the poor. Later, the Metropolitan Life Insurance Company offered these services to their clients; and in the 1940s, Montefiore Hospital in New York City provided holistic home health care. Medicare mandated home health care, and Medicaid, allows minimum home health care to be a part of state plans.

LICENSURE, CERTIFICATION, AND ACCREDITATION

Home health care is licensed by several organizations, such as the Joint Commission on Accreditation of Hospitals (JCAH) and the National League of Nursing (NLN).

PURPOSE/INTENT

"Home health care can be defined as all the services and products that maintain, restore, or promote physical, mental, and emotional health provided to clients in their homes. The purpose of home health care is to preserve the quality of life for the individual at home by increasing the client's level of independence and reducing the effects of existing disabilities through noninstitutional supportive services" (p. 23).

CLIENT SERVICES

    High technology services
    Client or family care services
    Personal care
    Standard health services
    Advanced physician, dental, and pharmaceutical services
    Hospice care

SOURCE: Adapted from "Home Health Services," by Beverly E. Holland, 1996, in W. Crimando and T. F. Riggar (Eds.), *Utilizing Community Resources: An Overview of Human Services*, pp. 21–28. Boca Raton, Florida: St. Lucie.

meet those needs. The worker may use services that are already known or may investigate other possibilities. Both formal and informal networks (described later) are useful in determining what services are available and appropriate to meet the client's needs.

Home health services, a popular alternative today to hospitalization, depends on its referral resources. The goal of these services is increasing client independence and minimizing the limitations of illness or disability. In many cases, this means knowing where needed services and products can be located. Home Health Source, described here, is an example of this community-based service.

EVALUATING THE REFERRAL

The referral process does not end once the referral has been made; it continues with systematic follow-up. The helper can call the agency to learn whether the client has kept the appointment, and can call the client to get the client's evaluation of the service. The worker needs to know whether the service was effective and whether the help received matched the worker's assessment of the problem. Such follow-up can be very time-consuming for the helper but will be valuable not only for this client but for others in the future. It is especially good feedback for the professional and increases the client's faith in the system. The follow-up also reinforces the professional's care for and commitment to the client.

Making referrals is difficult for several reasons. Agencies are constantly changing, and maintaining an accurate picture of an agency, its current staff, and the services it provides is difficult. Sometimes services are not designed to meet the exact needs of the client, and the referring worker cannot guarantee treatment to the client. Each agency must independently assess the client's needs and the agency's ability to meet those needs. The service may not be provided because the client does not meet the eligibility criteria, because the services needed may not exist, or because there is a waiting list for assistance. The agency may not cooperate fully with the referring agency in the referral process or the follow-up. Many agencies also are so understaffed that they simply do not have the staff to provide follow-up (see Table 8-4).

TABLE 8-4 ◆ SUMMARY POINTS: REFERRALS

- The agency to which the client is referred must be able and willing to provide the service, be accessible geographically, and have reasonable eligibility criteria.
- A referral may be appropriate when the professional cannot provide the needed service or when the professional believes another helper might be more effective.
- When referring, the helper explains the purpose of the referral, describes the services, talks with the agency to identify a contact person, and sends appropriate client information to the agency receiving the referral.
- It is necessary to identify the client's problem prior to deciding where to refer.
- Follow-up to evaluate the success of the referral completes the referral process.

Building an Information Network

To make successful referrals, the human service professional must make effective use of all human service agencies in a community. First, the helper must know what services are available. The beginning professional is at a particular disadvantage because of a lack of experience in the system, a lack of personal contacts with other professionals in the system, and a lack of knowledge about the many problems that clients may have. Therefore, the helper must develop a systematic way of building a file of information about the human service network for referral purposes. The worker must first decide how to categorize the information to be gathered. Whether services are being organized by the physical, social, and emotional needs of the clients, the specific populations served, or one of the other organizational frameworks mentioned, the categories will help the worker think about how services are delivered in the community.

The helper can then begin to collect information and record it using computer software, a card file, a file box, a loose-leaf notebook, or any other storage device that allows for easy additions and revisions. In reality the helper is building a database. The summary information needed includes a description of the agency or service, the types of clients it serves, the payment required for the service, the phone number and address, the e-mail address, the URL for websites, and a contact person. The human service professional may collect information about community services from colleagues, clients, handbooks of agencies, newspapers, professional meetings, the phone book, the Web, and any community service directories produced by other agencies. The internet has increased the access to information about other agencies; and e-mail and shared databases have facilitated communication between agencies.

Knowing more detailed information about each agency is helpful, including the purpose of the agency, eligibility requirements for services, location and hours of operation, organizational patterns of staffing, and the nature of the agency funding. Prior to using an agency for referral, a human service professional should know what services it provides, to whom they are provided (individuals or families), whether it uses case management services, and whether it has a good record as a client advocate. Other helpful information includes the qualifications of the staff, their caseload, and their experience with specific populations. The human service professional will have better knowledge of the agency after visiting the facility to determine its accessibility and its psychological and physical environment. Also critical is knowing how the agency receives referrals, if there is a waiting list, how long a client must wait for services, and what follow-up procedure is used to inform the referring agency of the disposition of the referred client's case (Crimando & Riggar, 1996). All this requires a detailed understanding of the organization and represents quite a bit of information to gather, but once you have this information, updates it can be done with relative ease.

Understanding that creating the file is only one part of building a network, the worker should also begin to make personal contacts with other human service professionals. The worker should then try to establish communication as a cooperative effort—sharing information with other agencies, following up on referrals, and providing feedback to other agencies that have made referrals. These efforts will begin to build the new helper's credibility as a serious professional interested in building and maintaining networks among agencies.

Network building takes time, but it makes the referral process more effective. The better the worker knows the services available, the more appropriate the referrals will be. A network is difficult to maintain: It is a never-ending project, no matter how long the human service professional has been serving the community, because agencies are constantly in flux.

Knowing the Formal and Informal Networks

According to *Webster's New World Dictionary of the American Language,* a network is "a fabric or structure of threads, cords, or wires that cross each other at regular intervals and are knotted or secured at the crossings" (1986, p. 1520). In human service settings, the fabric of the system is formed by the elaborate channels of communication among the agencies and the workers. The securing takes place when both parties confirm that they wish to communicate, engage in two-way communication, and establish channels of communication. Human service delivery is a complex system containing two networks of communication: the formal and the informal. Both must be mastered if professionals are to participate fully in the system.

The formal network consists of organizations such as public and private human service agencies, self-help groups, schools, churches, businesses, and federal, state, and local government agencies. To understand this network, the worker must discover the answers to certain questions: What are the politics of these organizations? Who bears the major responsibilities within each? What are the formal ways to "hook up" the client to the services and resources available?

Beyond the formal network is a valuable informal network that is more difficult to recognize. It is not described in agency policy, formal reporting, or organizational diagrams. It is determined by an established history of agencies working together, personal friendships among workers, and political pressures, and it is maintained by mutual satisfaction and support. The informal network may also include informal helpers such as family and friends who provide needed support. Understanding this informal network is difficult, and accessing it takes time and effort.

There are three types of formal and informal networks: personal, professional, and organizational networks. Personal networks consist of individuals, families, and groups of people who are part of the helper's family or part of his or her social support. Individuals in this context often know the helper very well and can also reach out to a variety of others who can help in the referral process, including people in church, social clubs, and exercise and other activity-based environments. Professional and organizational networks consist of individuals with whom you work and include colleagues, teachers, and supervisors. Networking with these individuals can help reduce duplication and fragmentation of services and eliminate service gaps.

One example of formal and informal networks that human service professionals find in the client population is in the description of service needs and support networks of members of the Prairie Band Potawatomi elders (John, 1986). This elderly population, which lives in a Native American reservation community, has housing, transportation, employment, income, health, medical, social, and recreational needs. Both formal and informal networks play major roles in meeting those needs. The elderly depend on the professionals in the formal network for financial and medical support, but individuals within the informal network provide services in all the areas mentioned. Children most often assume the care of the elders, especially during times of illness, death, or divorce. Siblings and other family members also play a supporting role.

A human service worker who wants to help the elderly in this Native American population would need in-depth knowledge of the two networks. A special knowledge of the informal system allows the worker to build on the services that are already present rather than duplicate or attempt to replace them with formal services. The worker may learn about the special relationships between helpers in the informal and the formal networks by asking the following questions: What formal services are available? How do the informal and formal systems communicate? Who are the key individuals in both networks who provide services effectively or who assist the elderly in accessing the services?

Promoting Change in a Dynamic World

One continuous theme throughout this text is that the world is changing rapidly. We are experiencing the globalization of the economy, increased immigration, the development of new technologies, and the emergence of new methodologies to approach the problems in this third millennium. For a human service professional to be effective with and responsive to clients and knowledgeable of and sensitive to community needs, it is increasingly important to function as a change agent. Becoming involved in change is often difficult for the beginning professional. This section will present three contexts in which professionals can promote change. The first is within the arena of the local community, becoming involved in developing specific services in response to community needs. The second is also within the context of the community, initiating and participating in community organizing. The focus on this type of change occurs with the development of a new vision or a new focus for the community. Community organizing occurs when the development of a coalition of individuals and communities is powerful enough to continue to create and promote change. The third approach centers around the empowerment of a specific population previously with little status or power. The empowerment occurs once the population is identified and a team of professionals and other interested individuals work with that population to build the skills that allow them to advocate for themselves and facilitate their own change. A description and examples of each of these three approaches follow.

Developing Services in Response to Human Needs

In developing, maintaining, and reevaluating human service delivery, a primary consideration is the response to community needs. The community has a dual role in the causation and resolution of client problems. On one hand, the community is a source of client problems. On the other hand, it provides many of the resources needed for resolving problems. A housing project in New Zealand for older Maori people, called Kaumathua housing, illustrates a community need and its resolution. Two issues, advocacy for nonexistent services and planning based on community needs, were probably integral to its success. These two activities are discussed next.

Advocating the establishment of services that are nonexistent is one of the most difficult responsibilities of the human service professional. The advocate is one who speaks up for the rights of others and defends those who cannot defend themselves. When helpers discover that their clients have needs that cannot be met through the human service delivery system, they have a responsibility to work with others to develop alternative ways of meeting those needs. To do so requires skills that incorporate working with the individual, agencies, and legal and legislative bodies. Regardless of the type of advocacy, the process is much the same:

- Identify the needs of the individual or the population.
- Identify how to meet the needs.
- Work with a network of individuals or agencies to provide the services.
- Identify the barriers that must be overcome.
- Teach clients about the advocacy process and give them a role.
- Negotiate to meet goals and objectives.
- Develop a framework that continues the success of the advocacy process.

Many professionals are successful in acting as advocates for their individual clients and can use their networking skills to find food where no food services exist, glasses and other special medical needs where resources are unavailable, and housing for those who temporarily need shelter. More difficult is the advocacy as an individual that involves developing a political voice for the larger issues that require community, state, or national attention. Ralph Nader lobbying for consumer protection, Maggie Kuhn championing the rights of the elderly, and Betty Ford heightening awareness of breast cancer are examples of individuals who are advocates in the community, state, and national arenas for issues of concern.

According to Moroney (1976), four types of needs should be considered when services are being developed. The first is the *informative* need—what

INTERNATIONAL FOCUS
Kaumathua Housing: A Special Housing Scheme for Older Maori People

In New Zealand there is an effort to address the problems of the aging population. Their focus has been on developing community-based care with a special emphasis on providing quality services and empowering the elderly. Much attention has been given to developing services that make sense according to the culture of the elderly populations instead of developing a program nationwide that must fit everyone. Government policy has been to support care of the elderly with the family or religious, voluntary, and community groups. The housing needs of the aging Maori population have been addressed with the following program:

> The Maori population has historically been a youthful population characterized by high fertility and high mortality. During the 1920s and 1930s about half the Maori populations were children under fifteen years of age. Since 1971 there has been a marked decrease in fertility so that by 1986 under 40% of the Maori populations were in this age group. What has received less attention are the changes which are taking place in terms of ageing. In 1986 Maori comprised 4% of those over sixty years of age and only just over 2% of those aged over sixty-five years, compared with 12.4% of the total population being Maori . . . beneath these figures however is a pattern of rapid increase in the numbers of Maori surviving into old age. Between 1986 and 1991 the number of Maori aged sixty to seventy-four increased by over a fifth and between 1981, 1986, and 1991 the number aged seventy-five and over increased by over 50% in each census period . . .
>
> The building of blocks of housing for older Maori people began in the late 1960s through a Special Maori Housing Fund administered by the Department of Maori and Island Affairs. The siting of this housing was focused around the *marae* (meeting house). This allowed some elderly Maori to remain in their home communities and be close to the focus of communal life on the *marae*. Another group for whom the scheme was attractive were those who had moved into urban areas and now wished to spend their old age back in their original tribal communities. Legislation was passed to allow Maori land to be gifted to the Crown for this kind of housing and to allow Maori trusts and incorporations to play a part in such development. The programme became formally referred to as "kaumathua housing." (pp. 179–180)

SOURCE: From "New Zealand and Community Care for Older People: A Demographic Window of Opportunity," by S. Uttley, 1995, in T. Scharf and G. C. Wengar, *International Perspectives on Community Care for Older People,* pp. 171–189. Brookfield, Vermont: Avebury.

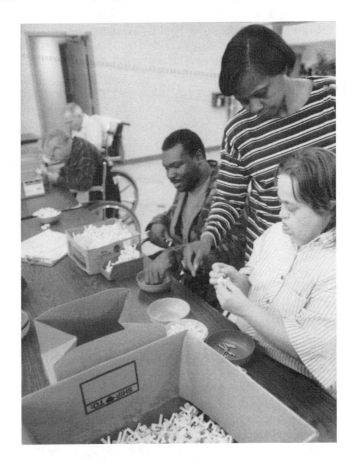

professionals and experts in the human service field have determined is necessary for effective service delivery. Professionals usually make this determination after study of and experience with the problem. The second kind is the *perceived* or *expressed* need—what the community itself defines as the services that would best serve it. Third, the expressed need of the *individuals* seeking the services is also important to consider; they may have opinions very different from those of the experts or the community at large. Fourth, *relative need*—the difference between what the community could use and what it already has available—is also important to consider. Often in planning service delivery, some services are already available. How the new services fit into the network of the existing services is an important question for planners to answer when building an effective service network.

It is important to consider all four types of needs so that planning can occur within the context of the environment. One principle to follow in developing services was proposed by Kreitner (1983): The development of services should follow the guidelines of Maslow's hierarchy, with services to meet basic needs developed first (see Chapter 5). If basic service needs go unmet, other services will not succeed. Following Maslow's hierarchy, physical needs must receive attention first, before planning for safety and security needs takes place. The needs assessment for the elderly described in Table 8-5 is based on Maslow's hierarchy.

A critical component in developing services is knowing both the needs and the characteristics of the populations in need. The following case study illustrates the importance of being able to identify the problems and develop programs that address those specific problems when planning for services (Butterfield, 1996).

In 1996, the city of Boston recorded a substantial drop in homicide rates. Researchers believe that this progress in reducing deaths by violence is attributed to a new cooperative arrangement between the juvenile court and the criminal justice system, two systems that do not usually work together. Two critical needs were identified prior to the program's implementation with the discovery that three-quarters of juvenile killers and victims had been involved with gangs. These were repeat offenders with established criminal records. Specifically, 75% of killers and victims had been to court at least once. Half these youths had been on probation before and one-third of them had been previously incarcerated. In addition, firearms dealers were selling guns to these juveniles. The central concepts that support the new program were these: letting probation officers ride in patrol cars, and reducing the number of firearms sold to youth (Butterfield, 1996).

The first program allowed the probation officer to arrest youths who had broken parole by violating their 8 P.M. curfew. The beginning of the experiment paired Bill Stewart, a probation officer, with city detective Robert Fratalia. The first night they worked together they received a call that a boy had been shot. When they arrived at the scene, Mr. Stewart discovered that the victim was on his caseload, he also saw 35 other youths who were on probation and violating curfew.

The benefits to the probation system are numerous with this new partnership. Many probation officers see their work as worthless, for there is a revolving door in the criminal justice system; it allows many of their clients to go free and later commit other crimes. They also have difficulty enforcing the rules of probation because they do not carry guns themselves and cannot safely arrest their clients for breaking parole or curfew. The police also benefit from this new arrangement. They are armed and have the power to arrest, but they do not know all the youths on probation so they cannot identify those who are breaking curfew. Because these youths are on probation, they can be incarcerated without a new trial and parole officers do not need probable cause to talk with them or to visit them in their homes. Since this program was implemented, the number of youths arrested for breaking curfew has tripled and compliance with conditions of probation has risen from 15% to 70% (Butterfield, 1996).

The second program focused on reducing arms sales. Several strategies were used. City officials made clear that they have zero tolerance for guns, and

TABLE 8-5 ✦ COMMUNITY SERVICE IDENTIFICATION USING THE
IDENTIFICATION OF NEEDS

WIDOWS AGED 85+ LIVING ALONE IN WEST KINGSTON

Type of need	Services typically designed to meet need	Services available in this community
Self-actualization needs	Education programs Volunteer opportunities	Available at Kingston Senior Center
Esteem needs	Support groups Psychosocial counseling Mental health centers	Two support groups Mental health center has limited services
Social needs	Recreational and social Groups Senior centers Home visitors	One senior center
Safety and security needs	Emergency response system Adult family homes Congregate care facilities Senior housing Continuing care retirement Communities Wellness clinics Telephone contact	No emergency system Three unlicensed homes One congregate facility No senior housing No retirement community Public health department has wellness clinic Church runs telephone Reassurance program
Survival needs	Home delivered meals Senior discounts Mobile meals Transportation Homemaker Home health Personal care Medical care	Limited delivered meals program Twenty mobile meals slots No bus system, one senior van available One licensed homemaker program No home health provider Two licensed personal care agencies One community hospital and one nursing home

SOURCE: From *Social Work Macro Practice*, Second Edition, by F. E. Netting, P. M. Kettner, and S. L. McMurtry, p. 164. Copyright (c) 1998 Allyn & Bacon. Reprinted by permission.

they called in gang members to talk to them about the tougher policies. These meetings included representatives from the United States District Attorney's office; the county District Attorney's office; the Federal Bureau of Alcohol, Tobacco and Firearms; and the state Department of Probation and Division of Youth Services. Also attending were school police and city employees who work with gangs. One major arrest was made of 23 gang members who refused to heed the warnings.

Boston has not had a single juvenile death since July 1995. This statistic speaks to the success of providing services based on identified needs and target population. It is also a good example of human service professionals working together to develop services in response to community needs.

Suppose you are a human service professional planning services to reduce youth-related violence in your city or rural area. What needs must be considered? How would you discover what those needs are? What problems might you anticipate in implementing new programs in the community? What actions might you take to ensure successful planning and implementation?

In answering these questions, you may realize how difficult planning is. Your responses should consider a variety of viewpoints and take into consideration how the services fit within the context of the current environment.

Organizing to Promote Community Change

Promoting community change relies on the development and use of a network or larger confederation to advance the cause, mobilize individuals and agencies in the community, and create a financial resource base and a willing workforce of professionals and volunteers. Although promoting community change is a broader activity than just creating services, the change that you want to create must be defined; and numerous issues could benefit from the effort and focus. Read any national or local newspaper, listen to conversations between friends, tape dialogues in a teacher's lounge, or monitor the exchanges in a human service agency and organization lounge. In all of these settings you will hear numerous issues being raised. Unfortunately, most of these communications end with frustration, hopelessness, some humor, but no hope for action. The difficulties seem too challenging to overcome.

Community organizing can be effective when there is an awareness of issues. In fact, community organizing is based on the principle of like-minded people joining together to promote change (Green Ontario, 2000). Important concepts that are foundation principles of community organizing are as follows:

- Individuals and organizations identify a common goal.
- Like-minded individuals and organizations consolidate themselves to have a more effective voice in the community.
- All individual members of the community are welcome to participate in the effort including politicians, business leaders, citizens, and others.
- Organizations and agencies are welcome to form a network of the concerned. This network includes schools, financial institutions, social service organizations, political organizations, nonprofit organizations, and others.
- The combined efforts of many voices has the power to facilitate change.
- Basic to the work is organizing as a team and gathering information to understand the community and its needs.
- Basic to the work is developing an action plan.

TABLE 8-6 ✦ SUMMARY POINTS: PROMOTING CHANGE

- Promoting change is an important role for the human service professional.
- One way of supporting change is to develop services in response to community needs including establishing services that are nonexistent.
- The process to promote change involves identifying needs, deciding how needs can best be met, working with a network of individuals or agencies to provide services, identifying barriers that must be overcome, and teaching clients the advocacy process.
- Negotiating the meeting of goals and objectives and developing plans for future services are also part of the process.
- Community involvement to promote change uses a confederation of individuals and organizations committed to the same cause.
- One model of client empowerment focuses almost entirely on supporting clients to develop their own agenda, support structure, plan for change and evaluation, and the recruitment of new members.

The process of community action begins with a community action plan (CAP). The Presidents' Summit for America's Future prepared material that outlines the steps in developing a community action plan (Iowa Summit America's Promise . . . Iowa Style, 2000). It is during the development of this plan that the concerned coalition answers the question, "How will this initiative be carried out?" To answer that question fully, the following questions adapted from the Iowa Summit America's Promise . . . Iowa Style, 2000 Work Pages, must be addressed:

- What will be community effort focus?
- Where can we find the resources we need?
- What knowledge and skills do we need to support our effort?
- What offices, technology, and equipment do we need?
- How will we gather support?
- What are the benefits of being in this coalition?
- How do we promote ourselves?

The CAP will address these questions, develop a plan of action, make assignments, and create a time line to ensure that the plan will be implemented.

The development of the CAP focuses on meeting the goals and objectives. It begins to bring people together to talk about issues. For the first time, individuals from every corner of the community are talking together. The action plan becomes the forum for the conversation; a strong community network is being built. Not all conversation has to occur when individuals are meeting together. There are new models of community organizing that use technology to bring people together to discuss major issues and develop CAPs. Numerous training packets, similar to the one created by Community Action Program for Children (http://www.opc.on.ca/CAP/index.html), are available on the internet. These programs are developed to teach organizers how to effectively use technology to allow individuals in remote areas to participate in the community action process.

The following is an example of a community organizing effort within the Baltimore community whose goal was to improve the health and safety of children. Individuals and organizations joined together to form "Safe and Sound," focusing on enhancing services and providing equal access to services for all of Baltimore's children (Safe and Sound, 2000). Baltimore received a planning grant from the Robert Woodruff Foundation in 1994 and spent two years planning this community effort. The result was an action plan spotlighting the areas of family support, after-school programs, literacy, gun homicide, and community promises. Strategies concentrated on efforts that make involvement of Safe and Sound very much a public process.

One area of focus for Safe and Sound is family support, defined by this group as "providing a network of services to increase self-sufficiency of families with young children" (Safe and Sound, 2000). To date, the success of the Safe and Sound efforts has been measured by school performance, socioeconomic status, percentage of low birth weights, and other factors. A report issued in December 1999 stated that coordinated human services delivery plans had been developed to "provide family support to five Baltimore communities," and services to families of children age 0 to 6 had already increased (Safe and Sound, 2000).

In summary, work within the community to promote change is an important part of the human service professional's responsibility. It can be a rewarding way to improve client environments and services and can expand the helper's network to include many individuals and organizations outside the human service sector (see Table 8-6).

Using a Model of Client Empowerment

Throughout this text we have discussed the importance of both advocacy for the client and empowerment of the client. Using a model of client empowerment is another approach to facilitating change, a model that is commonly used in many developing countries. The primary goal of this model is to ultimately place the advocacy and empowerment in the hands and voices of the clients or those in need. The basic thrust of this model is to educate and train those in need to organize, establish their agenda, and work for their own cause by organizing campaigns, networking with government and business leaders, proposing legislation, and participating in the political, economic, and social processes of the community (Gordon, 2000; Woodside & McClam, 1998). How does an effort like this begin?

One such example is the Workplace Project, a worker center located in Long Island, New York (Gordon, 2000). The project, organized to address immigrant labor issues, founded by Jennifer Gordon, began its work in 1992. Over

● ● ● ● ● ● ● ● ●

 INTERNATIONAL FOCUS
The Council on the Ageing (Western Australia) Incorporated

ACTIVITY

The Council on the Ageing of Western Australia (COTA) was established in 1959, out of concerns for the ageing population in this state, and the associated needs and problems of seniors. The Council is a "peak" advocacy body, addressing issues confronting seniors living in the community. The COTA seeks to protect and promote the well-being of all older people through the improvement of policy and programs for seniors, through information, advice, and referral, along with general community education about all aspects of ageing. COTA is connected to the National Council on the Ageing based in Melbourne, which seeks to provide "the voice of older Australians" to the federal government in Canberra. The Council in Western Australia is staffed almost entirely by volunteer effort, though it has sometimes received a measure of governmental funding over the years.

HISTORY

In the four decades since its inception the Council has pioneered many initiatives, some of which have been subsequently mimicked by more formal governmental programs. In 1961, for example, the Council established a volunteer-based "Golden Age Visiting Service" to address the needs of frail and lonely older people, a program which is mirrored in recent federal and state activities. In the same year the Council invented "Old People's Week," which was the forerunner of the modern "Seniors' Week" promoting positive images of ageing, and organized by the State government now for over a decade. In 1974 the Council established the "Residential Aged Care Association," now relabelled as Aged Care Australia, which looks after the interests of those frail or sick seniors living in residential care facilities. In the same year the Council launched its "Guide to Services for Older People in WA," which in its many revised editions has been an invaluable resource for seniors and for those working with seniors in this state. In 1992 the Council conducted extensive consultations with Aboriginal and Ethnic elders in outback and metropolitan regions, and integrated this feedback into recommendations for the State Strategy on Ageing, which was designed to address seniors' issues into the twenty-first century. In the same year the Council also initiated and sponsored the now independently incorporated Intergenerational Activity Network, which seeks to promote exchange, empathy, and understanding between the generations.

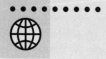

MISSION

Across the western world during the eighties and nineties, the Welfare State has been in retreat, and Western Australia has not been immune from this trend. The non-government organizations have had increasing tasks but less resources, and in the case of the Council it is now, as it was in the beginning, almost entirely supported through voluntary effort. Nevertheless, the Council looks forward to serving seniors in the future. At its recent AGM, President Bettine Heathcote spoke of "hope," "optimism," and "progress," and noted two recent programs in evidence. First, the "Be Wise with Medicines" seminars seek to educate seniors and the community about polypharmacy and its associated dangers, and constitutes a most worthwhile project in the "community education" tradition. Second, the establishment of the "Seniors Computer Centre" trains older citizens in the ways of computers and connects them with the modern world of the "information superhighway," in this way empowering older people to participate more completely in our rapidly changing technological society.

SUMMARY

Thus in terms of its helping agenda on behalf of seniors, its history of pioneering social programs later adopted by government, and its struggle to complete its mission for its clients while doing more with less, the Council on the Ageing of Western Australia provides a useful insight into the voluntary and informal human service sector within this country.

REFERENCES

Heathcote, B. (1996). President's Report, to the AGM of the Council on the Ageing (WA) Incorporated, held on Monday, 14 October, at the Auditorium Wesley Centre, Perth.
Hooper, J. (1990). The history of WACOTA: The origins and development of the WA Council on the Ageing 1959–1988. Perth: Murdoch University.

SOURCE: Prepared by David Wiles, Ph.D., Lecturer in Human Services and Gerontology, Edith Cowan University (Joondalup, Perth), School of International, Cultural, and Community Studies, 5 December 1996.

• • • • • • • • •

WEB SOURCES
Find Out More About Community Organizing

http://uac.rdp.utoledo.edu/comm-org/

This comprehensive community organizing online site is housed at the University of Toledo. The mission of this organization is to help connect people who care about the craft of community organizing. This organization is also committed to finding and providing information that organizers, scholars, and scholar-organizers can use to learn, teach, and do community organizing.

http://www.uwm.edu:80/Library/arch/findaids/mss011.htm

This website provides a fascinating history of a community organizing effort in Milwaukee, Wisconsin, of the Eastside Housing Action Committee. The records of activities were kept from 1972 to 1978.

http://www.gamaliel.org/

This is the website of The Gamaliel Foundation, originally established in 1968 to support the Contract Buyers League, an organization in the African-American community on Chicago's West Side. The league was fighting to protect homeowners who had bought their homes on contract because financial institutions had redlined the area. In 1986, the foundation was revamped as an organizing institute, with a mission to support grassroots leaders in their efforts to build and maintain empowerment organizations in low income communities. The purpose of this website is to link those in need with community organizing resources.

http://www.communities-by-choice.org/index.html

Community organizing efforts are strong in the area of sustainable development. This organization, Communities By Choice, supports a web page that describes their efforts and invites others to work with them to support the environment.

http://www.communitychange.org/CO.htm

Community Organizing is about building power among a broad membership base—either individual or institutional—of low and very low income people. The members provide the leadership, direction, and "troops" for the organization's activities. The group's work is centered around issues chosen by the members themselves and focuses largely on subjects that affect a broad swath of very low to moderate income people.

http://www.cflsl.org/organizing.html

Community Family Life Services in Washington, D.C., is active in making changes within the environments of those in need. The CFLS Community Organizing Program develops and implements strategies for neighborhood participation and revitalization in low income sections of Washington, D.C. Working closely with the residents and housing developers in the Galveston Place and Brandywine Street neighborhoods in Ward 8, CFLS has helped residents take pride in and take charge of their communities.

400,000 Latino immigrants from El Salvador, Central and South America, Mexico, and the Caribbean live on Long Island. About 150,000 of these are undocumented. Unions do not negotiate for these workers who literally provide sweatshop services, often for as little as $1.90 an hour, with no overtime, no benefits, and payments in cash. Many workers never receive payment for the long hours of service rendered (Gordon, 2000).

This project began its work with the immigrants through a study course that prioritized learning labor law, and immigration and labor history, and organizing techniques. A small staff works with the graduates of the course, teaching them how to run the center, organize campaigns, and recruit other members. The hierarchy includes workers' committees, membership committees, and a board of directors comprised of workers.

The first goal that the Long Island Workers Committee established was to change the New York State labor law. They worked with two other centers, the Chinese Staff and Workers Association and the Latino Workers Center, to increase the fine on employers for nonpayment of wages and to make the nonpayment a felony, rather than a misdemeanor. In the early planning, the committee believed that they could win the State Assembly, but they needed strong Republican backing in the Senate to ensure passage of the proposed bills there. The Workers Committee developed a plan to canvass the five Republican delegations from Long Island at a time when anti-immigration sentiment was high and anti-immigrant legislation was pending in the state government.

The immigrants developed a political strategy, effectively used the media, gathered allies from churches and social service organizations, massed a petition campaign, and presented a convincing case to the Long Island delegates that these delegates sponsored the bill. On a personal level, since the immigrants presented their case combining personal stories with statistics and immigration history, the delegates were able to relate to them through their own families' histories of immigration. It was obvious that these workers were not looking for a free meal or free housing, rather fair treatment and fair wage in return for hard work.

This success has had its reward beyond the passage of the labor bill. Workers have begun to think of themselves as activists, able to impact the social, economic, and political process. Two have begun new workers' organizations; three have begun similar efforts in their own home countries; several have begun national immigration efforts. They have been able to promote change even though many of them are undocumented and most cannot vote.

What are the guidelines for this type of empowerment? The key is fivefold: relevant education and training; knowledge about how to turn information into action; development of a structure that supports the empowerment efforts; efforts are client run; development of an environment where organizing efforts are encouraged and continued (Gordon, 2000).

Education and training   Key to the beginning of the empowerment efforts, education and training is an ongoing process. The education must be relevant to the needs of the clients and must include information concerning the history of the problems, legal history, current laws, and the process of change.

Knowledge about how to turn information into action   This knowledge begins during the education phase and continues when the clients decide on their issues of focus. The clients are the ones who run the organizations, serve on the board of directors, and establish other centers. They become active in the political process and they serve as their own spokespersons.

Development of a structure that supports the empowerment efforts   This critical aspect of the activity ensures that individuals have a way in which to participate in the efforts. There can be a board of directors, committee staff, smaller worker committees (by neighborhoods, professions, or other relevant groupings), coordinating committees, and the like. The key here is that all participants have a place to work for the established causes.

Efforts are client run   Such efforts are important and a critical factor that distinguishes this empowerment model from others in which clients are "partners." Here the clients are the "owners" of the efforts.

Development of an environment where organizing efforts are encouraged and continued   The empowerment model is not a one-issue model. All of the education, training, and established organizational hierarchy promotes long-term commitment to activism.

Becoming involved in change is a important way that the human services professional can influence the life and the environment of the client. Where does one begin? Homan (1999) suggests the following ways to promote change:

Neighborhood empowerment—help members of the same geographical area work together to improve their surroundings.

Community problem solving—bring lots of different individuals and groups together to solve one particular problem.

Developing community support systems—helping isolated or lonely individuals to connect with each other to provide mutual support.

Community education—provide education to citizens so they understand the issues.

Developing a broad-based community organization—becoming part of a group that is active in redistributing the community resources. (Homan, 1999, pp. 21–22)

There are many ways the human service worker can become involved in change. You do not have to spearhead a movement or fight single handed for your clients. Just look around your neighborhood, city, or organization to find efforts you wish to support to ultimately improve the lives and environments of your clients.

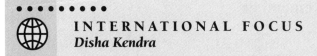

Disha Kendra was established in 1978 by Jagrut Bhaubandhi Sangatana to help village tribal people in India fight their socioeconomic and political oppression. Tribals are indigenous people who live in remote rural areas in India. Each tribe has a different culture, speaks a unique dialect, and lives according to long-standing traditions.

The first phase of the organization's work (1978–1983) focused on economic and human rights development. One example of this work was the two-year process of breaking the economic hold of the money lender on the 35-household village of Chadhawadi and substituting a six-year bank-loan program to support local farming efforts. During this initial phase, education was also enhanced with the formation of preschool and adult education programs. From 1983 to 1991—the second and third phases of the organization's history—the effort determined long- and short-term needs of the village and assessed the outcomes of past efforts. In addition, the organization promoted the tribal people's ability to lead their own political organizations as they struggled to increase the availability of water, electricity, and employment opportunities.

The fourth phase of the agency's work is underway and includes strengthening political organization and leadership training, improving community organization, and improving the lives of tribal women. The emphasis is on helping tribals help themselves. During the authors' visit to the village, the agency's political action director, Bunsi, conducted a meeting of the village committee, a group of six men from surrounding villages. Their task was to prepare for a meeting the following week with the police superintendent inspector who would rule on a land-access dispute. A wealthy Mumbai businessman had bought a large track of land near the village and was denying access to their farmland, water supply, and firewood. Bunsi asked those in attendance to decide who would speak for the committee, and he explained the hearing process. They then role-played what the spokesman would say at the hearing.

The agency workers visit the villages weekly or live in the villages themselves. They are available to help with whatever issues arise that affect the rights of tribals as a protected class of people in India.

Things to Remember

1. The activities of the human service professional do not occur in a vacuum but are performed with clients within the context of their own environments and within the context of the human service delivery system.
2. Systems theory focuses on the interaction of elements in a system, including their relationships, their structures, and their interdependence.
3. One characteristic of a system is that any change in one part affects another part.
4. The worker must be aware of the many influences on the client, and the many influences on the human service delivery system which can be represented in a diagram of systems involved.
5. There are many influences that impact the life of the client.
6. Human service delivery occurs within an environment of agency, community, and global influences.
7. One of the most important roles of a human service professional is brokering, or referring a client to another agency or service.
8. The referral process involves the worker, the client, and the other agency to which the client is referred.
9. In referral, the beginning human service professional is at a disadvantage because of a lack of experience in the system, a lack of personal contacts with workers in the system, and a lack of knowledge about the many problems that clients may have.
10. The beginning professional must develop a systematic way of building a file of information about the human services network for referral purposes.
11. Human service delivery is a complex system containing two networks of communication: the formal and the informal.
12. An important responsibility of the human service professional is to be an advocate for change.
13. In developing, maintaining, and reevaluating the delivery of human services, it is important to consider human services as a response to community needs.
14. Empowering clients to advocate for their own change is one model of responding to client needs.

Additional Readings: Focus on Organizations

Bolman, L. G., & Deal, T. E. (1997). *Reframing organizations: Artistry, choice, and leadership*. San Francisco: Jossey-Bass.
A consistent bestseller, this book offers practical ways of thinking about today's challenges.

Homan, M. S. (1999). *Rules of the game: Lessons from the field of community change*. Pacific Grove, CA: Brooks/Cole.

The author offers practical wisdom and 135 guidelines for community change as readers explore what they need to know about themselves, others, and the change process.

Keidel, R. W. (1995). *Seeing organizational patterns: A new theory and language of organizational design.* San Francisco: Berrett-Koehler.
The author explains that most organizational issues are a balance of three variables: individual autonomy, hierarchical control, and spontaneous cooperation. By learning to frame issues as trade-offs among these design variables, one becomes able to see the underlying patterns.

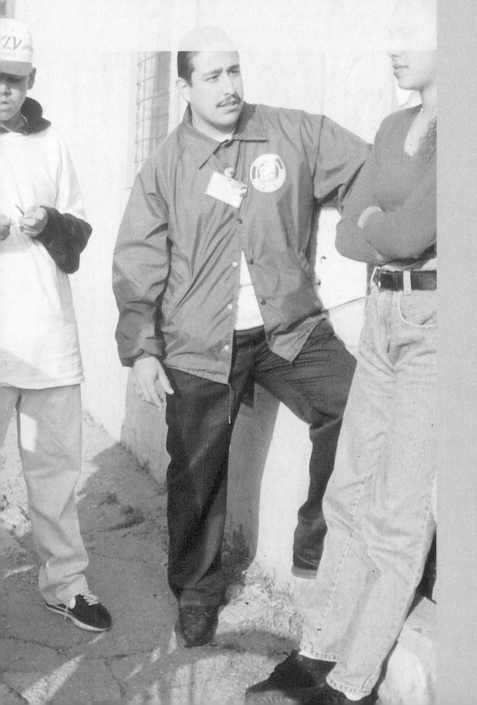

Chapter 9

Professional Concerns

This final chapter focuses on the ethics of human service practice. The helper is continually faced with ethical decisions. Sometimes these issues arise between the professional and the client and other times there are multiple individuals and even agencies with a stake in the decisions made. The helper's responsibilities are not simply to recognize an ethical situation and make the "right" decision. In fact, ethical practice and decision making require that the helping professional consider the situation from all points of view, develop a list of issues that represent multiple viewpoints, generate possible decisions, and weigh carefully the consequences of each decision. This type of ethical practice demands that the helper have knowledge of the professional code of ethics, critical thinking skills, an understanding of human behavior, good communication skills, the ability to establish rapport, and decision-making skills. It also challenges the professional to examine the ethics involved with carrying out the day-to-day work of helping.

In this chapter you will use your knowledge of the history of human services, the work of the professional, and the nature of clients and settings to imagine yourself in the role of the helper. The professional concerns highlighted in this chapter are divided into two areas. The first includes an introduction to codes of ethics, definitions of competence and responsibility, a discussion of confidentiality, a description of the client's rights, ethical standards of human service professionals, and a model for ethical decision making. This section describes what we traditionally think of as the study of ethics. The second focus will be on the ethics of the professional decisions that are woven into the fabric of the professional work. These decisions often receive little or no attention and are rarely considered a matter of "ethics." Ms. Bailey, the case manager for Almeada who you met in Chapter 1, also presents her view of professional ethics and discusses the many ethical decisions that she makes as she works within the human service delivery system.

 ## Ethical Considerations

As you deliver human services, situations will arise in which you may be unsure about the appropriate action to take. A third party requests information about a client; you observe a colleague joking about a client in the break room at work; a client requests information about obtaining an abortion, but your agency opposes providing this type of information. These situations represent ethical dilemmas for the human service professional. Even though education and training in human services emphasize the values of confidentiality, acceptance, individualism, self-determination, and tolerance, situations will inevitably occur in which simply possessing these values will not be enough to determine the right course of action.

In the past decade, increased public awareness of professional behavior, coupled with the passage of federal and state legislation controlling the helping professions, has underscored the importance of ethical concerns in service delivery. Stadler (1986) cites the Family Educational Rights and Privacy Act of 1974, state legislation requiring the reporting of child abuse, and *Tarasoff* v. *Regents of the University of California* (1976), which imposed a duty to warn potential victims, as examples of government action that directly affects the ethics of service provision. The human service professional must obey the law and also be cognizant of the implications of the law.

In this section, we explore codes of ethics or statements of standards of behavior as guides for professional behavior, as well as some major areas of ethical concern for the human service professional. Then we describe an ethical decision-making model that can be applied to dilemmas for which there is no relevant guideline. Vignettes are used to illustrate the range of dilemmas that may arise.

Codes of Ethics

Professionals have responded to the dilemmas of service provision by developing *codes of ethics* or *statements of ethical standards of behavior* for the members of their profession. Codes of ethics or ethical standards reflect professional concerns and define the guiding principles of professional activities. As an aid to ethical decision making in dilemmas arising in service delivery, such standards or codes help clarify the professional's responsibilities to clients, to the agency, and to society. Typically, a code of ethics includes items that state the goals or aims of the profession, that protect the client, that provide guidance to professional behavior, and that contribute to a professional identity for the helper. A complete understanding of a code of ethics or ethical standards requires knowledge of the code's strengths and purposes as well as its limitations.

PURPOSES AND LIMITATIONS

The primary functions of a code of ethics or ethical standards are to establish guidelines for professional behavior and to assist members of the profession in establishing a professional identity (Corey, Corey, & Callanan, 1998; Welfel, 1998). Other purposes include providing criteria for evaluating the ethics of a professional's practice, and serving as a benchmark in the enforcement of ethical standards (Kenyon, 1999).

Ethical codes do have limitations; they cannot cover every situation. They do, however, present a framework for ethical behavior, although their exact interpretation will depend on the situation to which they are being applied. As a result of this vagueness, codes may have a limited range, and some codes of ethics will likely conflict with others regarding some standard of behavior. Such conflicts pose problems for professionals who are members of more than one professional organization.

Parallel standard-setting entities may also issue ethical standards that conflict. For example, a code may not include a statement relating to the duty to warn, but the California Supreme Court has ruled in *Tarasoff* (1976) that there is a duty to warn potential victims of danger. Members who are bound by a

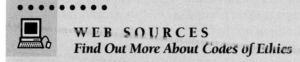

WEB SOURCES
Find Out More About Codes of Ethics

http://csep.iit.edu/codes/

This site, prepared by the Illinois Institute of Technology, provides links to over 850 codes of ethics. The site focuses on professional ethics and includes ethics within the helping professions.

http://courses.cs.vt.edu/~cs3604/lib/WorldCodes/WorldCodes.html

This site describes in detail the computer codes of ethics. As helping moves more into the technological world, these sites will be important to the consultant as one reflects about ethical use of the medium.

http://www.britannica.com/bcom/eb/article/6/0,5716,108566+2,00.html

The *Encyclopedia Britannica* describes the history of codes of ethics and moral codes of conduct. This article describes the history and moral source of our professional codes that we use today.

http://www.mapnp.org/library/ethics/ethics.htm

Although focused on business, this helpful site outlines how to develop and maintain an ethical workplace. It will be helpful for those who want to work in an ethical organization.

http://www.counseling.org/resources/codeofethics.htm

This site details the Code of Ethics of the American Counseling Association.

http://www.apa.org/ethics/code.html

This is the site for the Code of Ethics of the American Psychological Association.

http://www.ssc.msu.edu/~sw/ethics/nasweth.html

The site includes the social worker's code of ethics.

http://www.breadcasters.com/code.html

This site of BreadCasters International presents the ethical principles for online counseling adapted from the Standards for the Ethical Practice of Web Counseling established by the National Board for Certified Counselors (NBCC).

http://www.nbcc.org/ethics/wcstandards.htm

This site provides the complete standards of Web Counseling published by the National Board for Certified Counselors (NBCC).

http://www.nohse.org

The site of the National Organization for Human Service Education includes the Ethical Standards of Human Service Professionals.

code of ethics must be alert to the possibility that other forums may reach conclusions that differ from their code. Of course, this is especially critical when the other forum is a court of law or a legislative body.

Some other limitations of codes of ethics are beyond the scope of this text; however, human service professionals must be aware that such limitations exist. The professional must develop ethical reasoning skills to help resolve ethical dilemmas that may arise. A first step in this process is differentiating ethical dilemmas from situations in which the guidelines are clear. For resolving problem situations for which there are no specific guidelines, an ethical decision-making model is presented later in this chapter.

ETHICS AND THE PROFESSION

A code of ethics is binding only on the members of the group or organization that adopts it. Several organizations in human services have issued codes of behavior expected of their membership—organizations such as the American Counseling Association, the National Council for Social Work Education, and others in the fields of corrections, mental health, gerontology, and education. Most codes of ethics stipulate that the worker's first responsibility is to enhance and protect the client's welfare. Codes also give guidance about the helper's responsibilities to employers, to colleagues in the profession and other fields, and to society in general.

Ethical codes adopted by a professional association are usually based on the premise that a profession polices itself. Members of helping professions are assumed to be responsible, sensitive persons who are accountable for their behavior and the behavior of their colleagues. Self-regulation involves two types of discipline: informal and formal. Informal discipline is seen in the subtle and not-so-subtle pressure that colleagues exert on one another in the form of consultations, client referrals, and informal and formal discussions. Formal discipline occurs when professional associations publicly criticize or censure their members—in extreme cases, barring them from membership.

CODES OF ETHICS AND THE LAW

The law is generally supportive of, or at least neutral toward, ethical codes and standards. It is supportive in that it enforces minimum standards for practitioners through licensing requirements and generally protects the confidentiality of statements and records provided by clients during service provision. It is neutral in that it allows each profession to police itself and govern the helper's relations with clients and fellow professionals. The law intervenes and overrides professional codes of ethics only when necessary to protect the public's health, safety, and welfare. One instance of legal intervention occurs when the profession's standards of confidentiality (deemed necessary to ensure effective treatment) call for the suppression of information that government authorities require to be disclosed to prevent harm to others.

TABLE 9-1   ✦   SUMMARY POINTS: CODES OF ETHICS

Reflect professional concerns
• Define guiding principles of professional activities
• Clarify responsibilities to clients, the agency, and society
• Do not cover every situation
• Are binding only on members of the group that adopts it

The California Supreme Court's ruling in the case of *Tarasoff* (1976) legally supported a "duty to warn" possible victims of clients once counselors have this information. The court stated that

> when a therapist determines, or pursuant to the standards of his profession should determine, that his patient presents a serious danger of violence to another, he incurs an obligation to use reasonable care to protect the intended victim against such danger. The discharge of this duty may require the therapist to take one or more steps, depending on the nature of the case. Thus, it may call for him or her to warn the intended victim or others likely to apprise the victim of the danger, to notify the police, or to take whatever other steps are reasonably necessary under the circumstances (p. 340) (see Table 9-1).

Competence and Responsibility

Before any involvement with clients, helpers must concern themselves with two areas: their competence as professionals and their responsibility to the individuals, groups, or organizations with whom they are affiliated or whom they serve as clients. Ethical concerns of competence and responsibility pervade all areas of professional practice.

Competence is a difficult concept to define from an ethical standpoint. One way to define it is by identifying the standards for practice within the profession. Most codes of ethics in helping professions include statements about academic training, practical training or supervised experience, and areas of specialization in which the helper is most knowledgeable or competent. During their training, human service professionals must acquire knowledge about the helping process, professional ethics, the limits of professional practice, and the pertinent legislation that governs practice.

In addition to the competence acquired through preparation to be a professional, the human service worker in practice also has an obligation to ensure that available services meet acceptable standards. Workers have a further obligation to improve services and skills through activities such as involvement in ongoing research and study, participation in peer consultation, and review of the current professional literature. All these activities contribute to the competence of the helper (see Table 9-2).

The second concept that pervades all phases of service delivery is *responsibility*. Rinas and Clyne-Jackson (1988) defined it as "an obligation to pro-

TABLE 9-2   ✦   SUMMARY POINTS: COMPETENCE

Standards for professional practice include:
* Academic training
* Supervised experience
* Areas of specialization
* Obligation to improve services and skills

Ethical Standards for Psychologists
American Psychological Association

PRINCIPLE TWO: COMPETENCE

Psychologists strive to maintain high standards of competence in their work. They recognize the boundaries of their particular competencies and the limitations of their expertise. They provide only those services and use only those techniques for which they are qualified by education, training, or experience. Psychologists are cognizant of the fact that the competencies required in serving, teaching, and/or studying groups of people vary with the distinctive characteristics of those groups. In those areas in which recognized professional standards do not yet exist, psychologists exercise careful judgment and take appropriate precautions to protect the welfare of those with whom they work. They maintain knowledge of relevant scientific and professional information related to the services they render, and they recognize the need for ongoing education. Psychologists make appropriate use of scientific, professional, technical, and administrative resources.

SOURCE: Material from "Ethical Principles of Psychologists and Code of Conduct." Copyright © 1992 by the American Psychological Association, Inc. Reprinted by permission.

mote and safeguard the dignity, well-being, and growth of clients, colleagues, the . . . profession itself, and society as a whole" (p. 3). The idea that helpers have obligations to others in addition to the client may present dilemmas for the helper in cases of conflict. It is important for the helper to understand the nature of the conflict and be able to explain to the client how this may limit the client–helper relationship.

To fulfill their commitment to be responsible, helpers must know the ethical and legal procedures that are pertinent to their service delivery functions. These include the profession's code of ethics, its standards of behavior, and the consequences of failure to conform to codes and standards.

In many instances, ethical standards of competence and responsibility are compatible. For example, human service professionals are obligated to

• • • • • • • • • •

Ethical Standards for School Counselors
American School Counselor Association

F. RESPONSIBILITIES TO THE PROFESSION

The school counselor:

1. Conducts herself/himself in such a manner as to bring credit to self and the profession.
2. Conducts appropriate research and reports findings in a manner consistent with acceptable educational and psychological research practices. When using client data for research, statistical or program planning purposes, the counselor ensures protection of the identity of the individual(s).
3. Actively participates in local, state, and national associations which foster the development and improvement of school counseling.
4. Adheres to ethical standards of the profession, other official policy statements pertaining to counseling, and relevant statutes established by federal, state, and local governments.
5. Clearly distinguishes between statements and actions made as a private individual and as a representative of the school counseling profession.
6. Contributes to the development of the profession through the sharing of skills, ideas, and expertise with colleagues.

SOURCE: Reprinted from *The ASCA Counselor,* 29(4), April 1992, pp. 13–16. Copyright ACA. Reprinted by permission.

provide high-quality service to their clients. Discharging this obligation relies to a certain extent on the competence of the worker, as the worker is expected to provide only those services he or she is trained and qualified to deliver. If the client has needs beyond the competence of the worker, then the worker has a duty, according to codes and standards of professional behavior, to locate alternative services from a coworker or another agency. In this situation, the competence of the human service professional is reflected in an awareness of available services and knowledge of how those services relate to the client's problems.

The responsibility of the helper extends beyond client contact. The helper is also concerned with having sufficient time to work with a client and the resources necessary for effective practice. Should these not be present, the helper is responsible for locating or developing resources such as grants for additional funding or increased staff for specialized caseloads. The overriding concern, of course, is the obligation and commitment to provide good-quality services to whomever needs those services (see Table 9-3).

The vignettes that follow illustrate some of the dilemmas that a helper might face while working with human service clients. The primary issues in these vignettes are competence and responsibility.

TABLE 9-3   ✦   SUMMARY POINTS: RESPONSIBILITY

Helpers must know the ethical and legal procedures, including:
- Profession's code of ethics
- Standards of behavior
- Consequences of failure to uphold codes of ethics and ethical standards

---

Case 1
Carmen is a night counselor for a cerebral palsy group home. She works five nights a week, arriving at 4 P.M. and staying until 7 A.M. the next day. Right now the group home is in the process of hiring three new staff members: a van driver, an evening visiting nurse, and a day teacher/counselor. Until these professionals are hired, much of the responsibility falls to Carmen. She does not mind doing all that she can for the group home and the clients, but she feels that she is not qualified to do some of the things asked of her.

Case 2
George has a job as a caseworker for a mental health outpatient service. He provides individual and group counseling for adult clients. One of his clients, Kim, is having trouble relating to her husband, her son, and her father. George suggests to Kim that she practice various forms of sexual intimacy with him as a part of her therapy to improve her relationships with men.

Case 3
Dim Su is a social service worker in a health care facility for the elderly. He is in a dilemma because several of his clients are requesting that he provide them with cigarettes even though smoking has been discouraged by the doctor. Dim Su's colleague, Betty, laughs when he tells her of his dilemma. She tells him that there is no dilemma. She has provided cigarettes for patients for the past three years.

Case 4
Jim, the sports program director for the Millerville Home for Boys, walks by a group of new workers who are discussing their recent orientation session. They mention the newest rule that prohibits workers from transporting a client in a private car. Jim had heard about the new rule, but so far he has ignored it, hoping to plead ignorance if someone were to challenge his behavior. Many of the relationships he forms with the children are established during one-on-one private outings to the mall, movies, and out to dinner. He hates to give them up.

Case 5
Bradley's job as coordinator of the hospice program in a local hospital is very demanding. His hours are 8 to 5, Monday through Friday, but the needs of the

clients do not follow these regular hours. He is operating the program with little help: one half-time secretary to answer the phone and one hospice nurse.
He often works 15 to 18 hours a day. He feels committed to his work, but is often so tired that he is afraid he cannot be effective

---

Case 6

Susan Deerpath is a traveling health department worker in a rural area. She
is the only worker serving clients in 12 counties. Once every two weeks, she
meets with other health department officials from the district, but for the most
part she has limited contact with other professionals. She read her last professional magazine two years ago, and she has attended only one in-service meeting in the past five years.

Case 7

Luis works for an outpatient AIDS clinic whose major goals include prevention and therapeutic counseling. Luis feels that meeting the demands of his
clients is the most important service he provides, and he has difficulty ignoring the clients. Consequently, he is booked solid each day, seeing individual
AIDS victims and their families. The director thinks he should spend more time
on preventive efforts to promote the agency's other main goal.

Case 8

Enrique is an intake worker for a local community development corporation.
He screens individuals for eligibility for housing, seeing more than 70 clients
a week. A majority of them qualify for the services, but only two to five housing units become available each week. There are few alternatives for the other
clients. Enrique worries about the welfare of these clients, who remain on a
waiting list for as long as six months. The dilemma occurs because his job responsibilities do not include referral.

In each of these situations, the helper faces a dilemma regarding worker
competence and responsibility for which there is no easy solution. *Competence*
is a personal issue that demands professional self-assessment and then commitment to professional development. *Responsibility* involves the interpersonal relationships the helper has with individual clients or groups and human
service agencies. The common ground between responsibility and competence
is the helper's primary commitment to serving the client.

Confidentiality

Confidentiality is the helper's assurance that information the client divulges
will remain between the two of them. If information is to be shared, it will be
shared only with those designated by the client. These two statements regard-

ing the concept of confidentiality provide only general guidelines for the helper. In some situations, laws require confidentiality to be breached: Parents have the legal right to information about their offspring in most circumstances; courts may require the disclosure of information that would otherwise be confidential; and helpers have a duty to alert authorities if they suspect child abuse (Rinas & Clyne-Jackson, 1988). The concept is a complex one. This section provides an introduction to confidentiality and gives examples of the complex situations workers may encounter in human service practice.

Confidentiality is a complex concept. For example, a term often associated with confidentiality is *privileged communication.* Both terms address the commitment to keep a client's identity and communications secret. There is a basic difference. Confidentiality is a moral obligation grounded in values and ethics (Welfel, 1998); privileged communication is a legal term that allows practitioners to legally refuse to release certain information in response to a subpoena. The term *legally* is used because privileged communication is a right granted to a group of professionals by state law-making bodies. Examples of situations in which helpers are ethically or legally obligated to breach confidentiality include but are not limited to the following:

1. When the client is dangerous to self or others
2. When there is suspicion of abuse or neglect
3. When the client brings charges against the counselor
4. When the client has already introduced privileged material into litigation

A second example of the complexity of confidentiality is a type often called *relative confidentiality.* This term refers to the informal sharing of information that occurs in an agency or organizational setting among coworkers or treatment team members and supervisors. The client's permission is not required for this type of exchange to take place. Typically, agency policy will also guide this sharing by determining who has access to confidential information. The Federal Privacy Act of 1974, which governs confidentiality in federally funded and administered programs such as the Department of Veterans Affairs and the Social Security Administration, states that clients have access to their records and establishes procedures for this to occur. It also supports the concept of relative confidentiality by providing for the sharing of information among those workers within the agency who need the information in the performance of their duties.

In summary, privileged communication and relative confidentiality illustrate the complexity of confidentiality. Privileged communication rarely exists for the beginning human service professional, but relative confidentiality is a concept that deserves the worker's attention. Agency guidelines, the profession's code of ethics, and the laws of the state in which one practices are important considerations in the delivery of services. A professional should be familiar with all three as guides to circumstances that may arise. The following vignettes provide examples of confidentiality dilemmas that you may face as a beginning human service professional.

Case 1
Sue Lee works for the Department of Human Services in Child Protective Services and visits families once a week to review the status of the home environment. Yesterday she received a subpoena and will be required to testify in court that the father in one of the families in her caseload was not at home the last two times she visited. He is charged with armed robbery and states in his defense that he was at home during the time of the crime. That time coincides with her visit.

Case 2
Joe Cullinane works in a small agency that provides educational services to children with developmental disabilities. He promises clients that his records are confidential and is very careful not to divulge the names of the clients or the nature of their problems. The mother of one of his young clients reports to him that "someone at her church" had heard that her child was receiving his services. If it was not Joe who breached confidentiality, it might be the secretary who answers the phones or the typist who keeps the records.

Case 3
Faye Goldstein is a counselor/recreation specialist working in an after-school recreation facility. One of her favorite teenagers has just told her "in confidence" that she is pregnant. Should she keep this confidential?

Case 4
Freda Tehaar is a group therapist for a grief group at the local mental health center. She has explained to the group the importance of confidentiality. One of the members asks, "How can I place my trust in a bunch of strangers?"

Case 5
David Root is a recovering alcoholic and has not had a drink in the last two years. He understands and practices confidentiality in his human service work, but he cannot help but wonder how well he would do in this regard if he were to go on a drinking binge.

Case 6
Cynthia Loomis works in a high-stress hospice program. Working with the dying patient and family and friends is emotionally draining, and she often "takes her work home." To help her relieve the stress, can she tell her friends and family anything about her work without breaching her promise of confidentiality?

Case 7
Jefferson Smith works with adults on probation and has just heard one of his clients tell how she abuses her six-month-old child. Does he report this information? To whom does he report it?

Case 8
Raphael Sanchez is a vocational rehabilitation counselor working with a Vietnam veteran. His client has been very depressed during the last month, and during his last individual conference with Raphael, he talked of "ending all the agony." Raphael wonders what he should do and whom he should tell.

These are just a few examples of the many conflicts that can arise over the issue of confidentiality. Many of the troublesome dilemmas result from the constant tension between worker responsibilities, agency policies, and client needs. Privileged communication and relative confidentiality are difficult principles to follow. The preceding cases illustrate the problems helpers may encounter as they translate their values into action in the workplace. An equally complex issue that human services professionals encounter concerns clients' rights.

Clients' Rights

Clients are first and foremost citizens of a democratic society; as such, they have certain rights and privileges. In a helping situation, the client's trust in the helper is important for the development of the helping relationship. In exchange for the trust of the client, the helper is ethically obligated to protect the rights of the client. Two examples of clients' rights are the right to privacy and informed consent.

Clients have the right to share whatever information they wish with a helper. They also have the right to withhold information they do not want to share. The helper is ethically bound to respect clients' *right to privacy* by not pressuring them to reveal things they do not wish to reveal.

Informed consent is another example of the rights of clients involved in the helping process. It is the client's right to know about the qualifications of the helper, treatment procedures, costs of services, confidentiality, and access to records. The concept of informed consent extends beyond simply telling the client about such matters. The client must comprehend this information and consent voluntarily. In some cases, the helper must educate the client about his or her rights with regard to consent.

Informed consent is a particularly critical aspect of client rights with respect to decision making. In the helping process, the client is an active participant who has a voice in what is happening. In the absence of informed consent, the client's right to self-determination is compromised. The helper has an ethical obligation to ensure that clients receive and understand the appropriate information.

Code of Professional Ethics for Rehabilitation Counselors: Confidentiality

CANON 6—CONFIDENTIALITY

Rehabilitation counselors shall respect the confidentiality of information obtained from clients in the course of their work.

Rules of Professional Conduct

R6.1 Rehabilitation counselors will inform clients at the onset of the counseling relationship of the limits of confidentiality.

R6.2 Rehabilitation counselors will take reasonable personal action, or inform responsible authorities, or inform those persons at risk, when the conditions or actions of clients indicate that there is clear and imminent danger to clients or others after advising clients that this must be done. Consultation with other professionals may be used where appropriate. The assumption of responsibility for clients must be taken only after careful deliberation and clients must be involved in the resumption of responsibility as quickly as possible.

R6.3 Rehabilitation counselors will not forward to another person, agency, or potential employer, any confidential information without the written permission of clients or their legal guardians.

R6.4 Rehabilitation counselors will ensure that there are defined policies and practices in other agencies cooperatively serving rehabilitation clients which effectively protect information confidentiality.

One way the client can become informed about the helper is for the helper to write and to share with the client a *professional disclosure statement.* This form should include information about the worker and the worker's credentials, which will allow the client to make an informed assessment of the worker's competence. In addition to name, business address, and telephone number, other information may include education and training competency areas, and the name, address, and telephone number of the state government agency that regulates human service delivery.

Developing a personal professional disclosure statement has several benefits. As the helper shares the statement with the client, it promotes the development of a helping relationship. Not only does it signal to the client that this relationship is different from informal helping relationships, but it also acquaints the client with the person in whom the client will soon place his or her trust. While working out the statement, the helper has an opportunity to think about and put into

R6.5 Rehabilitation counselors will safeguard the maintenance, storage, and disposal of the records of clients so that unauthorized persons shall not have access to these records. All non-professional persons who must have access to these records will be thoroughly briefed concerning the confidential standards to be observed.

R6.6 Rehabilitation counselors, in the preparation of written and oral reports, will present only germane data and will make every effort to avoid undue invasion of privacy.

R6.7 Rehabilitation counselors will obtain written permission from clients or their legal guardians prior to taping or otherwise recording counseling sessions. Even with guardians' written consent, rehabilitation counselors will not record sessions against the expressed wishes of clients.

R6.8 Rehabilitation counselors will persist in claiming the privileged status of confidential information obtained from clients, where communications are privileged by statute for rehabilitation counselors.

R6.9 Rehabilitation counselors will provide prospective employers with only job relevant information about clients and will secure the permission of clients or their legal guardians for the release of any information which might be considered confidential.

SOURCE: Material from "Code of Professional Ethics for Rehabilitation Counselors." Reprinted by permission of the Commission on Rehabilitation Counselor Certification.

words exactly who he or she is as a human service professional. It also allows the worker to define himself or herself as a professional and links the individual to the common knowledge, skills, and values of the profession (see Table 9-4).

The following sample professional disclosure statement was written by Carmen Rodriguez, the vocational evaluator introduced in Chapter 6.

My name is Carmen Rodriguez, and I am involved in vocational rehabilitation of the handicapped. My purpose is to help my clients understand who they are and what they can do to make their lives more satisfying. Specifically, I evaluate clients to determine what knowledge, skills, and abilities they possess and explain to them what potential work opportunities are available for them.

Once a client meets the eligibility requirements established by the agency, there is no charge for my services. I have worked for this agency for four years

American Counseling Association Code of Ethics and Standards of Practice: Clients' Rights

A.3. CLIENT RIGHTS

a. *Disclosure to Clients.* When counseling is initiated, and throughout the counseling process as necessary, counselors inform clients of the purposes, goals, techniques, procedures, limitations, potential risks and benefits of services to be performed, and other pertinent information. Counselors take steps to ensure that clients understand the implications of diagnosis, the intended use of tests and reports, fees, and billing arrangements. Clients have the right to expect confidentiality and to be provided with an explanation of its limitations, including supervision and/or treatment team professionals; to obtain clear information about their case records; to participate in the ongoing counseling plans; and to refuse any recommended services and be advised of the consequences of such refusal. (See E.5.a. and G.2.)

b. *Freedom of Choice.* Counselors offer clients the freedom to choose whether to enter into a counseling relationship and to determine which professional(s) will provide counseling.

c. *Inability to Give Consent.* When counseling minors or persons unable to give voluntary informed consent, counselors act in these clients' best interests. (See B.3.)

SOURCE: Material from "American Counseling Association Code of Ethics and Standards of Practice." Reprinted by permission of the American Counseling Association.

TABLE 9-4 ✦ SUMMARY POINTS: PROFESSIONAL DISCLOSURE
STATEMENTS

- Promotes the development of a helping relationship
- Introduces the helper to the client
- Provides opportunity for the helper to clarify his/her professional identity

---

as a vocational evaluator. I received training in college for this work and frequently attend workshops to update my knowledge.

Evaluations can take from two weeks to six weeks. This may depend on the client, the disability, and what we want to know. I often refer my client to other team members in my agency and to other professionals in the community. The clients I see usually have such complex problems that I cannot address them all by myself, so I work with a team. Because my agency uses this team approach, I may share information about clients with coworkers within the agency but not with outsiders or other clients.

Now that you have read Carmen's statement, can you write one of your own? It may be easier to write such a statement if you imagine that you work in a specific agency with a well-defined population.

Protection is another of the helper's obligations to clients. Clients have the right to expect the helper to protect them from harm. It is the helper's responsibility to be sensitive to situations in which the client risks economic or physical harm, and, if possible, to prevent harm from occurring. If there is a clear and imminent danger to a third party, the helper has a duty to take action to protect the individual at risk. Determining when a situation warrants action may be difficult for the human service professional; when questionable occasions arise, consultation with colleagues or supervisors will be helpful in deciding on a course of action.

The following cases provide examples of dilemmas that a human service professional may encounter in relation to clients' rights. Several of the cases present ethical situations in which the human service professional is confronted with a difficult decision about what action to take. In other cases, the dilemma is one over which the worker has little or no control.

Case 1

Susan Yew and her client, Mr. Rodriguez, have agreed on what referral information should be sent to a local educational reading clinic. The clinic, however, wants more information. Specifically, they want to know whether Mr. Rodriguez is a veteran, but he feels they will treat him "special" if they know that he fought in Vietnam. Susan has agreed that the file to be sent should include a short note explaining why he does not want to answer that particular question.

Case 2

Once a week, the staff members at the battered women's shelter discuss the cases in which they are involved. One client, age 56, told the worker "in confidence" that she had an abortion when she was 13. She asked the worker not to tell the other staff members.

Case 3

The local mental health institution has a new professional worker: the patient advocate, who has been hired by the mental health association to protect the rights of the clients in the institution. The patient advocate explains to each patient his or her rights when he or she enters the institution, but many patients forget or are unable to comprehend how they might use the services of the advocate. Sometimes Ron, a social worker on a treatment team serving the men's locked ward, sees clients' rights being abused, but to recommend that a client see the advocate might cause trouble for the treatment team to which Ron belongs.

Case 4

Youvella is a patient in a health care facility. She wants to see her medical records before they are examined by the team of specialists who will decide what protocol to prescribe for the treatment of her cancer-ridden pancreas. Although Youvella is entitled to review these records, the nurse questions the wisdom of this decision because of Youvella's emotional instability. The nurse requests assistance from the hospital social service worker in this dilemma.

Case 5

Emile is a human service student working with rehabilitation services. For the next two weeks, he will be administering vocational aptitude tests to new clients. He is unsure whether he should tell his clients that he is a student. He wants them to trust him and have confidence in him, as they would if he were a seasoned worker.

Case 6

The adoption agency is reviewing the files of a young couple considering adoption. Unfortunately, the adoption counselor has received some damaging information from the couple's landlord of 10 years ago that will make it impossible for the agency to consider them suitable as parents. The counselor really likes this couple and believes that they would make wonderful parents, but she also knows that the information cannot be withheld. The adoption counselor must tell the couple of the agency's decision not to consider them "fit" to adopt and must tell them of the negative recommendation.

Case 7

The Annas are involved in marital therapy; the stated purpose of the counseling is to "save the marriage." They receive individual counseling once a week, and once a month they participate in counseling sessions together. Ms. Anna has recently told the counselor of her desire to harm Mr. Anna. The counselor wonders how to handle this information, since it was given in confidence and also may jeopardize the goal of saving the marriage.

In clients' rights issues, the helper's judgment and the agency's judgment are often not the only considerations. Legal rulings must also be taken into account. Sometimes legal pronouncements, ethical standards, and personal commitments conflict, presenting a difficult dilemma for the worker. The worker then must decide what action is most ethical.

Ethical Standards of Human Service Professionals

During 1990 and 1991, both the National Organization for Human Service Education (NOHSE) and the Council for Standards in Human Service Education (CSHSE) recognized the need for the development of a separate and distinct ethical code for human service professionals. Previously, students and graduates were guided by the codes of ethics or ethical standards of various other professions, some of which have been excerpted in this chapter. These codes did not reflect the unique history or philosophy of the human service profession.

In 1990, the governing boards of NOHSE and CSHSE expressed the desire to enhance the professional identity of human service professionals; this resulted in the appointment of a committee by NOHSE to develop a code of ethics. Developing a code of ethics or ethical standards for a profession is a lengthy process. In this case, there was a review of the code of ethics of related professions: the American Counseling Association (ACA), the National Association of Social Workers (NASW), and the American Psychological Association (APA). An examination of literature on ethical guidelines followed. These steps led to written ethical guidelines that were eventually approved by the boards of two human service organizations and their memberships in 1995. As you read these ethical standards, you will note that they address the topics discussed at the beginning of this chapter. The preamble introduces the goals or aims of the profession. The ethical standards then divide professional responsibilities in six areas: to clients, to the community and society, to colleagues, to the profession, to employers, and to self.

These ethical standards and those in other helping professions provide guidelines only. They do not provide answers to all ethical dilemmas. The ethical decision making that follows the ethical standards is helpful when these situations arise.

Ethical Decision Making

Clearly, no code of ethics or statement of standards can provide a course of action for every situation that might arise in the practice of human services. What does the human service professional do in situations for which there are no guidelines or guidelines that conflict? In such *ethical dilemmas,* the conflict is in determining the right thing to do regarding obligations to two or more constituencies. They occur in situations when a choice exists between contradictory directives or standards or "when every alternative results in an undesirable outcome for one or more persons" (Loewenberg & Dolgoff, 1996, p. 8). The areas of confidentiality, role conflict, and counselor competence frequently present ethical dilemmas. Rather than attempt to provide possible solutions to every situation that comes to mind, this subsection will introduce a model for ethical decision making that can be applied to many dilemmas to determine a course of action.

The key question in the decision-making model is, "What is the best action under the circumstances and with the individuals involved?" In asking this question, the helper must assume an attitude of *moral responsibleness.* This should be distinguished from the kind of responsibility discussed earlier. That responsibility is imposed by some higher authority, such as the profession or

Ethical Standards of Human Service Professionals

National Organization for Human Service Education Council for Standards in Human Service Education

PREAMBLE

Human services is a profession developing in response to and in anticipation of the direction of human needs and human problems in the late twentieth century. Characterized particularly by an appreciation of human beings in all of their diversity, human services offers assistance to its clients within the context of their community and environment. Human service professionals and those who educate them, regardless of whether they are students, faculty or practitioners, promote and encourage the unique values and characteristics of human services. In so doing human service professionals and educators uphold the integrity and ethics of the profession, partake in constructive criticism of the profession, promote client and community well-being, and enhance their own professional growth.

The ethical guidelines presented are a set of standards of conduct which the human service professionals and educators consider in ethical and professional decision making. It is hoped that these guidelines will be of assistance when human service professionals and educators are challenged by difficult ethical dilemmas. Although ethical codes are not legal documents, they may be used to assist in the adjudication of issues related to ethical human service behavior.

SECTION I—STANDARDS FOR HUMAN SERVICE PROFESSIONAL

Human service professionals function in many ways and carry out many roles. They enter into professional–client relationships with individuals, families, groups and communities who are all referred to as "clients" in these standards. Among their roles are caregiver, case manager, broker, teacher/educator, behavior changer, consultant, outreach professional, mobilizer, advocate, community planner, community change organizer, evaluator and administrator (SREB, 1967). The following standards are written with these multifaceted roles in mind.

THE HUMAN SERVICE PROFESSIONAL'S RESPONSIBILITY TO CLIENTS

STATEMENT 1 Human service professionals negotiate with clients the purpose, goals, and nature of the helping relationship prior to its onset as well as inform clients of the limitations of the proposed relationship.

STATEMENT 2 Human service professionals respect the integrity and welfare of the client at all times. Each client is treated with respect, acceptance and dignity.

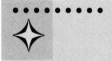

STATEMENT 3 Human service professionals protect the client's right to privacy and confidentiality except when such confidentiality would cause harm to the client or others, when agency guidelines state otherwise, or under other stated conditions (e.g., local, state, or federal laws). Professionals inform clients of the limits of confidentiality prior to the onset of the helping relationship.

STATEMENT 4 If it is suspected that danger or harm may occur to the client or to others as a result of a client's behavior, the human service professional acts in an appropriate and professional manner to protect the safety of those individuals. This may involve seeking consultation, supervision, and/or breaking the confidentiality of the relationship.

STATEMENT 5 Human service professionals protect the integrity, safety, and security of client records. All written client information that is shared with other professionals, except in the course of professional supervision, must have the client's prior written consent.

STATEMENT 6 Human service professionals are aware that in their relationships with clients power and status are unequal. Therefore they recognize that dual or multiple relationships may increase the risk of harm to, or exploitation of, clients, and may impair their professional judgment. However, in some communities and situations it may not be feasible to avoid social or other nonprofessional contact with clients. Human service professionals support the trust implicit in the helping relationship by avoiding dual relationships that may impair professional judgment, increase the risk of harm to clients or lead to exploitation.

STATEMENT 7 Sexual relationships with current clients are not considered to be in the best interest of the client and are prohibited. Sexual relationships with previous clients are considered dual relationships and are addressed in Statement 6 (above).

STATEMENT 8 The client's right to self-determination is protected by human service professionals. They recognize the client's right to receive or refuse services.

STATEMENT 9 Human service professionals recognize and build on client strengths.

continued

Ethical Standards of Human Service Professionals (continued)

THE HUMAN SERVICE PROFESSIONAL'S RESPONSIBILITY TO THE COMMUNITY AND SOCIETY

STATEMENT 10 Human service professionals are aware of local, state, and federal laws. They advocate for change in regulations and statutes when such legislation conflicts with ethical guidelines and/or client rights. Where laws are harmful to individuals, groups or communities, human service professionals consider the conflict between the values of obeying the law and the values of serving people and may decide to initiate social action.

STATEMENT 11 Human service professionals keep informed about current social issues as they affect the client and the community. They share that information with clients, groups and community as part of their work.

STATEMENT 12 Human service professionals understand the complex interaction between individuals, their families, the communities in which they live, and society.

STATEMENT 13 Human service professionals act as advocates in addressing unmet client and community needs. Human service professionals provide a mechanism for identifying unmet client needs, calling attention to these needs, and assisting in planning and mobilizing to advocate for those needs at the local community level.

STATEMENT 14 Human service professionals represent their qualifications to the public accurately.

STATEMENT 15 Human service professionals describe the effectiveness of programs, treatments, and/or techniques accurately.

STATEMENT 16 Human service professionals advocate for the rights of all members of society, particularly those who are members of minorities and groups at which discriminatory practices have historically been directed.

STATEMENT 17 Human service professionals provide services without discrimination or preference based on age, ethnicity, culture, race, disability, gender, religion, sexual orientation or socioeconomic status.

STATEMENT 18 Human service professionals are knowledgeable about the cultures and communities within which they practice. They are aware of multiculturalism in society and its impact on the community as well as individuals within the community. They respect individuals and groups, their cultures and beliefs.

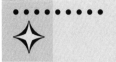

STATEMENT 19 Human service professionals are aware of their own cultural backgrounds, beliefs, and values, recognizing the potential for impact on their relationships with others.

STATEMENT 20 Human service professionals are aware of sociopolitical issues that differentially affect clients from diverse backgrounds.

STATEMENT 21 Human service professionals seek the training, experience, education and supervision necessary to ensure their effectiveness in working with culturally diverse client populations.

THE HUMAN SERVICE PROFESSIONAL'S RESPONSIBILITY TO COLLEAGUES

STATEMENT 22 Human service professionals avoid duplicating another professional's helping relationship with a client. They consult with other professionals who are assisting the client in a different type of relationship when it is in the best interest of the client to do so.

STATEMENT 23 When a human service professional has a conflict with a colleague, he or she first seeks out the colleague in an attempt to manage the problem. If necessary, the professional then seeks the assistance of supervisors, consultants or other professionals in efforts to manage the problem.

STATEMENT 24 Human service professionals respond appropriately to unethical behavior of colleagues. Usually this means initially talking directly with the colleague and, if no resolution is forthcoming, reporting the colleague's behavior to supervisory or administrative staff and/or to the professional organization(s) to which the colleague belongs.

STATEMENT 25 All consultations between human service professionals are kept confidential unless to do so would result in harm to clients or communities.

THE HUMAN SERVICE PROFESSIONAL'S RESPONSIBILITY TO THE PROFESSION

STATEMENT 26 Human service professionals know the limit and scope of their professional knowledge and offer services only within their knowledge and skill base.

STATEMENT 27 Human service professionals seek appropriate consultation and supervision to assist in decision-making when there are legal, ethical or other dilemmas.

STATEMENT 28 Human service professionals act with integrity, honesty, genuineness, and objectivity.

continued

Ethical Standards of Human Service Professionals (continued)

STATEMENT 29 Human service professionals promote cooperation among related disciplines (e.g., psychology, counseling, social work, nursing, family and consumer sciences, medicine, education) to foster professional growth and interests within the various fields.

STATEMENT 30 Human service professionals promote the continuing development of their profession. They encourage membership in professional associations, support research endeavors, foster educational advancement, advocate for appropriate legislative actions, and participate in other related professional activities.

STATEMENT 31 Human service professionals continually seek out new and effective approaches to enhance their professional abilities.

THE HUMAN SERVICE PROFESSIONAL'S RESPONSIBILITY TO EMPLOYERS

STATEMENT 32 Human service professionals adhere to commitments made to their employers.

STATEMENT 33 Human service professionals participate in efforts to establish and maintain employment conditions which are conducive to high quality client services. They assist in evaluating the effectiveness of the agency through reliable and valid assessment measures.

STATEMENT 34 When a conflict arises between fulfilling the responsibility to the employer and the responsibility to the client, human service professionals advise both of the conflict and work conjointly with all involved to manage the conflict.

THE HUMAN SERVICE PROFESSIONAL'S RESPONSIBILITY TO SELF

STATEMENT 35 Human service professionals strive to personify those characteristics typically associated with the profession (e.g., accountability, respect for others, genuineness, empathy, pragmatism).

STATEMENT 36 Human service professionals foster self-awareness and personal growth in themselves. They recognize that when professionals are aware of their own values, attitudes, cultural background, and personal needs, the process of helping others is less likely to be negatively impacted by those factors.

STATEMENT 37 Human service professionals recognize a commitment to lifelong learning and continually upgrade knowledge and skills to serve the populations better.

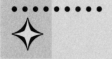

SECTION II—STANDARDS FOR HUMAN SERVICE EDUCATORS

Human service educators are familiar with, informed by, and accountable to the standards of professional conduct put forth by their institutions of higher learning; their professional disciplines, for example, American Association of University Professors (AAUP), American Counseling Association (ACA), Academy of Criminal Justice (ACJS), American Psychological Association (APA), American Sociological Association (ASA), National Association of Social Workers (NASW), National Board of Certified Counselors (NBCC), National Education Association (NEA), and the National Organization for Human Service Education (NOHSE).

STATEMENT 38 Human service educators uphold the principle of liberal education and embrace the essence of academic freedom, abstaining from inflicting their own personal views/morals on students, and allowing students the freedom to express their views without penalty, censure or ridicule, and to engage in critical thinking.

STATEMENT 39 Human service educators provide students with readily available and explicit program policies and criteria regarding program goals and objectives, recruitment, admission, course requirements, evaluations, retention and dismissal in accordance with due process procedures.

STATEMENT 40 Human service educators demonstrate high standards of scholarship in content areas and of pedagogy by staying current with developments in the field of human services and in teaching effectiveness, for example, learning styles and teaching styles.

STATEMENT 41 Human service educators monitor students' field experiences to ensure the quality of the placement site, supervisory experience, and learning experience towards the goals of professional identity and skill development.

STATEMENT 42 Human service educators participate actively in the selection of required readings and use them with care, based strictly on the merits of the material's content, and present relevant information accurately, objectively, and fully.

STATEMENT 43 Human service educators, at the onset of courses, inform students if sensitive/controversial issues or experiential/affective content or process are part of the course design; ensure that students are

continued

• • • • • • • • • •

Ethical Standards of Human Service Professionals (continued)

offered opportunities to discuss in structured ways their reactions to sensitive or controversial class content; ensure that the presentation of such material is justified on pedagogical grounds directly related to the course; and differentiate between information based on scientific data, anecdotal data, and personal opinion.

STATEMENT 44 Human service educators develop and demonstrate culturally sensitive knowledge, awareness, and teaching methodology.

STATEMENT 45 Human service educators demonstrate full commitment to their appointed responsibilities, and are enthusiastic about and encouraging of students' learning.

STATEMENT 46 Human service educators model the personal attributes, values and skills of the human service professional, including but not limited to, the willingness to seek and respond to feedback from students.

STATEMENT 47 Human service educators establish and uphold appropriate guidelines concerning self-disclosure or student-disclosure of sensitive/personal information.

STATEMENT 48 Human service educators establish an appropriate and timely process for providing clear and objective feedback to students about their performance on relevant and established course/program academic and personal competence requirements and their suitability for the field.

STATEMENT 49 Human service educators are aware that in their relationships with students, power and status are unequal; therefore, human service educators are responsible to clearly define and maintain ethical and professional relationships with students, and avoid conduct that is demeaning, embarrassing or exploitative of students, and to treat students fairly, equally and without discrimination.

the government; it may be interpreted as one's duty. Moral responsibleness, on the other hand, comes from within the individual, who assumes that there is a course of action that is morally right (Tennyson & Strom, 1986). A commitment to rational thinking and a knowledge of moral principles are necessary components of moral reasoning.

The ethical decision-making model proposed by Van Hoose and Paradise (1979) consists of five steps. The first is identification of the problem or dilemma. Second is an examination of existing rules or guiding principles that may be applied to resolve the dilemma. If none are found, the helper proceeds

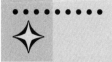

STATEMENT 50 Human service educators recognize and acknowledge the contributions of students to their work, for example, in case material, workshops, research, and publications.

STATEMENT 51 Human service educators demonstrate professional standards of conduct in managing personal or professional differences with colleagues, for example, not disclosing such differences and/or affirming a student's negative opinion of a faculty/program.

STATEMENT 52 Human service educators ensure that students are familiar with, informed by, and accountable to the ethical standards and policies put forth by their program/department, the course syllabus/instructor, their advisor(s), and the Ethical Standards of Human Service Professionals.

STATEMENT 53 Human service educators are aware of all relevant curriculum standards, including those of the Council for Standards in Human Service Education (CSHSE), the Community Support Skills Standards, and state/local standards; and take them into consideration in designing the curriculum.

STATEMENT 54 Human service educators create a learning context in which students can achieve the knowledge, skills, values, and attitudes of the academic program.

Southern Regional Education Board. (1967). *Roles and Functions for Mental Health Workers: A Report of a Symposium.* Atlanta, GA: Community Mental Health Worker Project.

SOURCE: Ethical Standards of Human Service Professionals. (2000). *Human Service Education,* 20(1), 61–68. Reprinted with permission of National Organization of Human Service Education.

to a third step: generating possible courses of action. The fourth step is consideration of the consequences of each proposed course of action, and the final step is selection of the best course of action.

We have discussed dilemmas that involve competency and responsibility, confidentiality, and clients' rights and have presented short cases to illustrate problems that might arise in actual practice. The following questions may be useful as you consider how you would respond to each case. These questions correspond to the ethical decision-making model proposed by Van Hoose and Paradise (1979) and illustrated in Figure 9-1.

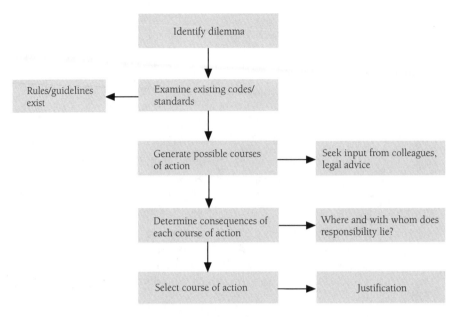

Figure 9-1 ✦ Ethical decision-making model

1. State the dilemma clearly. There may be more than one; if so, please think of all that you can.
2. What options are available to you?
3. What are the disadvantages and advantages of choosing each option?
4. What action do you choose?
5. What factor most influenced your decision?

Another place to use the ethical decision-making model is with dilemmas that are unique to a specific setting, for it provides a purposeful way of thinking about them. Human services in a correctional setting provides examples of such ethical conflicts. The dilemmas that correctional workers face illustrate the conflict between human service professionals' responsibilities to the client, to the agency, and to society. As an officer of the court, the corrections worker has the primary role of ensuring that clients do not break the law or injure others. This role places the professional in the position of judge, evaluator, and reporter, making establishing and maintaining helping relationships difficult. The following two dilemmas arise from a conflict between this primary role of the corrections worker and the human service professional's overriding concern for the welfare of the client (Page, 1979).

One dilemma may arise when the courts mandate counseling sessions for public offenders. The fact that counseling is imposed will probably impede the helping relationship. The second dilemma, which further complicates the relationship, occurs when the worker explains what confidentiality means in the corrections setting. If a client has violated an institution's rules or any state or

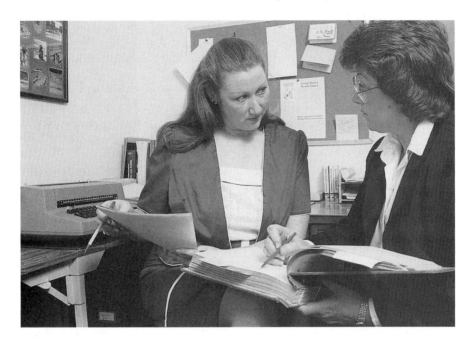

federal law and tells the worker of the violations, the professional is expected to report this information to the appropriate authorities. Many clients never develop the trust needed for a good helping relationship, refusing to share problems with the worker. Other clients may be reluctant to disclose real problems they are experiencing, as the worker is often in a position to provide information and make recommendations about clients. Thus, clients may tell the helper only good news, in hopes of securing a positive recommendation.

In situations like these, the professional should begin by identifying exactly what the conflict is. After reviewing ethical guidelines, the helper then considers possible courses of action and the consequences of each. It may be helpful at this point to ask coworkers for input and clarification as the professional explores what each course of action will mean to the client, to the agency, and to the helper. At some point, the helper will have to select a course of action. This ethical decision-making model provides only a structure for thinking about a dilemma; selecting a course of action may still be difficult. Apply what you have learned about ethical decision making to the following case.

The Ethical Dilemma of Counselor B

Background

Counselor B is working as a youth service counselor for the Child Welfare Board of an urban city. She has been asked by the court to see ten-year-old Nancy L. to determine if she should be returned to the custody of her mother. Nancy L. has been living with foster parents for the past two years.

The foster parents, Mr. and Mrs. S., have become quite attached to Nancy and have initiated legal proceedings to adopt her. Shortly after they informed the Child Welfare Board of their intentions, Nancy's natural mother, Mrs. L., hired a lawyer to regain custody of her daughter.

Nancy had been sent to live with her foster parents after her mother was convicted of prostitution. After serving six months, Mrs. L. was paroled and began working in a department store. She has recently married a former boyfriend. They have been married for almost a year and would like to have Nancy live with them.

For several weeks, Counselor B has been seeing all parties involved in the situation. The following background information has been obtained: Nancy has a loving relationship with her foster parents and does not want to be separated from them, even though she believes them to be very strict parents. During the first year that Nancy lived with them, her mother made no attempts to contact her or to see her. The foster parents believe that it was only after the mother learned of the impending adoption that she began to take an interest in her daughter. Counselor B has also learned through a former neighbor of Nancy's mother that the man Mrs. L. has married was also involved in the prostitution activities that caused her arrest. However, in talking with Mrs. L. and her husband, it was determined that both seem sincere in their desire to have Nancy in their home. Mrs. L. and her husband feel that Mrs. L. has paid for her past actions and that she has a right to have custody of her daughter. Mrs. L. states that prison was a very difficult adjustment for her and that it took some time for her to "get back on her feet." This is why she did not attempt to contact her daughter earlier. Mrs. L.'s husband claims he has a good job that will support Nancy and her mother and that Mrs. L. will be able to stay at home and devote her attentions to Nancy. Although he had some minor scrapes with the law as a juvenile, and although the police suspect him of continued involvement in prostitution, he has no police record.

The court would like the counselor's recommendation, as to whether Nancy should be returned to the custody of her natural mother, as soon as possible.

The Problem

Should the counselor recommend that Nancy be returned to her mother, overriding Nancy's wishes to remain with her foster parents? While Nancy's natural mother appears to be making a constructive change in her life, there is some suspicion as to whether this is really the case. Counselor B has just learned from the Child Welfare Agency that several unsubstantiated complaints have been filed against Mr. and Mrs. S., the foster parents, for the apparent harsh discipline they have exercised on previous children in their care.

The Dilemma

Should a mother be deprived of her child? Should Counselor B act on her suspicions about Nancy's mother and stepfather? Does Mrs. L. deserve to be pun-

ished again for past actions? What would you recommend? Why? To help you decide what Counselor B should do, answer the following questions:

1. *Exactly who is Counselor B's client?*
2. *What are the counselor's responsibilities to Nancy?*
3. *What are the counselor's responsibilities to Nancy's natural mother?*
4. *What impact do the wishes of ten-year-old Nancy have on Counselor B's recommendations?*
5. *What are the counselor's responsibilities to the court?*
6. *What are the counselor's responsibilities to society (i.e., the welfare of this child and others like her)?*
7. *Generate possible alternative courses of action stating why they were chosen.*
8. *What are the possible and probable consequences of the actions that Counselor B could take?*
9. *As Counselor B, what would you do and why? Which ethical standards support your decision?*

SOURCE: From Ethics in Counseling and Psychotherapy: Perspectives in Issues and Decision Making, by William H. Van Hoose and Louis V. Paradise, 1979, pp. 65–68. New York: Sulzburger & Graham.

 ## Day-to-Day Human Service Work

As stated earlier, human service professionals make many ethical decisions during the day that influence their work, their clients, and their agencies. At the time, many do not seem to be serious decisions; they appear to be merely choices about how professionals organize their work and spend their days. Many times there is little consideration as to the impact of the word or deed. Let us examine some of the issues and their potential effect on those involved in the helping process.

Allocation of Resources

The resources in the human service delivery system include staff, buildings, and money. Traditionally, administrators and boards of directors are responsible for allocating resources. It follows then that direct service professionals are solely involved in providing services once administrators have determined which services, where, and to whom they are to be provided. In reality, however, human service professionals are also involved in resource allocation. Often they determine how they will spend their time, how much time they will spend with each client, and which services the client needs or is eligible to receive. Since resources are limited and the demands for resources often exceed their availability in many agencies and organizations, the decisions made by human service professionals determine the type of services that each client receives.

In Chapter 1 you met Ms. Bailey, Almeada's first case manager. We were able to see her work with Almeada and appreciated her ability to support

Almeada—providing her information, services, and support during her prenatal care and after the birth of little Anne. In that chapter we had only one
view of Ms. Bailey, that of Almeada's helper. In the following paragraphs she
talks about her work during the days when she had Almeada as a client.

---

*Sometimes I think about my job during the time that I met Almeada. It was all
that I could do to keep my head above water, I was so busy. I was serving adolescents in the schools and also I was working with teenage dropouts. In addition, I was providing support for at-home young mothers. This was another
program that was run by the city. With these three responsibilities I had over
65 girls on my caseload at one time. Every day I tried to maintain a chart on
each of my clients, just so that I keep track of all of them. Looking back, I am
sure that it was an impossible task. In fact, I knew it even then, but I didn't
want to admit it.*

*But as I was saying, I would start every day and make a list of everything
I had to do, not things that I wanted to do. For example, I had minimum requirements for the young women whom I worked with in the home. For the first
month that they were on the program I was supposed to visit them once a week.
After the first three weeks, I was supposed to see them every month for the next
six months. Then they would be reevaluated to see if they could be referred to
another service. Also, during that time, the schools wanted me to act as a case
manager for any girls who were pregnant. I was to make a full assessment of
the situation—in another words, conduct an in-depth intake interview. Then I
would provide a list of goals and make appropriate referrals. The school referred about four girls to me each week. I tried hard to see all four during the
week that they were referred. I knew if I didn't do this, then I would be so behind that I would never catch up. And finally I worked with teenage dropouts
in a special program that identified irregular attendees who showed potential.
I received about 10 referrals a week, both boys and girls. Sometimes I would
discover that these girls were pregnant or that the boys were fathers-to-be.*

*I had two offices, one at the school and one at the welfare agency. I made
it a point to begin each day at the school. That way I could check in with the
office to see if I could gather any additional information about the students
that I was helping. Unfortunately when I began my work at the school, I did
not get to hear the early morning cries for help that I would occasionally receive from my young mothers. I also missed out on the "talk" with my colleagues at the welfare agency. For them, each morning was important. They
all checked in with each other at the coffee pot early in the day to discuss professional as well as personal business. So what I gained in helping my students
at the school, I lost in helping my clients at the welfare office.*

*The day that I received the referral about Almeada, I also received seven
other referrals. Almeada was the first student on the list, so I decided that I
would try to find her first. Taking the first person on the list was a technique
of mine that I used to try to decide where to start on my day. I would look
through the list of referrals and the list of students left from the day before for*

crisis situations; and I would check with the assistant principal to see if he had any information about the students or if there were any problems that I needed to attend to immediately. I was so alarmed when I first talked with Almeada's parents that I became determined to find her. They told me that she was pregnant and they resented this inconvenience. I knew that she needed my help; it was obvious that she had no support from her parents. Usually in the afternoon I worked with the welfare mothers or I looked for my dropouts. That afternoon, I found Almeada at the grocery store. I canceled an appointment that evening so that I could meet her after work.

As Ms. Bailey describes her work, it becomes obvious that she is involved in a daily allocation of her own resources. One resource is time. She is like many other human service professionals for she is not able to spend as much time as she would like with each client. She constantly makes decisions about how she allocates her time. In general she has decided that the pregnant teens and dropouts are a priority, so she spends the mornings of each day seeking them out and helping them plan for the future. When she began to gather information about Almeada, she discovered a very difficult situation. She determined that Almeada needed her immediate attention. She canceled an appointment with another client, so she could begin her work with Almeada. This meant that another client did not receive Ms. Bailey's services that evening (see Table 9-5).

Ms. Bailey also describes some of the resources that Almeada received at the expense of some of her other clients.

If you asked me about the most difficult part of my job, I would tell you not being able to give my clients all of the services that they need. So many times I discover programs that can serve my students or dropouts, especially the girls. At least ostensibly they can serve them. Often the girls are not eligible for the services or there are not enough services for all of the girls who need them. During the time that I spent with Almeada, I worried about her and her little girl, Anne. I tried to find several options for her to continue her education. I had a friend who ran a night program and she made an exception for me to accept Almeada. Almeada did not really have enough credits to quality for the

---

TABLE 9-5 ✦ SUMMARY POINTS: ALLOCATION OF RESOURCES

- Resources include staff, buildings, and money.
- Human service professionals are involved in resource allocation.
- When human service professionals determine how they will spend their time, they are involved in resource allocation.
- Decisions about implementation of a client plan also involves resource allocation.
- Special favors, extra attention, or concessions to clients also indicate involvement in resource allocation.

night classes. In the end Almeada did not participate in the class; but the fa-
vor was granted and now I owe my friend the next favor.

I took Almeada to a family-planning clinic. She was really scared to go.
Before the appointment she and I stopped at a fast-food restaurant to have a
soda and talk about the appointment and what she could expect. The school
believes that we should not buy our clients food—it is not a rule but a sugges-
tion. The school personnel think that sharing food constitutes "friendly" rela-
tionships with students and it is a use of time that cannot be documented. Hon-
estly, Almeada was so worried about the appointment that I thought if we could
just sit and talk in a place where she felt comfortable, then she might feel bet-
ter about going. It worked, but it was not time that I could account for in my
records.

The staff at the family-planning clinic really liked Almeada and they spent
almost twice as long as usual with her. She had so many questions and she was
so enthusiastic about everything they told her about pregnancy and prenatal
care. Rarely have they had such an attentive client. They asked her to partic-
ipate in an educational group that was meeting the next hour. It was for moth-
ers over 40 years of age and the class was full, but Almeada was ready for any
kind of class that they could offer. I went with her to the class, just to provide
her support. And I was her transportation home.

It is obvious that Almeada received quite a bit of special treatment from
Ms. Bailey and other professionals. Almeada brought an intensity and interest
to the helping process, and many professionals worked hard and "bent their
rules" to help her. Again, decisions were made to provide Almeada with resources—resources that could have been provided to someone else. Ms. Bailey
"breaks" the school suggestion not to take students "out" for lunch or a snack.
She is aware that she is violating this protocol, but feels that it was absolutely
necessary to help Almeada prepare for her appointment at the family-planning
clinic.

The staff at the family-planning clinic are completely taken with Almeada
and her enthusiasm for prenatal issues. They place her into a class that is already
full with clients who have little in common with her. It is their decision to serve
Almeada, perhaps at the expense of other people in the class. Ms. Bailey stayed
with Almeada at the family-planning clinic, since she was to provide Almeada
transportation. This was time that she could have used helping other clients.

Paperwork Blues

Paperwork is a part of the human service practice. It serves many functions including providing a permanent record for the services that are received by the
client. It documents client history in the human service delivery system to be
read by professionals who serve the clients in the future. A thorough written
record includes an intake interview, a social history, and medical, educational,
and mental health records. Paperwork also involves a record of referrals and

notes for client–helper meetings and documents the time that has been spent by an agency or professional which is used for billing and accountability audits. Paperwork is becoming increasingly important in this time of strict professional accountability and scarce resources. Work with insurance and managed care has not only intensified and complicated the need for paperwork, but has also created additional work for each professional who struggles with managing it all. Clearly, the task of doing the paperwork signifies less time for client contact. Ms. Bailey struggles with this exact problem.

I have always liked to do my paperwork. Most of the people that I work with really do not like it and some of them absolutely hate it. When I do my paperwork, it gives me a time to think about my clients, their problems, and how I can help them. I will admit that some of the paperwork drives me crazy, especially when I have to fill out the same forms with the same information. Thank heavens for computers. They do make the paperwork easier. When I was working with Almeada, the paperwork had actually become a nightmare for me because I was not used to it being such a challenge. Since I was working in three programs, I had to keep three sets of records. Each record-keeping system was not developed by me, so the forms and the information needed were very different. Sometimes I would try to fill out one form for the right person in the wrong program. I would catch myself before I did too much damage. Because I had two offices, it was also difficult to always have the things that I needed at the right office.

I have always been one to come early or stay late to do paperwork, but with three jobs, I had to do my paperwork in chunks during the day. I would actually get my activities mixed up and my plans would become fuzzy if I didn't stop and do the paperwork. So I did it in my car. What I regret is the amount of time that I spent with my papers. I had so many clients that could have used my help.

Each professional learns the importance of paperwork; and learning how to handle it represents an ethical decision. Some helpers are very well organized and they manage their paperwork beautifully and still manage to see a large number of clients. For most, the nature of the job with its crises and unexpected client requests works against any set time for paperwork. The best plans are often left unfulfilled. There is no doubt that the paperwork takes valuable time that could be used with the client. To solve that problem, workers often take their paperwork home, working long after hours so that they can spend more time with their clients. They then shortchange themselves on time to focus on self, families, and others. Some helpers shorten the time they spend on paperwork, not being as thorough as they might. Incomplete or spotty records do not help the agency or the client in the long run. Still others take the time to keep excellent records and accept this as part of the job, but then they have less client contact (see Table 9-6).

TABLE 9-6 ✦ SUMMARY POINTS: THE IMPORTANCE OF PAPERWORK

- Paperwork has a variety of functions that include establishing a permanent client record, documenting client history, writing important assessments and reports, documenting referrals and billing units, and providing a record for accountability purposes.
- Professionals determine how much time and effort will go into their paperwork and report writing.
- Intensive time spent with paperwork means less time with clients.

The Encapsulated or Burned-Out Professional

Working as a human service professional is challenging and rewarding. Unfortunately, the enthusiasm can fade as workers become disenchanted, experience disequilibrium, and behave in ways that are less than professional. One reaction to the stresses and strains experienced by workers in helping professions is becoming encapsulated—retreating from the engagement of helping and becoming rigid, insensitive, uncaring professionals. Another result of the pressures of the job may be burnout, a syndrome that can result in poor work performance or a decision to leave the profession. As the states of encapsulation or burnout effect the human service professional, ethical issues arise as these professionals interact with their clients and their coworkers in less than positive ways.

Helpers who become encapsulated may become static in their work as they face the difficulties of working within the human service delivery system. They may feel so threatened and frightened by the difficult tasks they are asked to perform that they quit learning, growing, and trying—thus becoming encapsulated. Such workers relate to clients in characteristic ways. First, they become rigid and inflexible, believing that there are enduring truths that must be upheld. Such truths can take many forms, such as "The system's rules are always right and just" or "Individuals who are unemployed do not deserve to be helped." If human service workers are not static but dynamic, their personal and professional experiences modify their ideas about clients and the entire delivery system. They grow, learning about the system and how it operates as well as learning about the self. To cling to the "truths" workers have at the beginning of their professional careers limits what they can learn from their experiences.

Ms. Bailey talks about a time when she was encapsulated as a worker. She learned a lot during this time and believes that she is now a more committed professional as a result of the experience.

Earlier I talked about my incredible schedule and workload. What I did not talk about was how much I enjoy my work. Working with adolescents is a great job. The preceding year, though, was a time of professional crisis for me. At this point I am able to see how much I have grown as a professional. I was once fairly rigid as a human service professional. Today it is almost impossi-

ble to believe that I could have been an effective helper. Maybe you should be the judge. Let me tell you a little bit more about it.

This trauma happened early in my career. I had been working with teenagers in a girls and boys club setting. I was so excited about my work when I began. I would get up and head to work about 7 A.M., just to be the first person in the building. By the time that the young children arrived at 7:30 A.M. I was ready for them. I became involved in the lives of many of the families of my clients and I worried about each and every one of them. I also was absolutely sure what would be best for them. I had a wonderful family life and was raised by loving and gentle parents. I was appalled by what I thought was the inadequate and sometimes frightening parenting that I saw. Many of the parents were not at home for their children; babies were left with older siblings while parents worked. Some of the parents had extreme ways of disciplining their children. I tried to change the behaviors of these parents and became so frustrated when they refused to change. When I look back now, I think the only thing that saved my relationship with these parents was my absolute dedication to helping them. They knew that they could depend upon me, even if I was constantly trying to show them a better way to raise their children. But by the end of the school year, I was frustrated and really did not like the parents. I was not sure that they deserved my attention since they were not changing their ways.

Change came slowly to me. During the summer I enrolled in two graduate classes. My supervisor understood how frustrated I was and she suggested that I work my eight hours on the afternoon shift and go to school each morning. These courses opened up a whole new world to me. My professionals challenged me to think about social problems in new ways. But it was talking with my classmates that had the greatest effect. Three students in my classes had been on welfare while raising their children. They spoke with some bitterness about the treatment they received from some professionals who assumed there was a "right" way to raise kids and that it was shameful to be on welfare. I listened and learned about the painful effects of the judgments of others.

Even when working with Almeada, I found I wanted to take her home, to give her the stable and safe environment all children should have. But I know now that it's okay to feel that way. I just can't act on those feelings. It's important to recognize the feelings and to behave in a professional manner that is good for the client and good for me as the helper.

In the vignette, Ms. Bailey describes another characteristic of encapsulated human service professionals, that of retaining the beliefs of the traditional culture. Ms. Bailey is sure that she understands the best ways of child rearing. Her ideas come from her own culture and her own experience. She is not open to alternative ways of caring for children. She describes being encapsulated and accepting the values of the times unquestioningly, no matter what pain those values may cause clients. She listened carefully and with great concern to clients, and then asked them to conform to the social norms. What she did not realize is that many people who seek help are not part of the traditional culture. To ask them to give up their own beliefs, lifestyles, and culture is to violate the values of human services. To demand that clients conform to the traditional culture is hardly a sign of tolerance and concern for individual clients and respect for their self-determination. Encapsulation had lead to unethical behavior and unfair treatment of clients. It can also impair the helping process.

Encapsulated workers depend only on their own personal experiences and frames of reference, which limits their understanding of clients. There are many different types of clients and client situations, and it is difficult for workers to be familiar with all of them. As a result, workers should constantly read, discuss, and observe clients so as to broaden the base from which they understand clients' experiences. Workers who do not expand their knowledge remain limited in the types of clients they can serve. Ms. Bailey certainly learned from her earlier experience at the boys and girls club. When she was working with Almeada, she did not suggest to her what specific action she should take after the birth of her daughter. Ms. Bailey provided Almeada with information, support, and a network of support services to use during her pregnancy and after baby Anne was born.

One way to address the problem of encapsulation is through a commitment to lifelong learning. Part of learning is making changes in behaviors and attitudes; change and growth can be very exciting parts of the learning process, though difficult at times. Part of the change process is *unlearning,* which can counteract the encapsulated workers' tendencies to cling to truths and to accept the values of the traditional culture. To avoid or counteract encapsulation, workers must constantly try to develop professionally by revising and updating the knowledge, skills, and values of the profession. Ms. Bailey's experience in graduate school opened up new ways of thinking for her. Because she was able to listen carefully to the experiences of her classmates and identify her own behaviors, she was able to be more objective about her own assumptions and begin to hold them in check as she worked with the parents at the boys and girls club (see Table 9-7).

As mentioned, another result of the stress and strain new professionals experience is burnout. This condition results from negative changes in attitudes and behavior that are precipitated by job strain (Cherniss, 1980). Like encap-

---

TABLE 9-7 ✦ SUMMARY POINTS: ENCAPSULATION AND BURNOUT

Encapsulation occurs when:
   Professionals become static in their work;
   Professionals become rigid and inflexible and uphold their own beliefs or truths;
   Professionals support the beliefs of the traditional culture; and
   Clients are asked to accept norms of the traditional culture.
Burnout occurs when:
   There are multiple pressures at work over a long period of time;
   Professionals have unrealistic expectations about their job outcomes;
   Professionals begin to miss work, arrive late, denigrate their clients; and
   The bureaucracy does not support the professional or the client.

sulation, burnout effects the day-to-day work of the professional and results in unethical behavior that has negative effects on the helping relationship and the helping process. There are identifiable pressures that lead to burnout. Loss of idealism and disappointment in client motivations may result in a loss of commitment to both job and clients. Professionals who experience burnout may also be reacting to a less-than-perfect work setting—one that is too demanding, too frustrating, or too boring.

Some symptoms of burnout are a change in attitude about work, lower expectations of performance, severe emotional detachment from work, reduced psychological involvement with clients, and an intense concern with self. As professionals burn out, they are likely to perceive work more negatively, resulting in sick days, tardiness, and clock watching. The syndrome also affects how workers perceive clients. They may call them names behind their backs, become angry with them, or feel that they are irresponsible and ungrateful for the help that is given them. These behaviors all impact negatively on the helper's ability to assist the client. They violate many of the basic values of helping such as tolerance and acceptance of the client. In addition, individuals who are themselves involuntary clients are less likely to respond positively or see helpers in a positive light.

There are also some physical symptoms of burnout, such as chronic fatigue, frequent colds, serious illness, stomach trouble, lower back pain, and perhaps even substance abuse. Burnout may also affect the person's relationships with others outside of work, and the helper may be unable to take up new hobbies or concentrate on anything for long periods of time.

Ms. Bailey has only experienced periodic burnout, but she has worked with a number of professionals who have experienced severe cases. During the time she was working with Almeada, she showed signs of the syndrome. It was because she was working such long hours. Although she was never late or tardy, she began to resent her large caseload. She would complain about her job to her friends and family; but she never took it out on her clients, or so she thought.

Ms. Bailey had begun to notice little things that denoted signs of burnout. As a result, she began immediately to correct her pattern of long days and long nights. It is easy to lose your way when so many clients need so much.

Burnout is not temporary strain, but rather a pattern of being and thinking that cannot easily be interrupted unless specific efforts are made to alleviate it. It is not just "poor adjustment" that can be corrected with increased time on the job. Recovery from burnout is a long process that necessitates many changes in the life and work of the professionals who are affected.

Burnout must be alleviated if the helper is to be effective. Changing one's career orientation, encouraging institutional change, increasing the intrinsic rewards of work, and improving the quality of life outside work are all ways professionals can counteract burnout. To develop a different career orientation, human service professionals adopt a more realistic view of what a career means to them, both personally and professionally. This also means realistically assessing what helpers can expect to do for clients, what they can expect from the organization, and how much fulfillment they should expect from their jobs. Part of this assessment is deciding what job activities are rewarding and then concentrating on those aspects. Because extrinsic rewards are not always available, workers must often depend on intrinsic rewards. They can learn to measure their performance by their own professional standards and begin to identify and articulate what they do well, rather than glossing over their successes in light of perceived failures.

The issues of realistic expectations and intrinsic rewards are also directly related to improving the quality of life outside of work. When work is an individual's major or only focus, it must fill psychological and social needs, such as the need to be close to others, to belong, to be creative, and to relax. Rarely can any one activity, even work in the human services, satisfy all these needs. Some can be met through well-chosen activities outside of work.

Ms. Bailey has always tried to have a life outside of work. It helps that she has a family of her own. They keep her in balance, not only because they demand a lot from her, but also because she wants to spend time with them and do things for them. They are also very supportive of her work. Her husband makes sacrifices so that she might help her clients. She has detected the signs of burnout before. To make the correction, she intentionally begins to refocus her energies on her family and herself. It always requires a major effort.

The human service organization can counteract burnout in other ways. Bureaucracies may not know how to protect their helpers; professionals may have to provide the leadership to promote these changes. One effective strategy is to establish a work structure that helps workers avoid boredom by varying work, responsibility, and routine. When individuals work in predictable patterns day after day, they get tired and begin to function like machines rather than human beings. A slight change in responsibility, timing, or setting may prevent boredom. Another strategy is to implement ways of recognizing and rewarding workers' efforts. Such extrinsic rewards as certificates of merit, small promotions, asking of workers' opinions, raises in pay, changes of job title, and support for education or professional development can all provide workers with formal recognition for jobs well done. Another approach is to provide a mechanism for workers to give feedback and effect even small changes in agency role, procedure, or policy. This provides professionals with evidence that they can make a difference and that the bureaucracy is not indifferent to those who are working on the frontline.

Ms. Bailey has always been employed by social service agencies. She has worked in a variety of circumstances. Some of the agencies support their pro-

fessionals, while others continue to make demands without caring for staff. At one point, Ms. Bailey worked for an agency that refused to allow its professionals to take vacation time. The director stated that the agency just could not operate with a reduced staff. In that agency Ms. Bailey helped other professionals to develop a plan to cover responsibilities that would allow others to take vacation time. Ms. Bailey admits that at times she has had to leave an agency because she was suffering both physically and mentally.

Another effective response to burnout is a focus on wellness—considering the well-being of individuals from the perspectives of their social, psychological, nutritional, safety, physical, and creative needs. The wellness movement is committed to educating individuals to take responsibility for their own lives, thus promoting a fuller, more satisfying lifestyle. The ultimate goal of the wellness movement is to promote the growth and development of individuals and to encourage them to strive for self-actualization, the highest stage of development in Maslow's hierarchy.

Ms. Bailey has firm ideas about using the concept of wellness in her work. Many times she chooses colleagues in her referral network who support the notion of wellness for themselves and for their clients.

Today I have some better ideas about how to sustain myself so that my day to day work with my clients is upbeat, positive and respectful. The concept of wellness is always with me. I see wellness as a proactive way of caring for ones' self. And that is the ultimate goal that I have with all of my clients. If I do not model the behavior and take care of myself, then how can I expect them to do so. One of the reasons that I took Almeada to the family planning clinic was because the concept of wellness is implicit in all that they do as they deliver their services. One specific goal that they have is for every client to walk away from the clinic believing that care for themselves is a priority. They try to teach that self-care is the first step in caring for others. I think that Almeada was such a willing participant, they wanted to help her all that they could right on the spot. That is one of the reasons that they immediately placed her in their class for mothers-to-be.

Professional Development

We believe one key to resolving the ethical issues that affect the day-to-day work of the helper is a commitment to professional development. We recommend such a commitment as a means of keeping the professional engaged and well supported in the delivery of services. Critical to improving one's professional standing is a commitment to developing new knowledge and skills. This is one goal of professional development that can also help counteract encapsulation and burnout. The ultimate goal is to be a more effective helper and to be able to respond to each helping opportunity in a way that positively supports the client.

The ethical dimensions of professional development are numerous. If a helper is not involved in learning new knowledge about clients, developing and improving skills, and reflecting on current practice, then the services provided may become less than adequate. Within the field of human services, new information is available about the problems clients experience. New methodologies are being developed to help professionals address client needs. As the field of human service delivery constantly changes, professionals also need to assess what these changes mean for their work with clients. We ask the question, Is it ethical to continue to serve clients in the same way, year after year, since their problems change, the world in which they live shifts, and new ways of helping continually emerge? We believe that continuing professional growth is critical.

Both formal and informal approaches to continuing education are important to professional growth. Returning to school for an advanced degree—whether it be an associate, baccalaureate, master's, doctorate, or specialist degree—is a legitimate way to continue professional education in the human services. Such formal education will also open alternative career paths and allow helpers to increase their qualifications and competence. The possibilities of formal education are many and include earning an associate of arts or science degree in human services or a more specialized program such as child care or mental health technology; earning a bachelor of arts or science degree in human services, social work, liberal arts, or education; or earning a master's or doctoral degree in social work, public health, rehabilitation, child and family studies, business, or law. Such degrees give professionals additional expertise and flexibility for future career moves and also enhance their performance in their current positions.

In-service training is also an excellent way to develop new expertise. Many workshops and conferences are available within an organization, or within the working radius of the professional, to broaden his or her understanding of client needs and the changing times. Other education opportunities may focus on developing one or two specific skills in greater depth. Ms. Bailey shares with us her own experiences with professional development.

I already described how indebted I am to my summer educational experience when I worked with the boys and girls club. My fellow students allowed me to see the "client experience" from another perspective. As they talked about their work with helpers and their frustrations with the helping process, I felt shame for the way in which I had treated the parents with whom I had worked. But we learned in class how to avoid treating clients in such a disrespectful way, so I was able to replace one set of thoughts and behaviors with another. Since that summer, I have continued to believe that professional development is a critical part of becoming a professional.

Sometimes it is easy to be involved in professional development. Other times it seems impossible to take the time to attend a workshop, lecture, or class. I know the times that I think I am too busy to go are the very times that

TABLE 9-8   ✦   SUMMARY POINTS: PROFESSIONAL DEVELOPMENT

- Ethical behavior includes a commitment to professional development.
- Helpers should continually be involved in new learning.
- Ways in which the helper can develop are by attending a college or university class, participating in in-service training, and becoming active in professional and community organizations.

I should quit what I am doing and sign up for that seminar or workshop. I am always so glad once I am there. There is an excitement when I am involved in learning. It is also a good way to share ideas with other professionals and to expand my professional network. The last workshop that I attended was three months ago. The focus was substance abuse, which is a common problem among my clientele. I learned how the very latest brain research impacts the way in which we now deliver treatment to this population. Three professionals in my discussion group volunteered to establish a "group counseling" experience for my pregnant girls.

Commitment to the profession is also a part of professional development. When human service professionals become active in an organization or become active members of the community, they expand their professional associations and their professional awareness. Any time they study political issues or become deeply involved in ethical situations that are difficult to comprehend, they are expanding their professional understanding. Even the continuous updating of their knowledge of the community, its workers, and its resources is an informal development process (see Table 9-8).

This chapter on professional ethics concludes your introduction to the field of human services. This material on professional ethics and ethical dilemmas should help you reflect on professional issues in light of your new understanding of human services. Understanding the more subtle ethical issues that permeate the helping process will help you think more clearly about your day-to-day work. Professional development represents a lifelong commitment to study and will help you as you reflect about your role and effectiveness in human service delivery. Whether the work involves resolving ethical dilemmas or focuses on meeting the challenges of demanding clients, thoughtful reflection and professional development support the human service professional.

 Things to Remember

1. In the course of delivering human services, the professional may encounter numerous ethical dilemmas; for some of these, the worker may be unsure of the appropriate action to take.
2. Professionals have responded to the dilemmas of service provision by developing codes of ethics or statements of ethical standards of

behavior for the members of their profession. Items are included that state the goals or aims of the profession, protect the client, provide guidance as to professional behavior, and contribute to a professional identity for the worker.

3. Most codes of ethics indicate that the helper's first responsibility is to enhance and protect the client's welfare.

4. Two areas with which helpers concern themselves are their *competence* as professionals and their *responsibility* to the individuals, groups, or organizations with whom they are affiliated or whom they serve as clients.

5. Confidentiality is the worker's assurance to the client that information divulged by the client will remain between the two of them.

6. Two examples of clients' rights are the right to privacy and informed consent.

7. The professional is also involved in making ethical decisions in the day-to-day work.

8. When helpers make resource allocation decisions, they are deciding how and what resources are to be given to whom. Evidence of this is how helpers spend their time. Time with one client limits the time that the helper can spend with another.

9. Paperwork is a necessary and important part of human service work. It serves a variety of functions. When the demands of paperwork are excessive, it is possible that work with the clients may suffer.

10. Professionals often become tired and frustrated with their work in human service delivery. Two ways in which they cope are encapsulation and burnout. Neither way is helpful to the client or the professional.

11. Professional development is one way that professionals actively avoid encapsulation and burnout and enhance their competence as professionals.

Additional Readings: Focus on Professionalism

Bollas, C., & Sundelson, D. (1995). *The new informants: The betrayal of confidentiality in psychoanalysis and psychotherapy.* Northvale, NJ: Aronson.
The authors survey, analyze, and attack the trend away from secrecy, which they attribute partly to the let-it-all-hang-out standard of contemporary culture.

Dickenson, D. T. (1995). *Law and the health and human services.* New York: Free Press.
This book focuses specifically on the law as it applies to the broad field of health and human services and on the legal issues that challenge its many professionals.

Douglass, M. E., & Douglass, D. N. (1993). *Manage your time, your work, yourself.* New York: American Management Association.
Covering every aspect of time management, this guide offers seven steps to transform time wasters to time masters.

Johnson, D. W. (1993). *Reaching out: Interpersonal effectiveness and self-actualization* (5th ed.). Boston: Allyn & Bacon.

This book outlines the theory and experience necessary to develop effective interpersonal skills such as building relationships, resolving interpersonal conflicts, and increasing communications skills.

Sykes, C. J. (1999). *The end of privacy.* New York: St. Martin's Press.

Privacy—the right to be left alone—is the most valued right enjoyed by Americans; but computer, video, and audio technology, marketing databases, and the media have us all under attack.

References

Administration on Aging. (1999, April 19). *Administration continues to address long-term care at local forum.* Retrieved December 19, 1999, from the World Wide Web: wysiwyg://421/http://www.aoa.dhhs.gov/pr/advo4199.

Afifi, A., & Breslow, L. (1994). The maturing paradigm of public health. *Annual Review of Public Health, 15,* 223–235.

Aguilera, D. C. (1998). *Crisis intervention: Theory and methodology.* St. Louis: Mosby.

Ahia, C. E., & Martin, D. (1993). *The danger-to-self-or-others exception to confidentiality.* Alexandria, VA: American Counseling Association.

Ainsworth, M. (1999). *E-therapy Mental Health Net.* Retrieved on December 9, 1999, from the World Wide Web: http://www.mentalhelp.net/guide/cyber.

Albee, G. W. (1961a). *Action for mental health.* New York: Basic Books.

Albee, G. W. (1961b). *Mental health manpower trends.* New York: Basic Books.

Alemangno, S., Frank, S., Mosavel, M., & Butts, J. (1998). Screening adolescents for health risks using interactive voice response technology: An evaluation. *Computers in Human Services, 15*(4). Retrieved October 23, 1999, from the World Wide Web: http://www2.uta.edu/cussn/jths/vol115.htm.

American Dietetic Association. (1999). *Position of the American Dietetic Association: Nutrition, aging, and the contin-uum of care.* Retrieved October 22, 1999, from the World Wide Web: http://www.eatright.org/adaposag.html.

American Psychological Association. (1999). *About the American Psychological Association.* Retrieved June 13, 1999, from the World Wide Web: http://www.apa.org/about.

Anderson, V. (1998, October 25). Teachers struggle to be "last safety net." *The Atlanta Journal Constitution,* p. A1.

Association for Specialists in Group Work. (1991). *Ethical guidelines for group counselors and professional standards for the training of group workers.* Alexandria, VA: Author.

Austin, C. (1983). Case management: A systems perspective. *Families in Society: The Journal of Contemporary Human Services, 79,* 451–459.

Axelson, J. A. (1999). *Counseling and development in a multicultural society* (3rd ed.). Pacific Grove, CA: Brooks/Cole.

Barker, B. (1996). *The management of information.* Presentation conducted at the Managed Care Institute: Future-care preparing for managed care and children's services, Nashville, TN.

Bartlett, R. C. (1994). *The direct option.* College Station, TX: Texas A&M University Press.

Bassoff, E. (1987). Mothering adolescent daughters: A psychodynamic perspective. *Journal of Counseling and Development, 65*(9), 471–474.

Beers, C. W. (1945). *A mind that found itself: An autobiography.* Garden City, NY: Doubleday, Doran & Co.

Blankertz, L. E., & Cnaan, R. A. (1995). Assessing the impact of two residential programs for dually diagnosed homeless individuals. *Social Service Review, 68*(4), 536–560.

Boland, T. (1998, December 13). *HUD: $850M homeless local assistance/ continuum of care grants. Arizona State Public Information Network.* Retrieved September 13, 1999, from the World Wide Web: http://aspin.asu.edu/hpn/ archives/Dec98/044.html.

Bosworth, K. (1994). Computer games and simulations as tools to reach and engage adolescents in health promotion activities. [Abstract]. *Computers in Human Services, 11*(1/2). Retrieved March 15, 1996, from the World Wide Web: http://www.uta.edu/cuss/ vol1.htm.

Bowler, M. (1974). *The Nixon guaranteed income proposal: Substance and process in policy change.* Cambridge, MA: Ballinger.

Boy, A., & Pine, G. (1968). *The counselor in the schools: A reconceptualization.* Boston: Houghton Mifflin.

Brammer, L. M. (1999). *The helping relationship* (7th ed.). Boston: Allyn & Bacon.

Brammer, L. M. (1978). Informal helping systems in selected subcultures. *Personnel and Guidance Journal, 56,* 476–479.

Brewin, B. (1999, January 29). Web link forces with families, services. *IDG.net.* Retrieved June 20, 1999, from the WWW: http://ww.edu. town.shibecha. hokkaido.jp:14966/-_-http://europe. cnn.com/TECH/computing/9901/29/ navyweb.idg/index.html.

Brill, N. I. (1998). *Working with people: The helping process* (6th ed.). New York: Longman.

Bronfenbrenner, U. (1979). *The ecology of human development.* Cambridge, MA: Harvard University Press.

Brown, D., & Srebalus, D. J. (1996). *An introduction to the counseling profession* (2nd ed.). Boston: Allyn & Bacon.

Brown, T. (1992, March 2). Why teams go bust. *Industry Week,* 20.

Burger, W. R., & Youkeles, M. (2000). *Human services in contemporary America* (5th ed.). Pacific Grove, CA: Brooks/ Cole.

Burns, B., Burke, J., & Ozarin, L. (1983). Linking health and mental health services in rural areas. *International Journal of Mental Health, 12,* 130–143.

Butterfield, F. (1996, November). In Boston, nothing is something. *The New York Times,* A8.

Cahill, J. M. (1994). HealthWorks: Interactive AIDS education mldeogrames. [Abstract] *Computers in Human Services, 11*(1/2). Retrieved March 15, 1996, from the World Wide Web: http://www.uta.edu/cuss/vol11.htm.

Cahill, M. (1993). Computer technology and human services in the 90s: Advancing theory and practice: Teleshopping and social services in the United Kingdom. In M. Leiderman, C. Guzetta, L. Struminger, & M. Monnickdam (Eds.), *Technology in people services: Research, theory, and application* (pp. 231–245). New York: Haworth.

Caring Company. (1998). *Appalachia: Journal of the Appalachian Regional Commission, 31*(2), 26.

Cathcart, J. (1990). *Relationship selling: The key to getting and keeping customers.* New York: Perigee Books.

Cherniss, C. (1980). *Professional burnout in human service organizations.* New York: Praeger.

Cimmino, P. (1999). Basic concepts and definitions of human services. In H. S. Harris & D. C. Maloney (Eds.), *Human services: Contemporary issues and trends* (pp. 9–21). Boston: Allyn & Bacon.

Clear, T. R., & Cole, G. F. (1997). *American corrections* (5th ed.). Belmont, CA: Wadsworth.

Clifford, P. J., Norcross, J., & Summer, R. (1999). Autobiographies of mental health clients. *Professional Psychology: Research and Practice, 30*(11), 56–59.

Clubok, M. (2001). The aging of America. In T. McClam & M. Woodside (Eds.), *Human services in the 21st cen-*

tury. New York: Council for Standards in Human Service Education, pp. 339–346.

Cohen, R., & Lavach, C. (1995). Strengthening partnerships between families and service providers. In P. Adams & K. Nelson (Eds.), *Reinventing human services: Community and family-centered practice* (pp. 262–277). New York: Aldine deGruyter.

Collier, R. (1965). *The general next to God: The story of William Booth and the Salvation Army.* New York: Dutton.

Collins, J. (1999). When good managers manage too much. *Inc., 21*(5), 31–32.

Combs, A. W. (1969). *Florida studies in the helping profession.* Gainesville, FL: University of Florida Press.

Committee Study of the Future of Public Health Institute of Medicine. (1988). *The future of public health.* Washington, DC: National Academy Press.

Cook, C., Selig, K., & Wedge, B. (1999). *Social Work, 44*(2), 129–139.

Cormier, M. (1979). From the council president. *Bulletin: Council for Standards in Human Services Education, 1*(1), 1.

Corey, G., Corey, M. S., & Callanan, P. (1998). *Issues and ethics in the helping professions.* Pacific Grove, CA: Brooks/Cole.

Council for Standards in Human Service Education (CSHSE). (1985). *Handbook* (2nd ed.). Atlanta, GA: Author.

Cranston, A. (1986). Psychology in the Veterans Administration. *American Psychologist, 41*(9), 990–995.

Crimando, E., & Riggar, T. F. (1996). *Utilizing community services: An overview of human service.* Del Ray Beach, FL: St. Lucia.

Crossette, B. (1996, June 11). New tally of world tragedy: Women who die giving life. *The New York Times,* A1, A7.

Crossette, B. (1995, December 11). UNICEF sees children as major victims of war. *The New York Times,* A7.

Desjarlais, R., Eisenberg, L., Good, B., & Kleinman, A. (1995). *World mental health: Problems and priorities in low-income countries.* New York: Oxford University Press.

Dewan, M. (1999). Are psychiatrists cost effective? An analysis of integrated versus split treatment. *The American Journal of Psychiatry, 156*(2), 324–326.

DeWitt, E. P. (1994, July 25). Battle for the soul INTERNET. *Time,* 50–56.

Dillon, N. (1999, June 14). Web should prepare for a non-English majority. *CNN Interactive.* Retrieved October 14, 1999, from the World Wide Web: http://www.edu.town.shibecha. hokkaido.jp:14966/-_-http://europe. cnn.com/TECH/computing/9902/12/ globalnet.idg/index.html/.

Dickerson, F. (1998). Strategies that foster empowerment. *Cognitive and Behavioral Practice, 5,* 255–275.

Dryfoos, J. (1994). *Full-service schools.* San Francisco: Jossey-Bass.

Egan, G. E. (1998). *The skilled helper: A problem management approach to helping* (6th ed.). Pacific Grove, CA: Brooks/Cole.

Ehrenreich, J. (1985). *The altruistic imagination.* Ithacca, NY: Cornell Press.

Ellis, S. J., & Noyes, K. H. (1978). *By the people: A history of Americans as volunteers.* Philadelphia, PA: Energize.

English, J. T., Kritzler, Z. A., & Scherl, D. J. (1984). Historical trends in the financing of psychiatric services. *Psychiatric Annals, 14*(5), 321–331.

Epstein, C. (1981). *Introduction to human services.* Englewood Cliffs, NJ: Prentice Hall.

Eriksen, K. (1981). *Human services today.* Reston, VA: Reston Publishing.

Erikson, E. (1963). *Childhood and society.* New York: Norton.

Farrell, M. (1997). Processing recyclables at correctional facilities. *Biocycle, 38*(8), 34.

Fetterman, D. (2000). Empowerment evaluation: Collaboration, action research, and a case Example. Retrieved September 3, 2000, from the World Wide Web: http://www.aepro.org/ inprint/conference/fetterman. html.

Foegen, J. (1999). Why not empowerment? *Business and Economic Review, 45*(3), 31–33.

For a healthy nation. (1988). Washington, DC: U.S. Department of Health and Human Services, Public Health Services.

Frager, D., Coyne, L., Lyle, J., Coulter, P., Graham, P., Sargent, J., & Allen, J. (1999). Which treatments help? The patient's perspective. *Bulletin of the Menninger Clinic, 63*(3), 388–400.

Franklin, R. M. (1995, September). Emotion and the physician–patient relationship. *Motivation and Emotion, 19*(3), 163–173.

Freddolino, P., & Han, A. S. (1998). Direct service application of videoconferencing technologies: Case example for Korea and the United States. *Computers in Human Services, 15*(6). Retrieved June 23, 1999, from the World Wide Web: http://www2.uta.edu/cussn/jths/vol116.htm.

Friedland, R., & Summer, L. (1999). *Demography is not destiny.* Washington, DC: National Academy on an Aging Society.

Friedman, D. (1996, March 24). Ahead: A very different nation. *U.S. News & World Report, 120,* 16.

Friedrich, O. (1976). *Going crazy: An inquiry into madness in our time.* New York: Avon Books.

Fujimura, L. E., Weis, D. M., & Cochran, J. R. (1985). Suicide: Dynamics and implications for counseling. *Journal of Counseling and Development, 63,* 612–615.

Fullerton, S. (1999). Theories as tools and resources for helping. In H. S. Harris & D. C. Maloney (Eds.), *Human services: Contemporary issues and trends* (pp. 71–78). Boston: Allyn & Bacon.

Galbraith, J. K. (1976). *The affluent society.* Boston: Houghton Mifflin.

Gardner, M. (1996, March 21). Tide shifts on how to protect abused children. *The Christian Science Monitor,* 12.

Gariti, P., Alterman, A. I., Holub-Beyer, E., & Volpicelli, J. R. (1995, May–June). Effects of an appointment reminder call on patient show rates. *Journal of Substance Abuse Treatment, 12*(3), 207–212.

Garrett, S. (1998). *Miles to go: Aging in rural Virginia.* Charlottesville, VA: University Press of Virginia.

Gaiske, G. (1999). The challenge of rehabilitation counselors: Work with people with psychiatric disabilities. *Journal of Rehabilitation, 65*(1), 21–25.

Ginsberg, L. H. (1998). Introduction: An overview of rural social work. In L. H. Ginsberg (Ed.), *Social work in rural communities* (pp. 1–22). Alexandria, VA: Council on Social Work Education.

Ginsberg, L. H. (1987). Economic, political and social context. In L. H. Ginsberg (Ed.), *Encyclopedia of Social Work* (18th ed.) (pp. xxxii–xxxvi). Silver Springs, MD: National Association of Social Workers.

Gladding, S. T. (1999). *Group work: A counseling specialty.* Upper Saddle River, NJ: Merrill.

Golden, T. (1996, August 1). People on welfare, too, find a 1st to criticize. *The New York Times,* A9.

Goodman, M., Brown, J., & Dietz, P. (1992). *Managing managed care.* Washington, DC: American Psychiatric Press.

Gordon, J. (2000, January 3). Immigrants fight the power. *The Nation, 270*(1), 16–20.

Gould, P. L. (1992). Adult developmental brief computer-assisted therapy. In J. L. Feldman & R. J. Fitzpatrick (Eds.), *Managed mental healthcare* (pp. 347–358). Washington, DC: American Psychiatric Press.

Granello, M. S. (1995, March/April). Creating links: Electronically. *The Advocate, 18*(7), 6.

Gray, J. I. (1994). Problem solving in case management (PIC): A computer assisted instruction simulation. [Abstract] *Computers in Human Services, 11*(1/2). Retrieved October 23, 1999, from the World Wide Web: http://www.uta.edu/cuss/vol11.htm.

Grebel, H. W. (1993). Information technology in the care of the mentally handicapped: An educational approach. In M. Leiderman, C. Guzetta, L. Struminger, & M. Monnickendam

(Eds.), *Technology in people services: Research, theory, and application* (pp. 329–335). New York: Haworth.

Green Ontario (2000). *Green Ontario.* Retrieved March 11, 2000, from the World Wide Web: http://www.green ontario.com/.

Grier, P. (1996, March 6). New Census Bureau portrait of the American landscape. *The Christian Science Monitor,* 3.

Gross, A., & McMullen, P. (1982). The help seeking process. In V. Derlega & J. Grzelak (Eds.), *Cooperation and helping behavior* (pp. 306–324). New York: Academic Press.

Gruber, M. (Ed.). (1981). *Management systems in the human services.* Philadelphia: Temple University Press.

Guardian for Scripps Howard News Service (The). (1998, Nov. 3). Computer sees climate catastrophe arriving by mid-century. *Knoxville News-Sentinel,* A5.

Haines, V., Petit, A., & Lefrancois, S. (1999). Explaining client satisfaction with an employee assistance program. *Employee Assistance Quarterly, 14*(4), 65–78.

Hamlin, P. (1985). *Experiences in mental institutions: Case studies.* Unpublished manuscript.

Harrington, M. (1962). *The other America.* New York: Macmillan.

Harris, H. S., & Maloney, D. C. (Eds.). (1999). *Human services: Contemporary issues and trends.* Boston: Allyn & Bacon.

Hazard, T. G. (1844, April 10). Astonishing tenacity of life. *Providence Journal,* 252–253.

Healthy people 2000: Midcourse review and 1995 revisions. (1995). Washington, DC: U.S. Department of Health and Human Services, Public Health Service.

Healy, M. (1998, December 2). *Welfare reform's success reaches inevitable slow-down those remaining on rolls will be harder to help.* Retrieved June 18, 1999, from the World Wide Web: http://www.sfgate.com/cgibin/article/ archive/1998/12/02/MN45270.DTL.

Hecht, D. (1996, July 25). Senegal's kid workers unite, demand rights. *The Christian Science Monitor,* 6.

Herlihy, B., & Sheeley, V. L. (1987). Privileged communication in selected helping professions: A comparison among statutes. *Journal of Counseling and Development, 65*(9), 479–483.

Hoff, L. A. (1995). *People in crisis: Understanding and helping.* San Francisco: Jossey-Bass.

Hoffman, D. L., & Novak, T. (1998). Bridging the racial divide on the internet. *Science, 17,* 390–391.

Holmes, S. (1996, March 14). Census sees a profound shift in ethnic U.S. *The New York Times,* A8.

Homan, M. (1999). *Promoting community change* (2nd ed.). Pacific Grove, CA: Brooks Cole.

Hook, M. P., & Ford, M. E. (1998). The linkage model for delivering mental health services in rural communities: Benefits and challenges. *Health & Social Work, 23*(1), 53–60.

Hornblower, M. (1996, June 3). It takes a school: A new approach to elementary education starts at birth and doesn't stop when the bell rings. *Time,* 37.

Huitt, W. G. (2000). *Psychology 702.* Retrieved February 7, 2000, from the World Wide Web: http://www.valdosta. edu/~whuitt/psy702/sysmdlhb.html/.

Human Services Research Institute. (2000). *Community support skill standards.* Retrieved September 1, 2000, from the World Wide Web: http:// www.hsri.org/skill/csss.html.

Husain, I. (1996, July 1). Global experience is bringing better antipoverty programs. *The Christian Science Monitor,* 19.

Hutchins, D. E., & Cole Vaught, C. (1997). *Helping relationships and strategies* (3rd ed.). Pacific Grove, CA: Brooks/Cole.

Independent Sector. (2000). Giving and volunteering in the United States: Findings from a national survey. Retrieved January 10, 2001 from the World Wide Web: http//www. independentsector.org.

Indritz, M. E. S. (1997). Examining the managed health care continuum. *Journal of*

Managed Care Pharmacy, 3(5). Retrieved September 18, 1999, from the World Wide Web: http://www.amcp.org/public/pubs/journal/vol3/num5.

Iowa Summit America's Promise . . . Iowa Style (2000). *Preparing for the Iowa Summit and beyond America's Promise . . . Iowa Style.* Retrieved March 13, 2000, from the World Wide Web: http://www.iowasummit.org/.

Ivey, A. E., & Ivey, M. B. (1999). *Intentional interviewing & counseling: Facilitating client development in a society* (4th ed.). Pacific Grove, CA: Brooks/Cole.

James, V. (1981, April). Mental health worker news: A forum for the mental health profession. *Bulletin: Council for Standards in Human Services Education, 4.*

Jamison, K. R. (1995). *An unquiet mind.* New York: Alfred A. Knopf.

Jansson, W., Almberg, B., Grafstroem, M., & Winblad, B. (1998). The circle model: Support for relatives of people with dementia. *International Journal of Geriatric Psychiatry, 13,* 674–681.

Jennifer, G. (1999). *Supportive souls mental health guide.* Retrieved August 27, 1999, from the World Wide Web: http://members.aol.com/zuzubaile/siteinfo.html.

John, R. (1986). Aging in a Native American community: Service needs and support networks among Prairie Band Potawatomi elders. *Dissertation Abstracts International, 47*(6), 23–32.

Johnson, D. (1996, July 31). One mothers's ordeal with life on welfare. *The New York Times,* A7.

Johnson, D. W. (1993). *Reaching out: Interpersonal effectiveness and self-actualization* (5th ed.). Boston: Allyn & Bacon.

Johnson, D. W., & Johnson, F. P. (1994). *Joining together: Group theory and group skills.* Boston: Allyn & Bacon.

Kane, R., Degenholtz, H., & Kane, R. (1999). Adding values: An experiment in systematic attention to values and preferences of community long-term care clients. *Journal of Gerontology, Series B: Psychological Sciences and Social Sciences, 54B,* 5109–5119.

Karger, H. J., & Levine, J. (1999). *The internet and technology for the human services.* New York: Longman.

Kelly, K., & Empson, G. (1999, May). Advocating for women in the criminal justice and addiction treatment systems. *Counseling Today,* 32–33.

Kennedy, J. F. (1964a). Remarks intended for delivery to the Texas Democratic State Committee in the Municipal Auditorium in Austin, November 22, 1963. *Public papers of the President of the United States: John F. Kennedy* (January 1–November 22, 1963), 897. Washington, DC: U.S. Government Printing Office.

Kennedy, J. F. (1964b). Remarks on proposed measures to combat mental illness and mental retardation. *Public papers of the Presidents of the United States: John F. Kennedy* (January 1– November 22, 1963), 50–51. Washington, DC: U.S. Government Printing Office.

Kenny, D. T. (1995, September). Determinants of patient satisfaction with the medical consultation. *Psychology and Health, 10*(5), 427–437.

Kenyon, P. (1999). *What would you do? An ethical case workbook for human service professionals.* Pacific Grove, CA: Brooks/Cole.

Kessler, K. (1989). Managed psychiatric care will continue to boom. *Clinical Psychiatry News, 17*(9), 6–7.

Kilborn, P. T. (1997, September 28). Dissatisfaction is growing with managed care plans. *The New York Times,* 12.

Korine, H. (1999). The new team organization: Learning to manage arbitrariness. *European Management Journal, 17*(1), 1–7.

Kreitner, R. (1983). *Management* (2nd ed.). Boston: Houghton Mifflin.

Kristof, N. D. (1996, April 14). Asian childhoods sacrificed to prosperity's best. *The New York Times,* 1, 6.

Kondrates, A. (1991). Ending homelessness: Policy changes. *American Psychologist, 46*(11), 1126–1136.

Le Francois, G. R. (1999). *The Lifespan* (6th ed.). Belmont, CA: Wadsworth.

Leiter, M. P., & Webb, M. (1983). *Developing human service networks*. New York: Irvington.

Levinson, D. (1978). *The seasons of a man's life*. New York: Ballantine.

Linn, N., McCreery, R., Kasab, D., & Schneider, S. (1998). Expert system for utilization review of alcohol and drug abuse cases. *Computers in Human Services 15*(4). Retrieved October 23, 1999, from the World Wide Web: http://www2.uta.edu/cussn/jths/vol115.htm.

Loewenberg, F. M., & Dolgoff, R. (1996). *Ethical dimensions for social work practice* (5th ed.). Itasca, NY: F. E. Peacock.

Long, L., Paradise, L. V., & Long, T. J. (1981). *Questioning: Skills for the helping process*. Pacific Grove, CA: Brooks/Cole.

Loveland-Cook, C., Selig, K., Wedge, B., & Gohn-Baube, E. (1999). Access barriers and the use of pre-natal care by low-income, inner-city women. *Social Work, 44,* 129–139.

Lyon, W., & Duke, B. J. (1981). *Introduction to human services*. Reston, VA: Reston Publishing.

Lyons, J., Libman-Minzer, L., & Kisiel, C. (1998). Understanding the mental health needs of children and adolescents in residential treatment. *Professional Psychology, Research and Practice, 29,* 582–587.

Macht, J. (1990). A historical perspective. In S. Fullerton & D. Osher (Eds.), *History of the Human Services Movement, 7,* 90–92.

Malinowski, B. (1984). *Argonauts of the Western Pacific*. Prospect Heights, IL: Waveland Press.

Maluccio, A. (1979). *Learning from clients*. New York: Free Press.

Mandell, B. R., & Schram, B. (1997a). *Human services: Introduction and interventions* (3rd ed.). New York: Wiley.

Mandell, B. R., & Schram, B. (1997b). *An introduction to human services: Policy and practice*. Boston: Allyn & Bacon.

Marino, T. W. (1996, January). Counselors in cyberspace debate whether client discussions are ethical. *Counseling Today,* 18.

Marino, T. W. (1999, December). New computer games help aid adolescents, counselors. *Counseling Today,* 2–3.

Marshall, H. (1937). *The forgotten samaritan*. Chapel Hill: University of North Carolina Press.

Masi, D. (1982). *Human services in industry*. Lexington, MA: Lexington Books.

Maslow, A. (1971). *The further reaches of human nature*. New York: Viking Press.

Mayer, J. E., & Timms, N. (1969). Clash in perspective between worker and client. *Social Casework, 50*(1), 32–40.

McBride, S. M. (1992). Rehabilitation case managers: Ahead of their time. *Holistic Nursing Practice, 6*(2), 67–75.

McClam, T., & Woodside, M. (1994). *Problem solving in the helping professions*. Pacific Grove, CA: Brooks/Cole.

McGinnis, J. M., & Foege, W. H. (1993). Actual causes of death in the United States. *Journal of the American Medical Association, 270,* 2207–2212.

Medicine On-line. (1999). *Mayo Clinic Women's Healthsource, 3*(9), 1–2.

Mehr, J. (1998). *Human services: Concepts and intervention strategies*. Boston: Allyn & Bacon.

Melson, G. F. (1980). *Family and environment: An ecological perspective*. Minneapolis: Burgess.

Mittler, J. (1999). Turning the elephant in a bathtub. *Industrial Management, 41*(1), 8–11.

Moroney, R. (1976). Needs assessment for human services. In W. F. Anderson, B. J. Friedem, & M. J. Murphy (Eds.), *Managing human services*. Washington, DC: International City Management Association.

Morse, G. A., Calsyn, K. J., Allen, G., & Kenny, D. A. (1994, October). Helping homeless mentally ill people: What variables mediate and moderate program effects? *American Journal of Community Psychology, 22*(5), 661–683.

NAACP targets minority gap in Internet use, TV roles. (1999, July 13). *CNN Interactive.* Retrieved May 20, 1999, from the World Wide Web: http:// www.edu.town.shibecha.hokkaido. jp:14966/-_-http://europe.cnn.com/US/ 9907/13/naacp.gap/index.html.

NAACP targets minority gap in Internet use, TV roles. (1999, July 13). *CNN Interactive.* Retrieved October 14, 1999, from the World Wide Web: http://www. edu.town.shibecha.hokkaido.jp:14966/ -_-http://europe.cnn.com/US/9907/13/ naacp.gap/index.html.

National Clearinghouse on Child Abuse and Neglect. (2000). *Databases.* Retrieved March 12, 2000, from the World Wide Web: http://www.cal.b. com:80/nccanch.

National Clearinghouse on Managed Care and Long-Term Support and Services for People with Developmental Disabilities and Their Families. (1999). *Participant-driven supports: Frequently asked questions and responses.* Retrieved September 3, 1999, from the World Wide Web: http:/www.mcare. net/briefs/pbrief4.html.

National Coalition for the Homeless. (1997). *Homelessness in America: Unabated and increasing.* Washington, DC: Author.

National Coalition of Mental Health Professionals & Consumers. (1999). *Mental health consumer protection manual: A guide to solving problems with insurance and managed care.* Retrieved September 2, 1999, from the World Wide Web: http:/www.nomangedcare.org/ consum.html.

National Commission for Human Service Workers. (1982). *Registration and certification of human service workers.* Atlanta, GA: Author.

National Institute of Mental Health (NIMH). (1971). *Mental illness and its treatment: Social issues resources issue series* (Vol. 1, Article 3; DHEW Publications No [HSM] 72–/9030). Washington, DC: Author.

National Law Center on Homelessness and Poverty. (1999). *Out of sight—out of mind? A report on anti-homeless laws, litigation, and alternatives in 50 United States cities.* Washington, DC: Author.

National Institute of Mental Health. (1985). *You are not alone: Facts about mental health and mental illness.* (DHHS Publication No. ADM 85–1178). Washington, DC: U.S. Government Printing Office.

Nebraska Network for Children and Families. (1999). *Eldercare.* Retrieved October 20, 1999, from the World Wide Web: http://www.nncf. unl.edu/eldercare/discuss/ discussion. html.

Neugebauer, R. (1979). Medieval and early modern theories of mental illness. *Archives of General Psychiatry, 36,* 477–483.

Neugeboren, B. (1991). *Organization, policy, and practice in the human services.* New York: Longman.

Neukrug. E. (1994). *Theory, practice, and trends in human services: An overview of an emerging profession.* Pacific Grove, CA: Brooks/Cole.

New interactive multimedia system for computerized cognitive therapy. (1995, June). *Counseling Today, 37*(12), 44.

Nifong, C. (1997, January 16). Welfare mom lays plans with an eye on the clock. *The Christian Science Monitor, 1,* 10–11.

Nifong, C. (1996, July 1). Work or else: Welfare moms strive to meet the ultimatum. *The Christian Science Monitor, 1,* 10–11.

Nirenberg, J. S. (1984). *How to sell your ideas.* New York: McGraw Hill.

Nooe, R. (2001). Mental illness and homelessness. In T. McClam & M. Woodside, *Human services in the 21st century.* New York: Council for Standards in Human Service Education, pp. 205–214.

Nord, M., & Luloff, A. E. (1995). Homeless children and their families in New Hampshire: A rural perspective. *Social Service Review, 69*(3), 461–478.

Oalcley, C. (1994). SMACK: A computer driven game for at-risk teens. [Abstract]. *Computers in Human Services,* 11(1/2). Retrieved March 15, 1996, from the World Wide Web: http://www.uta.edu/cuss/vol11.htm.

Occupational outlook handbook. (1998–1999). Washington, DC: U.S. Department of Labor, Bureau of Labor Statistics.

Occupational outlook handbook. (1998). Washington, DC: U.S. Department of Labor, Bureau of Labor Statistics.

Occupational outlook handbook. (1992–1993). Bulletin 2400. Washington, DC: U.S. Department of Labor, Bureau of Labor Statistics.

O'Donnell, M., Parker, G., Proberts, M., Matthews, R., Fisher, D., Johnson, B., & Hadzi/Pavlovic, D. (1999). A study of client–focused case management and consumer advocacy: The Community and Consumer Service Project. *Australian and New Zealand Journal of Psychiatry, 33*(5), 684–693.

Offer, J. (1998–1999). On sociological studies of interaction between social workers and clients and why they matter. *Social Work and Social Sciences Review, 8*(1), 5–24.

Okun, B. F. (1997). *Effective helping: Interviewing and counseling techniques* (5th ed.). Pacific Grove, CA: Brooks/Cole.

Okun, B. F., Fried, J., & Okun, M. L. (1999). *Understanding diversity: A learning-as-practice primer.* Pacific Grove, CA: Brooks/Cole.

Page, R. C. (1979). Major ethical issues in public offender counseling. *Counseling and Values, 24,* 33–40.

Pattison, E. M. (1984). Cultural level interventions in the arena of alcoholism. *Alcoholism, 8*(2), 160–164.

Paquet, C. (1999, February 12). Report counts 147 million global Net users. *IDG.com.* Retrieved September 30, 1999, from the World Wide Web: http://www.edu.town.shibecha.hokkaido.jp:14966/-_-http://europe.cnn.com/TECH/computing/9902/12/globalnet.idg/ index.html.

Perlman, H. H. (1979). *Relationship: The heart of helping people.* Chicago: University of Chicago Press.

Perlman, R. (1975). *Consumers and social services.* New York: Wiley.

Pichot, P. (1985). Remedicalisation of psychiatry. *Psychiatrial Fennica, 16,* 9–17.

Pilisuk, M. (1980, April). The future of human services without funding. *American Journal of Orthopsychiatry, 50*(2), 200–204.

Pinkstaff, E. (1985). An experience in narrative writing to improve public health practice by students. *Journal of Nursing Education, 24*(1), 25–28.

Pins, A. M. (1963). *Who chooses social work, when and why.* New York: Council on Social Work Education.

Ponterotto, J. G. (1985). A counselor's guide to psychopharmacology. *Journal of Counseling and Development, 64,* 109–115.

Poor nations have many of year's 100 million new people. (1995, December 28). *The Knoxville News-Sentinel,* A1.

Porter, B. (1998). Predicting active and effective agents for safety: Test of the actively caring approach. *Journal of Safety Research, 29,* 223–233.

Prentice Hall. (1999). *What is sociology?* Retrieved September 16, 1999, from the World Wide Web: http://www.macionis.com/whatis.htm.

Rapoport, L. (1962). The state of crisis: Some theoretical considerations. *Social Service Review, 36,* 211–217.

Raths, L. E., Harmin, M., & Simon, S. B. (1978). *Values and teaching: Working with values in the classroom.* Columbus, OH: Merrill.

Ray, J. R., & Warden, M. K. (1995). *Technology, computers, and the special needs learner.* Albany, NY: Delmar.

Reichert, D. (1998a, July). *Welfare return project: Where does the money go?* National Conference of State Legislatures. Retrieved May 15, 1999, from the World Wide Web: http://www.ncsl.org/statefed/welfare/moespend.htm.

Reichert, D. (1998b, October). *Welfare reform program: TANF appropriations.* National Conference of State Legislatures. Retrieved May 15, 1999, from the World Wide Web: http://www.ncsl.org/statefed/welfare/moememo.htm.

Reinhard, S. (1986). Financing long-term health care of the elderly: Dismantling the medical model. *Public Health Nursing, 3*(1), 3 22.

Resnick, H. (1994). Electronic technology and rehabilitation: A computerized simulation game for youthful offenders. [Abstract]. *Computers in Human Services, 11*(1/2). Retrieved March 15, 1996, from the World Wide Web: http://www.uta.edu/cuss/vol11.htm.

Richmond, M. (1917). *Social diagnosis.* New York: Russell Sage Foundation.

Rinas, J., & Clyne-Jackson, S. (1988). *Professional conduct and legal concerns in mental health practice.* Norwalk, CT: Appleton & Lange.

Ritchie, M. H. (1986). Counseling the involuntary client. *Journal of Counseling and Development, 64,* 516–518.

Rivlin, L. G. (1986). A new look at the homeless. *Social Policy, 16*(4), 3–10.

Rock, B., & Congress, E. (1999). The new confidentiality for the 21st century in a managed care environment. *Social Work, 44,* 253–262.

Rogers, C. (1958). The characteristics of a helping relationship. *Personnel and Guidance Journal, 37*(1), 6–16.

Rost, K., Humphrey, J., & Kelleher, K. (1994). Physician management preferences and barriers to care for rural patients with depression. *Archives of Family Medicine, 3,* 409–414.

Rothman, J. (2000). Alternative approaches to measuring neighborhood change. Retrieved September 1, 2000, from the World Wide Web: http://www.aepro.org/innprint/papers/fanniemae.html.

Sack, D. (1995, November 25). Volunteering made easier for busy young workers. *The New York Times,* A1, 9.

Sadler, C., & Morty, F. (1998). Socialization of hospice volunteers: Members of the family. *Hospice Journal, 13*(3), 49–68.

Safe and Sound. (2000). *Safe and Sound.* Retrieved March 12, 2000, from the World Wide Web: http://www.safeand sound.org/.

Schafer, K. (1996). *Managed care and children's services.* Presentation conducted at the Managed Care Institute: Futurecare preparing for managed care and children's services in Tennessee, Nashville, TN.

Schneider-Braus, K. (1992). Managing a mental health department in a staff model HMO. In J. L. Feldman & R. T. Fitzpatrick (Eds.), *Managed mental health care* (pp. 125–141). Washington, DC: American Psychiatric Press.

Schmolling, P., Jr., Youkeles, M., & Burger, W. R. (1997). *Human service in contemporary America* (4th ed.). Pacific Grove, CA: Brooks/Cole.

Sciolino, E. (1996, November 12). A painful road from Vietnam to forgiveness. *The New York Times,* A7.

Scott, C., & Jaffe, D. (1991). *Empowerment: A practical guide for success.* Menlo Park, CA: Crisp Publications.

Selfish managers are more likely to succeed. (1999). *Management Today,* 8–9.

Sheehy, G. (1995). *New passage: Mapping your life across time.* New York: Ballantine.

Sherman, R. E. (2000). Program evaluation: Its purpose and nature. Retrieved September 3, 2000, from the World Wide Web: http://www.grantstech.com/articles/programevaluation.html.

Shirreffs, J. H. (1982). *Community health: Contemporary perspectives.* Englewood Cliffs, NJ: Prentice Hall.

Sielski, L. M. (1979). Understanding body language. *Personnel and Guidance Journal, 57,* 238–242.

Smothers, R. (1996, July 1). As Olympics approach, homeless are not feeling at home. *The New York Times,* A11.

Snyder, W. T. (1996, February). *Opportunities for partnering between professional societies and universities.* Paper presented at the meeting of WATTEC, Knoxville, TN.

Southern Regional Education Board. (1979). *Staff roles for mental health personnel: A history and a rationale.* Atlanta, GA: Author.

Southern Regional Education Board. (1969). *Roles and functions for different levels of mental health workers.* Atlanta, GA: Author.

Stadler, H. (1986). Preface to the special issue. *Journal of Counseling and Development, 64*(5), 291–292.

Study: Most former Wisconsin welfare recipients now working. (1999, January 14). *CNN Interactive.* Retrieved May 19, 1999, from the World Wide Web: http://cnn.com/US/9901/14/work.welfare/index.html.

Study shows minorities less likely to own computers, use Internet. (1999, July 8). *CNN Interactive.* Retrieved September 23, 1999, from the World Wide Web: http://europe.cnn.com/TECH/computing/9907/08/digital.divide.ap/.

Survey: New rules leading cause of decline in welfare rolls. (1999, March 29). *CNN Interactive.* Retrieved May 15, 1999, from the World Wide Web: http://www.cnn.com/allpolitics/stories/1999/03/29/welfare .

Tarasoff v. Regents of the University of California. (1976). *Pacific Reporter,* 2nd Series, 551, 340.

Taylor, C. (1985). *Carl Rogers and client-centered therapy.* Unpublished manuscript. Knoxville, TN.

Taylor, M., Bradley, V., & Warren, R. (1996). *The community support skill standards.* Cambridge, MA: Human Service Research Institute.

Teague, D. (1970). *Background information.* Boulder, CO: WICHE Project for Manpower Utilization. Unpublished manuscript.

Tennyson, W. W., & Strom, S. M. (1986). Beyond professional standards: Developing responsibleness. *Journal of Counseling and Development, 64*(5), 298–302.

Tims, M. (1961). *Jane Addams of Hull House: 1860–1935: A centenary study.* London: Allen & Unwin.

Toczek-McPeake, A., & Matthews, M. (1995, September–October). Quality management: A survey of client and career satisfaction with speech pathology and physio-therapy services in a rehabilitation setting. *Journal of Cognitive Rehabilitation, 13*(5), 12–18.

Torrey, E. F. (1997). *Out of the shadows: Confronting America's mental illness crisis.* New York: John Wiley & Sons.

Trattner, W. I. (1999). *From poor law to welfare state: A history of social welfare in America.* New York: Free Press.

Treas, J. (1995). Older Americans in the 1990s and beyond. *Population Bulletin, 50*(2), 1–48.

Tuckfelt, S., Fink, J., Warren, M., & Travis, T. A. (1999). The psychotherapist's guide to managed care in the 21st century. *The American Journal of Psychiatry, 156*(5), 793.

Tweedie, J. (1999, January). *Welfare reform: Eight questions to ask about welfare reform.* Retrieved May 15, 1999, from the World Wide Web: http://www.ncsl.org/statefed/welfare/8quest.htm.

20 Hot Job Tracks: Career Guide 1999. (1998, October 26). *U.S. News & World Report, 125*(16), 84–90.

20 Hot Career Tracks: Career Guide 1998. (1997, October 27). *U.S. News & World Report, 123*(6), 96–98, 100, 104–106.

20 Hot Job Tracks: Career Guide 1997. (1996, October 28). *U.S. News & World Report, 121*(17), 95.

Tyson, A. S. (1995, December 6). Keeping it together—barely. *The Christain Science Monitor,* A10.

U.S. Census Bureau. (1996). *Population projections of the United States by age, sex, race and Hispanic origin: 1995 to 2050.* Washington, DC: U.S. Government Printing Office.

U.S. Census Population Survey. (1994). Washington, DC: U.S. Government Printing Office.

U.S. Congress, Office of Technology Assessment. (1990). *Health care in rural America.* Washington, DC: U.S. Government Printing Office.

Van Hoose, W. H., & Paradise, L. V. (1979). *Ethics in counseling and psychotherapy: Perspectives in issues and decision making.* Cranston, RI: Carroll.

Vatterott, M., Callier, J., & Hile, M. (1992). [Abstract]. *Computers in Human Services, 8*(3/4). Retrieved October 23, 1999, from the World Wide Web: http://www.uta.edu/cuss/vol11.htm.

Villani, S., & Sharfstein, S. (1999). Evaluating and treating violent adolescents in the managed care era. *The American Journal of Psychiatry, 156,* 458–464.

Vissing, Y. (1996). *Out of sight, out of mind: Homeless children and families in small town America.* Lexington: The University Press of Kentucky.

Volunteers: Numbers, hows and dollar values. (1997). Washington, DC: Independent Sector.

Von Bertalanffy, L. (1968). *General systems theory.* New York: Braziller.

Vreeland, E. (1991, July 14). Teachers: Social ills taking toll in class. *Knoxville News-Sentinel,* B1.

Wagner, M. (1994, June). *A healthy start for California's children and families: Early findings from statewide evaluations of school-linked services.* Menlo Park, CA: SRI International.

Webb, B. (1996). *The management of information.* Presentation conducted at the Managed Care Institute: Futurecare preparing for managed care and children's services, Nashville, TN.

Webster's New World Dictionary of the American Language (2nd college ed.). (1986). Springfield, MA: Merriam Webster.

Webster's third new international dictionary (1986). Springfield, MA: Merriam Webster.

Welfare rolls hit a 30-year low, but the decline is slowing. (1999, January 25). *The Salt Lake Tribune.* Retrieved May 15, 1999, from the World Wide Web: http://www.sltrib.com/1999/jan/01251999/nation%5fw/77743.htm.

Welfel, E. R. (1998). *Ethics in counseling and psychotherapy: Standards, research, and emerging issues.* Pacific Grove, CA: Brooks/Cole.

Whitley, D., White, K., & Kelley, S. (1999). Strengths-based case management: The application to grandparents raising grandchildren. *Families in Society, 80*(2), 110–119.

Williams, D. (1994). *Nobody nowhere.* New York: Avon.

Willis, R. (1999, November). Looking for sense in a senseless crime. *Counseling Today,* 16.

Wilson, S. J. (1978). *Confidentiality in social work: Issues and principles.* New York: Free Press.

Winefield, H. R., & Barlow, J. A. (1995). Client and worker satisfaction in a child protection agency. *Child Abuse and Neglect, 19*(8), 897–905.

Woodside, M., & McClam, T., (1998). *Generalist case management.* Pacific Grove, CA: Brooks/Cole.

Woodside, M., McClam, T., & McGarrh, K. (1993). Human service education: Perceptions of the past and the future. *Human Service Education, 13*(1), 3–11.

World Health Organization (1975). *Organization of mental health services in developing countries: Sixteenth report of the committee on mental health.* (World Health Organization Technical Report Series No. 564). Geneva: World Health Organization.

A world in need. (1996, June 24). *U.S. News & World Report, 120,* 20.

Yovovick, B. G. (1997, April 25). Demographics of web use: Two starkly different worlds. *E & P Interactive.* Retrieved June 24, 1999, from the World Wide Web: http:/www.medianinfo.com/ephome/news/newshtm/recent/042597n2.htm.

Zimbalist, S. E. (1977). *Historic themes and landmarks in social welfare research.* New York: Harper & Row.

Index

Photo Credits

TO THE OWNER OF THIS BOOK:

We hope that you have found *An Introduction to Human Services* , Fourth Edition, useful. So that this book can be improved in a future edition, would you take the time to complete this sheet and return it? Thank you.

School and address:_____

Department:_____

Instructor's name:_____

1. What I like most about this book is:_____

_____

_____

2. What I like least about this book is:_____

_____

_____

3. My general reaction to this book is:_____

_____

4. The name of the course in which I used this book is:_____

_____

5. Were all of the chapters of the book assigned for you to read?_____

   If not, which ones weren't?_____

6. In the space below, or on a separate sheet of paper, please write specific suggestions for improving this book and anything else you'd care to share about your experience in using the book.

_____

_____

_____

_____

Optional:

Your name: _____ Date: _____

May Brooks/Cole quote you, either in promotion for *An Introduction to Human Services,*
Fourth Edition, or in future publishing ventures?

Yes: _____ No: _____

Sincerely,

Marianne Woodside
Tricia McClam